Atlas of

Surface
Palpation

Anatomy of the

Publisher: **Sarena Wolfaard**
Commissioning Editor: **Claire Wilson**
Development Editor: **Claire Bonnett**
Project Manager: **Jess Thompson**
Design Direction: **Charles Gray**

The photographs were devised and staged by the author and taken by Charles Menge and Frederic Moix (osteopath) at the medical illustration department of the Faculty of Medicine at the University of Geneva.

Netter images reprinted with permission from Elsevier Inc.

Atlas of Surface Palpation

Anatomy of the Neck, Trunk, Upper and Lower Limbs

SECOND EDITION

By

Serge Tixa

Instructor in anatomy and palpatory anatomy at the Swiss School of Osteopathy, Lausanne, Switzerland

Translated by Louis Honoré and Elaine Richards

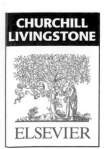

CHURCHILL LIVINGSTONE

ELSEVIER

Edinburgh   London   New York   Oxford   Philadelphia   St Louis   Sydney   Toronto   2008

CHURCHILL
LIVINGSTONE
ELSEVIER

An imprint of Elsevier Limited

The right of Serge Tixa to be identified as author/s of this work has been asserted by him/her/them in accordance with the Copyright, Designs and Patents Act 1988.

This English language edition is produced from two French language works originally published as:
Atlas d'anatomie palpatoire. Tome 1: Cou, tronc, membre supérieur. Investigation manuelle de surface © Masson, Paris, 1999, 2005
Atlas d'anatomie palpatoire. Tome 2: Membre inférieur. Investigation manuelle de surface © Masson, Paris, 1999, 2005.

French edition by Masson, Paris, 2005
English edition 2008

ISBN 978-0-443-06875-1

British Library Cataloguing in Publication Data
A catalogue record for this book is available from the British Library

Library of Congress Cataloging in Publication Data
A catalog record for this book is available from the Library of Congress

Note
Neither the Publisher nor the Author assumes any responsibility for any loss or injury and/or damage to persons or property arising out of or related to any use of the material contained in this book. It is the responsibility of the treating practitioner, relying on independent expertise and knowledge of the patient, to determine the best treatment and method of application for the patient.

The Publisher

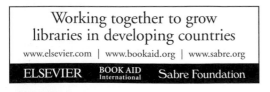

Working together to grow
libraries in developing countries
www.elsevier.com | www.bookaid.org | www.sabre.org

ELSEVIER   BOOK AID International   Sabre Foundation

The publisher's policy is to use paper manufactured from sustainable forests

ELSEVIER
your source for books,
journals and multimedia
in the health sciences
www.elsevierhealth.com
Printed in China

CONTENTS

CONTENTS

INTRODUCTION

This book presents a method of palpatory anatomy, which we have called Manual Exploration of Surface Anatomy (MESA). This is a method of locating anatomical structures (bones, ligaments, tendons, muscles, and neurovascular bundles). It is highly visual, as each structure studied is illustrated with a photograph; it also provides practical instruction, since each photograph is accompanied by a section of text describing a method of approach to the structure concerned.

Who is the book intended for?
It is aimed at all who need a method of applied anatomy in the performance of their profession.

How is the book organized?
This atlas consists of over 800 photographs of the neck, trunk, and upper and lower limbs. There are twelve chapters (The Neck, The Trunk and Sacrum, The Shoulder, The Arm, The Elbow, The Forearm, The Wrist and Hand, The Hip, The Thigh, The Knee, The Leg, and The Ankle and Foot). Each has up to four subsections, as appropriate, treating the various aspects of that region. These cover osteology, myology (musculotendinous structures), arthrology (joints and ligaments), and, lastly, nerves and blood vessels.

The nomenclature used is the most recent anatomical terminology. The text uses the recognized English terms followed by the internationally recognized Latin of the Terminologia Anatomica (the Latin is printed in italics and in brackets). Some synonyms in common use are added in brackets where appropriate.

The two types of photograph
- Descriptive photographs include:
  - An overall photograph at the start of each chapter
  - Topographical photographs showing a body region with its group of notable structures accessible to palpation
  - Structural photographs illustrating, wherever possible, an anatomical structure and its relationships with the adjacent structures. These are mainly photographs of muscle groups.
- The MESA photographs constitute the main body of the book. They display the structure to be studied. A descriptive note on the method of approach accompanies each photograph.

How is the book intended to be used?
There are two possible methods:

- To explore a particular region in its entirety (e.g. the shoulder) or part of a region (e.g. the bones of the wrist), simply turn to the relevant chapter or subsection, as indicated in the list of contents.
- To look at a specific structure in all its possible aspects, consult the index for a list of all the pages that treat that topic. The index gives the English nomenclature agreed by the Federative Committee on Anatomical Terminology and International Federation of Associations of Anatomists (Terminologia Anatomica; TA) and the Latin Terminologia Anatomica (TA) terms, the internationally recognized nomenclature. It also lists the Parisiensia Nomina Anatomica (PNA, later known as NA) terms.

What is new in this edition?
- *New methods of approach* illustrated by *new photographs*.
- *Anatomical dissection plates* culled from reference works by authors such as Netter, or Rouvière and Delmas. This use of visual illustrations enhances the instructional material by showing the location of a given muscle, its relationship to neighboring muscles, and its sites of origin and insertion. In the same way it aids the localization of bony structures, joint cavities, nerves, and blood vessels.
- *Information on the origins and insertions of muscles.* Informative notes follow the description of the corresponding technique of approach. They are presented clearly and distinctly for easy reference and use. Practitioners and students alike are well aware how easy it is to learn and forget anatomy many times before finally mastering it. It is primarily to address this concern that the information on muscle insertions has been included in this new edition. It is impossible to master palpatory anatomy without a thorough knowledge of theoretical anatomy.
- *Information on the actions of muscles.* In this new edition, this information is included on each page in which a muscle or muscle group is presented, as always in order to help the student master palpatory anatomy.

INTRODUCTION

Comments

- The boundaries of the regions studied in each of the ensuing chapters must not be viewed as strictly defined. When studying certain muscles, it is inevitable that the area under consideration will extend beyond that immediate region. The reason for this lies in the approach being taken. Each is viewed both in terms of a "transverse" approach that localizes it with respect to adjacent structures, and in terms of a "longitudinal" approach that looks at its proximal part, its main body, and its distal part.

- The terms *proximal hand* and *distal hand*, occasionally used in presenting methods of approach, need to be clarified. There is only one hand or one grip (that of the therapist) and *proximal* and *distal* refer respectively to the hand when it is closer to the site of attachment of the patient's lower limb and to the hand when it is farther away from that attachment site.

ACKNOWLEDGMENTS

My warmest thanks go to the many students who agreed to volunteer their time and their energy and to pose for photographic sessions that were often lengthy and tedious.

They are too numerous to mention by name here, but I must pay tribute to them all, both those whose photographs were used and those whose photographs were not.

To them all I wish to express my most profound gratitude.

I am anxious for them to know that I remember them all and will never forget them, since without them this book would not be what it is.

Serge Tixa

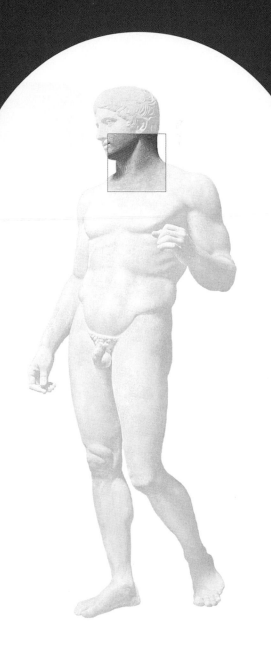

CHAPTER 1

THE NECK

TOPOGRAPHICAL PRESENTATION OF THE NECK

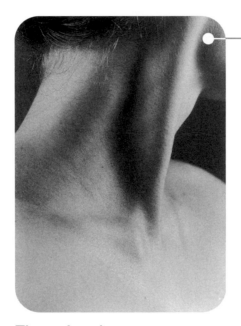

Fig. 1.1

The neck region

OSTEOLOGY

THE OSSEOUS SKELETON OF THE HEAD AND NECK[1]

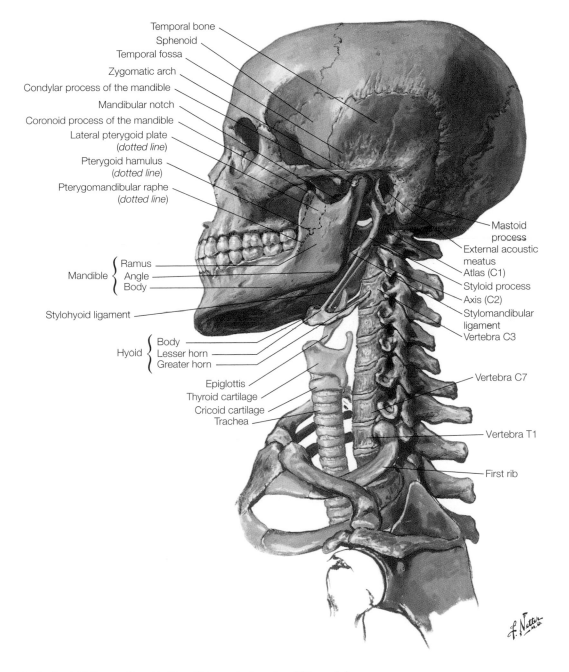

Temporal bone
Sphenoid
Temporal fossa
Zygomatic arch
Condylar process of the mandible
Mandibular notch
Coronoid process of the mandible
Lateral pterygoid plate
(*dotted line*)
Pterygoid hamulus
(*dotted line*)
Pterygomandibular raphe
(*dotted line*)

Mastoid process
External acoustic meatus
Atlas (C1)
Styloid process
Axis (C2)
Stylomandibular ligament
Vertebra C3

Mandible { Ramus
Angle
Body }

Stylohyoid ligament

Hyoid { Body
Lesser horn
Greater horn }

Epiglottis
Thyroid cartilage
Cricoid cartilage
Trachea

Vertebra C7

Vertebra T1

First rib

1. The plates by Frank Netter are from his *Atlas of Human Anatomy* (see Bibliography).

THE ANTERIOR CERVICAL REGION (ANTERIOR TRIANGLE OF THE NECK)

The notable structures that can be detected by palpation are:

- The thyroid cartilage (*cartilago thyroidea*) (Figs 1.3–1.6).
- The superior thyroid notch (*incisura thyroidea superior*) (Figs 1.5 and 1.6).
- The hyoid bone (*os hyoideum*):
    — Body of the hyoid (*corpus ossis hyoidei*) (Figs 1.3–1.6)
    — Median tubercle of the hyoid (Fig. 1.7)
    — Lesser horn (*cornu minus*) (Fig. 1.8)
    — Greater horn (*cornu majus*) (Fig.1.9).
- The cricoid cartilage (*cartilago cricoidea*) (Fig. 1.10).
- The trachea (Fig. 1.11).

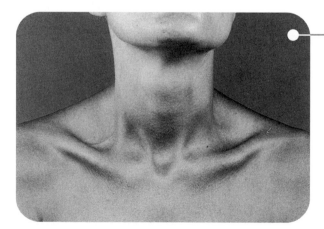

Fig. 1.2

Anterior view of the neck region

Fig. 1.3 | Visualization of the osseocartilaginous elements belonging to the larynx

The larynx, the essential organ of voice, is situated in the median anterior part of the neck. It opens superiorly into the laryngopharynx, the inferior part of the pharynx. It lies below the hyoid bone and above the trachea, and can be palpated between the hyoid above, and the superior border of the sternal manubrium. It is mobile, rising by approximately the height of one vertebra, when the subject is speaking, breathing, and especially swallowing.

The larynx is composed of a number of cartilages. The only ones discussed here are those providing support: the thyroid and cricoid cartilages.

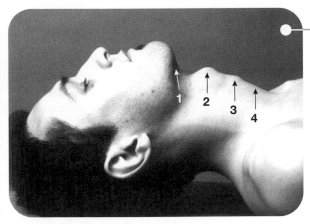

Note: Although the hyoid is attached to the thyroid cartilage by the thyrohyoid membrane, it does not form part of the skeleton of the larynx.

1. Position of the hyoid bone.
2. The laryngeal prominence (thyroid cartilage).
3. The cricoid cartilage.
4. The trachea.

Fig. 1.4 | The thyroid cartilage (*cartilago thyroidea*)

This can best be visualized if the subject's head is hyperextended. The thyroid cartilage is situated between the hyoid (Figs 1.3 and 1.6–1.9) above and the cricoid cartilage (Figs 1.3 and 1.10) below. The thyroid cartilage (indicated by the practitioner's index finger) is the largest of the cartilages of the larynx. Its name (from the Greek for a "shield") refers to both its shape and its position, since it covers or shields the other elements of the larynx anteriorly. It is much more prominent in males than in females.

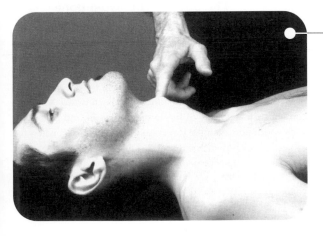

Note: Three of the eleven cartilages constituting the larynx are unpaired, median structures: the thyroid cartilage (which tends to ossify in adults and the elderly), the cricoid cartilage, and the epiglottis.

Fig. 1.5 | The superior thyroid notch Lateral aspect

The superior thyroid notch can be palpated at the point where the two lobes of the body of the thyroid join, above the prominence. In the adjacent figure it is very marked. The practitioner's index finger indicates the notch, which is situated in the median line, on the superior border of the thyroid cartilage, at the Adam's apple (laryngeal prominence).

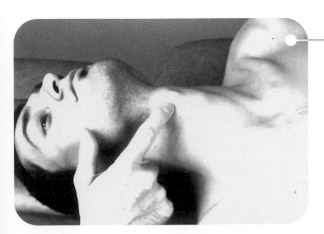

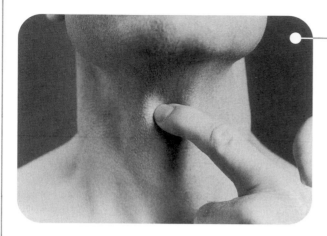

Fig. 1.6 | **The body of the hyoid bone (*os hyoideum*) Step 1**

Place your index finger on the superior thyroid notch, on the superior border of the thyroid cartilage (Fig. 1.5). This is the first stage in locating the body of the hyoid, which is situated immediately above.

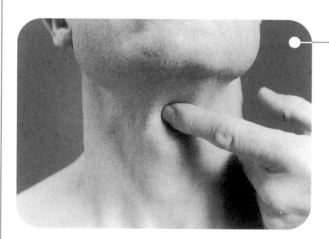

Fig. 1.7 | **The body of the hyoid bone (*corpus ossis hyoidei*) Step 2, and median tubercle of the hyoid**

When you have completed the first step in locating the hyoid (Figs 1.3–1.6), move your index finger upward to make contact with the body of the hyoid. You will find it one finger's width above, in the direction of the mandible, when the subject's neck is slightly extended. The median tubercle of the hyoid forms a bony projection that can be felt directly beneath the skin.

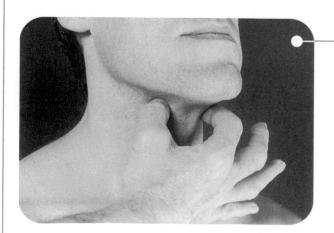

Fig. 1.8 | **The body of the hyoid bone: lesser horn (*cornu minus*)**

Once you have located the superior border of the thyroid cartilage (Figs 1.5 and 1.6), the body of the hyoid and the median tubercle of the hyoid (Fig. 1.7), use a thumb and index finger contact and gently shift the contact slightly to each side, continuing to follow the line of the body of the hyoid. You will then make contact with two small raised bony projections — tiny upwardly oriented horns.

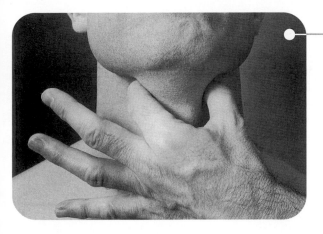

Fig. 1.9 | **The body of the hyoid bone: greater horn (*cornu majus*) and the posterior tubercle of the greater horn**

Having located the body of the hyoid (Figs 1.3–1.6) and the lesser horns (Fig. 1.8), simply shift your thumb and finger laterally, using the same contact, to make contact with the greater horns. These extend upward, posteriorly and laterally to the body of the hyoid, and end posteriorly in a tubercle that you can also feel beneath your fingers. Position the subject's head in extension to perceive these structures more clearly.

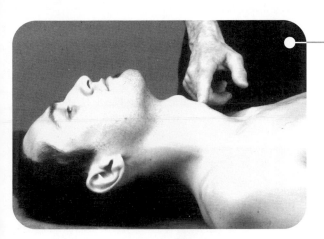

Fig. 1.10 | **The cricoid cartilage (*cartilago cricoidea*)**

This is the most inferiorly situated of the cartilages of the larynx. In this figure, the practitioner's index finger indicates the cricoid cartilage, which lies two finger-widths below the laryngeal prominence (see Fig. 1.3). The cricoid cartilage forms the base of the laryngeal pyramid and creates the transition between the larynx and the first tracheal cartilage.

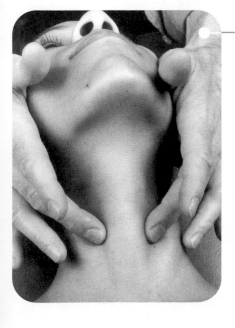

Fig. 1.11 | **The trachea**

The subject's head should be hyperextended to isolate this structure clearly.

The trachea extends from the inferior border of the sixth cervical vertebra to the fifth thoracic vertebra or a little beyond. It has the shape of a cylindrical tube which is flattened posteriorly. The cylindrical part has rings of cartilage, separated by spaces or interannular depressions, and can easily be palpated.

The trachea follows an oblique course running down from above and from anterior to posterior. The cervical portion of the trachea extends from the inferior border of the cricoid cartilage (level with intervertebral disc C6–C7) to the superior border of the sternum. It has an overall length of around 12 cm (5 in), varying according to the position of the larynx (which rises and descends in the living adult male). Its diameter is approximately 12 mm ($^{1}/_{2}$ in).

THE POSTERIOR AND LATERAL CERVICAL REGIONS (NUCHAL REGION AND POSTERIOR TRIANGLE OF THE NECK, *REGIO CERVICALIS POSTERIOR* AND *LATERALIS*)

The notable structures that can be detected by palpation are:

- The cervical spine (Fig. 1.13).
- The spinous process (*processus spinosus*) of the seventh cervical vertebra (*vertebra prominens*) (Fig. 1.14).
- The spinous process of the sixth cervical vertebra (Fig. 1.15).
- The posterior tubercle (*tuberculum posterius*) of the atlas (Fig. 1.16).
- The spinous process of the axis (Fig. 1.17).
- The transverse process (*processus transversus*) of the atlas (Fig. 1.18).
- The transverse process of the axis (Fig. 1.19).
- The transverse processes of the third to the seventh cervical vertebrae (Fig. 1.20).
- The articular processes (*processus articulares*) of the cervical vertebrae (Figs 1.21 and 1.22).

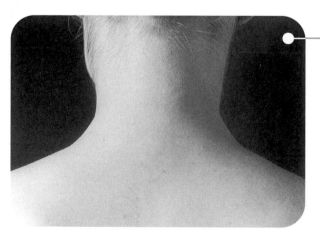

Fig. 1.12

The posterior cervical region (nuchal region)
(*regio cervicalis posterior*)

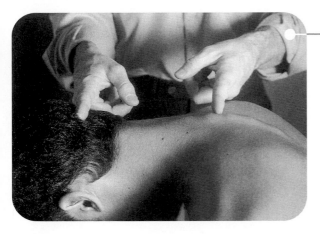

Fig. 1.13 | **The cervical spine**

The practitioner is indicating the general topographical location of the cervical spine, between the occipital bone and the first thoracic vertebra. It consists of seven cervical vertebrae arranged one above the other and each articulating with the next.

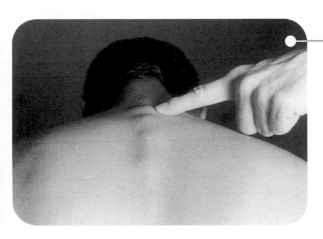

Fig. 1.14 | **The spinous process (*processus spinosus*) of the seventh cervical vertebra (*vertebra prominens*)**

This process is distinguished by its length and prominence and by having a single tubercle at its extremity. However, it is easy to confuse with the first thoracic vertebra. This figure should be carefully compared with Figures 2.34 and 2.35, so as to avoid any possible errors of identification.

Note: As a general rule, the spinous process of C7 is the most prominent of the spinous processes of the cervico–thoracic transition (C6–C7–T1).

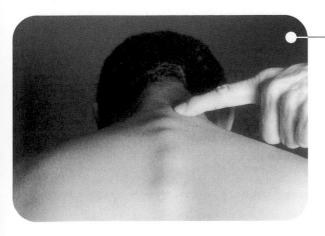

Fig. 1.15 | **The spinous process of the sixth cervical vertebra**

This structure is easy to find once you have clearly identified the spinous process of the seventh cervical vertebra (see Fig. 1.14 and Figs 2.32–2.34); the sixth is situated immediately above it. Identification can be confirmed by asking subjects to rotate their head repeatedly to left and right, when the process of C6 can distinctly be felt to shift beneath your fingers relative to the spinous process of C7.

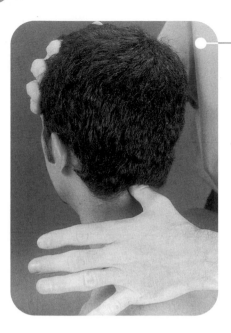

Fig. 1.16 | **The posterior tubercle of the atlas (*tuberculum posterius atlantis*)**

This can be found in the extension of the external occipital crest (*crista occipitalis externa*), on the exocranial surface of the occipital bone (*os occipitale*). The posterior border of the foramen magnum can be felt beneath your fingers, and just beneath this (in the caudal direction), you will detect a small depression. Within this depression the practitioner's thumb can be seen making contact with the posterior tubercle of the atlas.

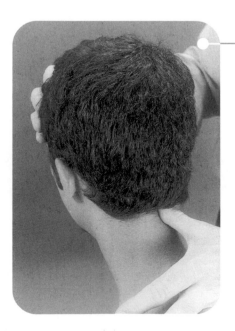

Fig. 1.17 | **The spinous process of the axis**

Below the small depression mentioned above (Fig. 1.6) (within which the posterior tubercle of the atlas is found) you can detect a bony structure beneath your fingers. This is the spinous process of the axis. It is very prominent, and can be revealed distinctly by slightly flexing and extending the subject's head, with a gentle movement using your fingers on the subject's forehead.

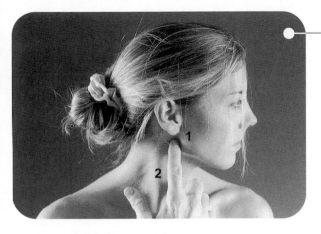

Fig. 1.18 | **The transverse process of the atlas**

Begin by locating the ramus of the mandible (*ramus mandibulae*) (1) and the sternocleidomastoid (2). The practitioner's index finger indicates the space between the two, and it is here that it is possible to palpate the transverse process of the atlas with its single tubercle. It is very prominent laterally.

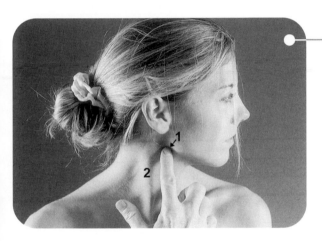

Fig. 1.19 | **The transverse process of the axis**

The point of reference in the approach to this structure is the angle of the mandible (gonion, *angulus mandibulae*) (1). The transverse process of the axis can be palpated either behind or in front of the sternocleidomastoid (2). It differs from the transverse process of the atlas in that it is very little defined.

Note: Great care should be taken in the approach to this structure. This need for caution applies to all the structures of the neck region.

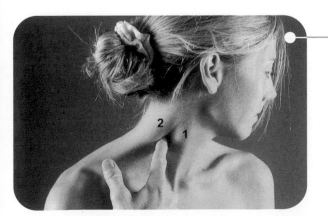

Fig. 1.20 | **The transverse processes of the third to seventh cervical vertebrae**

In the illustration opposite, the practitioner's index finger indicates the region between the sternocleidomastoid (1) and trapezius (2) muscles. These transverse processes can be located by sliding your contact into this region.

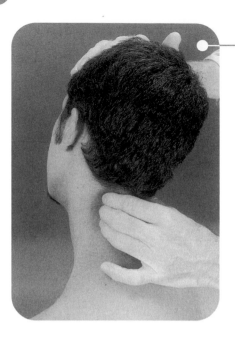

Fig. 1.21 | **The articular processes (*processus articulares*) of the cervical vertebrae**
Global approach

The practitioner has adopted a global contact, and is using a broad contact with the thumb and next three fingers to press the cervical portion of the trapezius muscle forward (Fig. 1.32) to make contact with the articular processes of the cervical vertebrae. The other hand should be placed on the subject's forehead, and used to bring about side-bending of the head to each side alternately. This causes the articular processes to appear distinctly beneath your fingers.

Note: Once the lateral border of the cervical portion of the trapezius has been located (Fig. 1.32), ensure that the muscle is thoroughly relaxed before beginning the palpation of the articular processes.

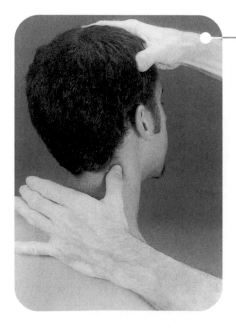

Fig. 1.22 | **The articular processes of the cervical vertebrae**
Global approach

The contact is identical to that described in Figure 1.21. This photograph illustrates the position of the practitioner's thumb in the contact shown there.

MYOLOGY

THE MUSCLES OF THE NECK, LATERAL ASPECT[1]

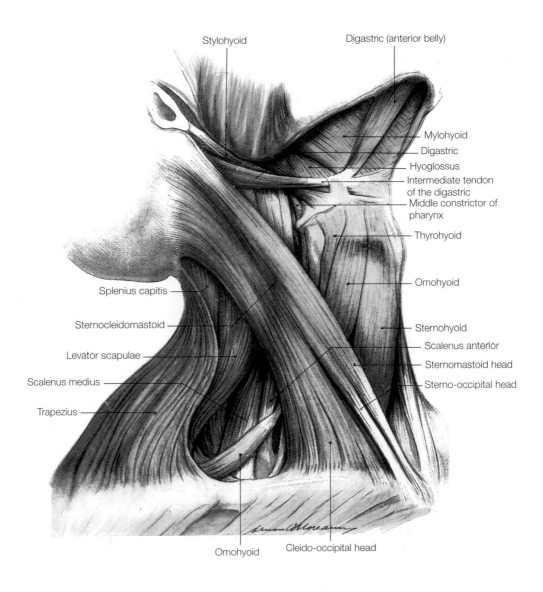

1. The plates by Henri Rouvière and André Delmas are from *Anatomie humaine, descriptive, topographique et fonctionnelle*, 15th edn. Vol. 1: *Tête et cou*; Vol. 2: *Tronc*; Vol. 3: *Membres*. Paris: Masson; 2002.

THE STERNOCLEIDOMASTOID REGION

The notable structures that can be detected by palpation are:

- The distal attachment of the sternal head of the sternocleidomastoid (*m. sternocleido-mastoideus*) (Fig. 1.24).
- The division of the sternal head of the sternocleidomastoid (Fig. 1.25).
- The body of the sternal head of the sternocleidomastoid (Fig. 1.26).
- The clavicular head of the sternocleidomastoid (Fig. 1.27).
- The mastoid insertion of the sternocleidomastoid (Fig. 1.28).

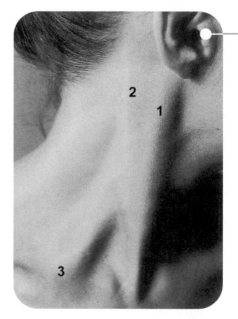

Fig. 1.23

Frontal view of the sternocleidomastoid (*m. sternocleidomastoideus*)

1. Sternal head of the sternocleidomastoid.
2. Occipital head of the sternocleidomastoid.
3. Clavicular head of the sternocleidomastoid.

Action
- Flexion.
- Inclination of the head and neck to the same side.
- Rotation of the head and neck to the opposite side.

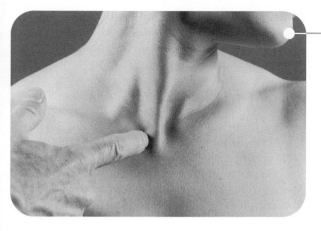

Fig. 1.24 | **The distal attachment of the sternal head of the sternocleidomastoid**
Method of approach and origin

The practitioner's index finger indicates the origin of this head, which is by means of a strong tendon on the sternal manubrium, medial to the sternoclavicular joint space. It can be made to protrude by asking the subject to rotate her head contralaterally (relative to the muscle concerned), slightly flexing it ipsilaterally.

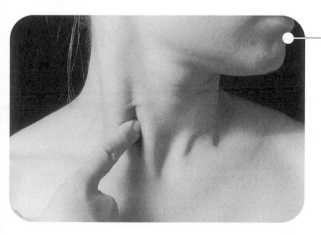

Fig. 1.25 | **Division of the sternal head of the sternocleidomastoid**
Method of approach and attachment

The sternal head is sometimes divided into two sets of fibers: the sternomastoid and the sterno-occipital. Where this is the case, these two sets of fibers attach to the sternum by two quite distinct tendons. The tendon of the sterno-occipital head is lateral to that of the sternomastoid head. The action required is exactly the same as that described above (Fig. 1.24). Where two heads exist, the practitioner's index finger can slide between them as shown in the adjacent figure.

Do not confuse the interstitium between the two heads with the triangular space that is easily palpable when the muscle is contracted (contralateral rotation with head inclined ipsilaterally), distinguishing the clavicular head from the sternal head (see 1 on Fig. 1.26).

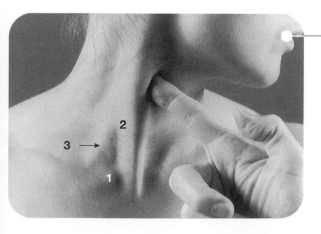

Fig. 1.26 | **The body of the sternal head of the sternocleidomastoid**

The body of the muscle takes shape a little above the sterno-clavicular joint, and runs in a cranio-posterolateral direction. Ask the subject to perform the same muscular action as that described for Figure 1.24.

Note: The number (1) indicates the triangular space between the sternal (2) and clavicular (3) heads of the sternocleidomastoid when the subject is asked to rotate the head and neck.

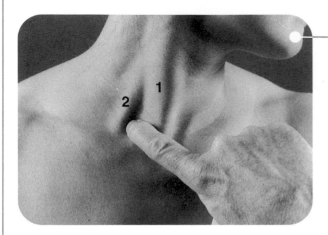

Fig. 1.27 | **The clavicular head of the sternocleidomastoid**
Method of approach and attachment

The practitioner's index finger indicates the cleido-occipital head, which is a superficial, oblique head arising distally on the medial third of the superior surface of the clavicle. It overlies the cleidomastoid head, which is aligned in a vertical direction. The muscular action requested of subjects is the same as that described for Figure 1.24. However, ask her this time to perform a more marked ipsilateral inclination of her head and to flex her head slightly.

Note: In the illustration opposite, the practitioner's index finger rests in an enclosed triangular space whose base lies inferiorly, separating the sternal (1) and clavicular (2) portions, the two main sets of fibers of the sternocleidomastoid.

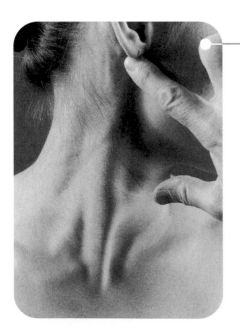

Fig. 1.28 | **The mastoid insertion of the sternocleidomastoid**
Method of approach and attachment

The sternocleidomastoid terminates on the cranium by means of four heads — two occipital, with their insertion on the lateral part of the superior nuchal line (*linea nuchae superior*) (not shown on the adjacent figure) — and two mastoid, which are inserted on the mastoid process of the temporal bone (*processus mastoideus*) (the structure indicated by the practitioner's index finger). The cleidomastoid head is inserted on the lateral surface of the mastoid process, and the sternomastoid on its apex.

THE LATERAL CERVICAL REGION (POSTERIOR TRIANGLE OF THE NECK, *REGIO CERVICALIS LATERALIS*)

The notable structures that can be detected by palpation are:

- The body of the scalenus posterior (posterior scalene) (*m. splenius posterior*) and scalenus medius (middle scalene) (*m. splenius medius*) muscles (Fig. 1.30).
- The splenius cervicis (*m. splenius cervicis; m. splenius colli*) (Fig. 1.30).

Actions

Posterior, middle, and anterior scalene muscles (scalenus posterior, medius, and anterior):

- When the fixed end is the cervical vertebral column: these muscles raise the first ribs and are inspiratory muscles.
- When the fixed end is on the thorax: these muscles bring about lateroflexion (side-bending) to the same side together with slight rotation to the opposite side.
  Splenius cervicis:
- Extension, inclination, and ipsilateral rotation of the head and neck.

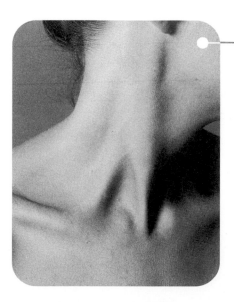

Fig. 1.29

Anterolateral aspect of the neck

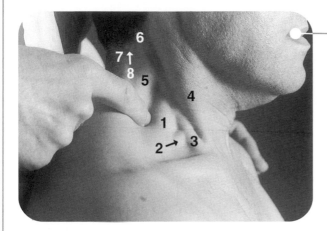

The scalenus muscles are classically described as being three in number; however, they can also be considered as proximally constituting a single muscular mass. The muscular mass (1) indicated by the practitioner's index finger is made up of the bodies of the scalenus posterior and medius muscles; the more posteriorly situated part could be considered as the scalenus posterior. To make this muscle mass appear, ask the subject to take several short, repeated in-breaths with the upper part of the thorax. This accessory inspiratory action is one of the actions of the scalenus muscles when the fixed end is on the cervical vertebral column.

Note: The scalenus posterior is inserted on the superolateral surface of the second rib. The scalenus medius is inserted on the superior surface of the first rib, behind the scalene tubercle (Lisfranc's tubercle, tuberculum musculi scaleni anterioris) and posterior to the groove for the subclavian artery.

1. Muscle mass made up of the bodies of the scalenus medius and scalenus posterior muscles.
2. Omohyoid, inferior belly (*m. omohyoideus, venter inferior*).
3. Sternocleidomastoid (clavicular head).
4. Sternocleidomastoid (sternal head).
5. Levator scapulae (*m. levator scapulae*).
6. Sternocleidomastoid (cleido-occipital head).
7. Trapezius (*m. trapezius*) (cervical portion).
8. Splenius cervicis (*m. splenius cervicis*).

SEQUENTIAL METHOD FOR THE EXPLORATION OF THE INDIVIDUAL MUSCLES OF THE LATERAL CERVICAL REGION

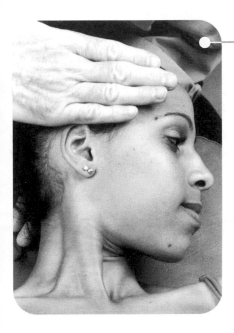

Fig. 1.31 | **Step 1: location of the sternocleidomastoid (*m. sternocleidomastoideus*)**

The subject is supine with the head turned to the left to cause the right sternocleidomastoid to become prominent. The practitioner takes up a position at the subject's head. Place one hand on the lateral surface of the subject's cranium, above the right ear, to cause the muscle to become prominent.

Attachments

The sternocleidomastoid can be described in terms of four heads: sterno-occipital, sternomastoid, cleido-occipital and cleidomastoid.

Inferiorly, the muscle arises from the pectoral girdle at two points; there is a clavicular and a sternal head.

- The clavicular head arises from the medial third of the superior surface of the clavicle, close to its posterior border. (The cleido-occipital head occupies a more superficial position than the cleidomastoid head, and lies closer to the anterior border of the clavicle.)
- The sternal head is attached inferiorly to the anterior surface of the sternal manubrium, below the sternoclavicular joint, by a strong tendon. In some cases this head is divided into two; in such cases this tendon is common to the sterno-occipital and the sternomastoid heads.

At the insertion, these four heads terminate in two occipital and two mastoid heads.

- The two occipital heads are inserted on the lateral part of the superior nuchal line (superior curved line of the occipital bone): the cleido-occipital head medially and the sterno-occipital head laterally.
- The two mastoid heads — cleidomastoid and sternomastoid — are inserted on the mastoid process of the temporal bone.

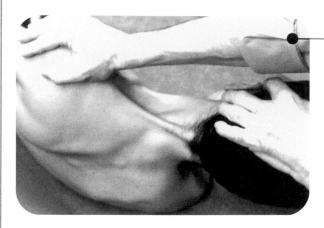

Fig. 1.32 | **Step 2: location of the trapezius (*m. trapezius*)**

The subject should lie on the right side. Hold down the subject's left shoulder with your right hand. At the same time, use your left hand on the inferolateral part of the subject's cranium to resist left side-bending of the head. This causes the clavicular portion of the trapezius, on the posterolateral part of the neck, to become prominent.

Note: See Attachments, Figure 2.58, p. 64.

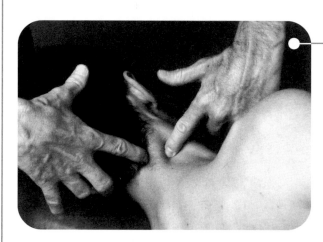

Fig. 1.33 | **Step 3: location of the levator scapulae (*m. levator scapulae*) Posterior view**

One method (not shown in the adjacent figure) of causing this muscle to become prominent, or to appear beneath your fingers, is to place one hand on the lateral surface of the subject's head to resist side-bending. This method calls for a starting position with the subject's head resting on the abdominal wall of the practitioner. Ask the subject to contract and relax the muscle repeatedly. This starting position enables you to control the period of relaxation between each set of alternating contraction and relaxation.

Another method (shown here) is to ask the subject to perform side-bending of the head and neck (with the weight of the head providing all the resistance required). This frees both your hands to take hold of the muscle to be investigated.

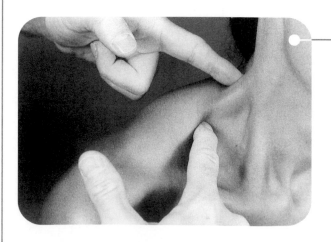

Fig. 1.34 | **Step 3 Alternative (anterior) view of the levator scapulae**

In the adjacent figure, the practitioner is holding the body of the levator scapulae between the two index fingers.

Attachments

- The origin of the levator scapulae is by means of four tendons on the posterior tubercles of the transverse processes of cervical vertebrae C1–C4.
- Its insertion is on the medial border of the scapula, above the spine of the scapula.

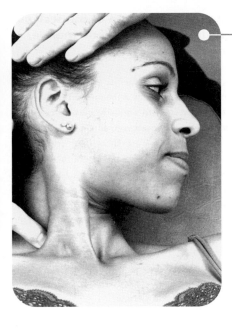

Fig. 1.35 | **Step 4**

The subject is supine, with the head turned to the left to make the right SCM appear prominently. The practitioner takes up a position at the subject's head. Place your left hand on the lateral surface of the subject's cranium, above the right ear. This makes prominent the posterior border of the clavicular head of the SCM. Locating this is important to enable the next step, in which you locate the scalenus anterior. This lies behind the SCM. Its position is indicated on the adjacent figure by the practitioner's index finger.

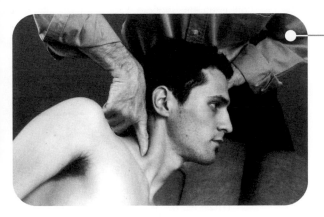

Fig. 1.36 | **Step 5: location of the scalenus anterior (anterior scalene muscle, *m. scalenus anterior*)**

The subject adopts a contralateral decubitus position. The practitioner's left hand supports the subject's head. Slide the index finger (perhaps also the middle finger) of your other hand behind the clavicular head of the SCM, so as to be able to palpate the scalenus anterior. This is more easily done if you also carry out passive side-bending of the subject's head and cervical spine. You can also ask subjects to take repeated short in-breaths to mobilize the upper part of the thoracic cage and so facilitate the perception of this muscle. This is one of the actions of scalenus anterior when its fixed end is superior (on the cervical spine).

Attachments
- The scalenus anterior arises superiorly, on the anterior tubercle of the transverse processes of vertebrae C3–C6.
- Its insertion is on the superior surface of the first rib (I), on the scalene tubercle (Lisfranc's tubercle) behind the subclavian vein and anterior to the subclavian artery. The phrenic nerve lies on its anterior surface.

Note: The phrenic nerve is situated in the sheath of the scalenus anterior, and connects with the subclavian nerve. It enters the thorax between the subclavian artery and vein.

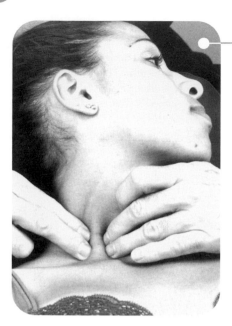

Fig. 1.37 | **Step 6: localization of the scalenus medius (middle scalene muscle, *m. scalenus medius*)**

Begin by locating the levator scapulae (*m. levator scapulae*) (Figs 1.33 and 1.34). Shift your contact anterior to that muscle. Your fingers roll into contact with a muscle mass of considerable volume; it lies directly beneath your fingers in the supraclavicular fossa. The adjacent figure shows the practitioner taking hold of this muscle, with a two-finger contact on each side. Ask the subject to flex the head and neck ipsilaterally, while you resist the side-bending action with one hand. The muscle is easier to detect beneath your fingers if you ask the subject to take repeated short in-breaths. (The subject should lie on the contralateral side, with the head resting on the practitioner's abdomen.)

Attachments
- The scalenus medius arises superiorly:
  - On the transverse process of the axis
  - On the anterior tubercles of the transverse processes of cervical vertebrae C3–C6
  - On the transverse process of C7.
- Its insertion is on the superior surface of the first rib, posterior to the scalene tubercle (Lisfranc's tubercle) and posterior to the subclavian artery.

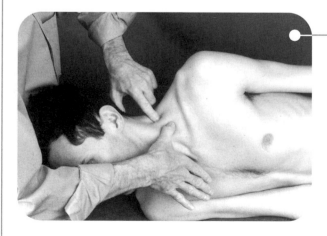

Fig. 1.38 | **Step 7: location of the scalenus posterior (posterior scalene muscle, *m. scalenus posterior*)**

The method is the same as that for the scalenus medius (Fig. 1.37). The adjacent figure shows the scalenus posterior between the practitioner's thumb and the index finger of the other hand. The bodies of the scalenus medius and scalenus posterior muscles sometimes fuse proximally so as to form a single muscle. In those cases where this has not happened, a depression can be felt between the two muscles.

Attachments
- The posterior scalenus arises on the posterior tubercle of the transverse processes of cervical vertebrae C4–C6.
- Inferiorly, it is inserted on the superolateral surface of the second rib.

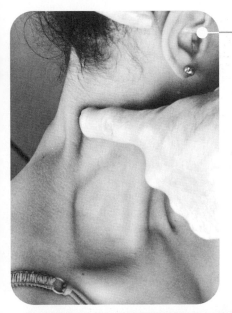

Fig. 1.39 | **Step 8: location of the splenius (*m. splenius cervicis, m. splenius colli*)**

This muscle is easy to locate once the levator scapulae has been found. Position your contact behind this muscle and you will make contact with the splenius; it is surrounded anteriorly and superiorly by the SCM, anteriorly and inferiorly by the levator scapulae, and posteriorly by the trapezius.

Attachments

The splenius arises inferiorly on the spinous processes of the middle cervical vertebrae and the inferior cervical and superior thoracic vertebrae (C4–T5). It then divides into two parts:

- The splenius capitis, with its insertion on the squama of the occipital bone and superior nuchal line, anterior to the SCM and on the mastoid process of the temporal bone.
- The splenius cervicis, which is inserted on the transverse processes of the atlas and axis and sometimes also the transverse processes of the third cervical vertebra (C3).

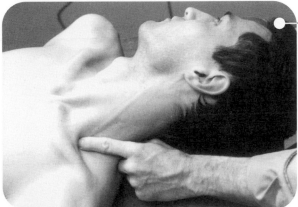

Fig. 1.40 | **Step 9: location of the omohyoid (*m. omohyoideus*)**
Method of approach and attachments

This muscle has two bellies and stretches from the hyoid to the superior border of the scapula. The practitioner's index finger indicates the inferior belly, at the inferior and lateral part of the supraclavicular fossa.

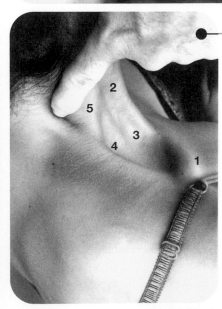

Fig. 1.41 | **Step 10: visualization and relations between the different muscles of the supraclavicular region**

In the adjacent figure, the practitioner's index finger indicates the position of the splenius muscle. It is also possible to visualize from this figure the relative positions of the muscles of the suprascapular region and the: clavicle (1): SCM (2), scalenus anterior (3) and scalenus medius (4) — sometimes fused together in its proximal part with the scalenus posterior — and the levator scapulae (5).

THE ANTERIOR CERVICAL REGION (ANTERIOR TRIANGLE OF THE NECK, *REGIO CERVICI ANTERIOR)*

The notable structures that can be detected by palpation are:

- The platysma (*platysma*) (Fig. 1.43).
- The mylohyoid muscle (*m. mylohyoideus*) (Fig. 1.44).
- The anterior belly of the digastric (*m. digastricus, venter anterior*) (Fig. 1.45).
- The sternohyoid (*m. sternohyoideus*). Topographical visualization (Fig. 1.46).
- The body of the sternohyoid muscle (*m. sternohyoideus*) (Fig. 1.47).
- The body of the superior (i.e. anterior) belly of the omohyoid (*m. omohyoideus — venter superior*) (Fig. 1.48).
- The sternothyroid muscle (*m. sternothyroideus*) (Fig. 1.49).

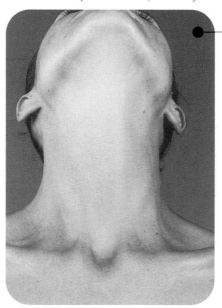

Fig. 1.42

The anterior cervical region

(See also anatomical plate p. 13.)

Actions

Suprahyoid muscles:

- The geniohyoid and mylohyoid muscles and the anterior belly of the digastric depress the mandible or elevate the hyoid. The action depends on which of these two bones is fixed.
- The posterior belly of the digastric, and the stylohyoid muscle, elevate the hyoid.

Infrahyoid muscles:

- These depress the hyoid bone.

All of the muscles acting on the hyoid also participate in lowering the mandible by fixing the inferior insertion of the suprahyoid muscles.

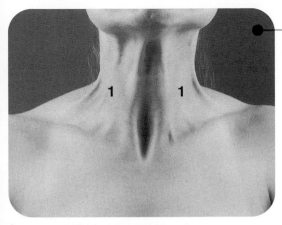

Fig. 1.43 | The platysma (*platysma*)

This structure (1) can be made to appear if you ask the subject to turn down the corners of the mouth, at the same time pulling them outward (laterally) and backward. The platysma stretches between the labial commissure and the inferior border of the mandible superiorly, and the skin of the pectoral and deltoid regions inferiorly. The platysma creates ridges in the deep layer of the skin.

Attachments

This is a very broad, thin, quadrate muscle, covering the anterolateral region of the neck and the inferior part of the face. It extends from the thorax to the mandible and cheek.

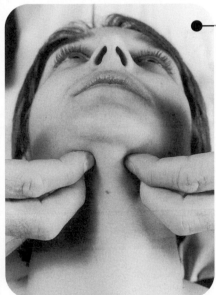

Fig. 1.44 | The mylohyoid (*m. mylohyoideus*)

This is the principal muscle of the floor of the mouth. Its inferior aspect is lined by the anterior belly of the digastric muscle (Fig. 1.45) and its superior aspect by the geniohyoid (*m. geniohyoideus*). Ask the subject to lower the mandible or open the mouth, or to swallow. This will enable you to sense contraction below and inside the free border of the mandible. (This action elevates the hyoid bone when the fixed end is on the mandible). (See plate p. 13.)

Attachments

- Superiorly, this muscle arises along the full length of the mylohyoid line of the mandible by means of tendinous fibers.
- Inferiorly, it is inserted on the body of the hyoid.

The two mylohyoid muscles intersect on the median line to form a median raphe.

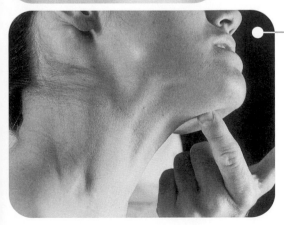

Fig. 1.45 | The anterior belly of the digastric (*m. digastricus, venter anterior*)

This muscle is situated superior to the hyoid bone (Figs 1.6–1.9); together with the mylohyoid it forms part of the muscles of the floor of the mouth (Fig. 1.44). Place your index finger in the interstitium between these two paired, symmetrical muscles, in contact with the raphe uniting the two mylohyoid muscles (see plate p. 13). The anterior bellies of the digastric muscles line the inferior surface of the mylohyoid muscles. The contraction can clearly be sensed if the subject is asked to lower the mandible.

The digastric is an elongated muscle made up of two bodies (the anterior and the posterior belly), which are joined by an intermediate tendon. It is situated in the superior, lateral part of the neck, and extends from the mastoid process to the mandibular symphysis.

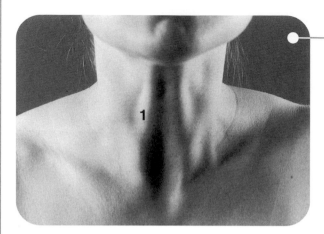

Fig. 1.46 | **The sternohyoid (*m. sternohyoideus*) Topographical visualization and attachments**

This muscle (1) arises on the posterior surface of the sterno-clavicular joint and adjacent parts of the clavicle and manubrium. It is inserted on the inferior border of the body of the hyoid bone, near the median line. These two muscles run superiorly and slightly medially (inward) in an oblique direction (see plate p. 13).

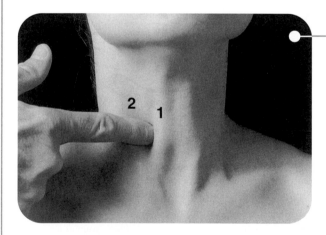

Fig. 1.47 | **The body of the sternohyoid**

In the adjacent figure the practitioner's index finger is separating the body of the sternohyoid (1) from the sternocleidomastoid (2).

Topographical relations: this is a thin muscle extending from the clavicle to the hyoid bone, anterior to the sternothyroid and thyrohyoid muscles.

Note: In some subjects, the muscle bodies are less easy to identify (see plate p. 13).

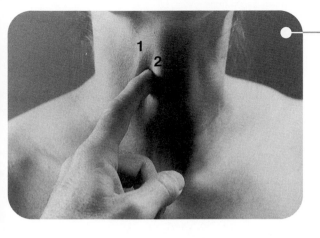

Fig. 1.48 | **The body of the superior belly of the omohyoid (*m. omohyoideus, venter superior*)**

This muscle (1) runs in a slightly oblique inferior and lateral (downward and outward) direction between the hyoid bone and the superior border of the scapula. The superior belly runs along the lateral border of the sternohyoid (2) (see also Fig. 1.46) and then continues via an intermediate tendon into the inferior belly (see Fig. 1.30). The tendon marks the change in direction of the muscle, and lies at the same depth as the internal jugular vein. The inferior belly arises on the anterior surface of the body of the scapula, close to the superior border and within the suprascapular notch (*incisura scapulae*) (see plate p. 13).

Attachments
The insertion of this muscle is by means of tendinous fibers on the inferior border of the body of the hyoid bone, behind the sternohyoid muscle.

Note: Contraction of the omohyoid may possibly affect the blood flow of the internal jugular vein (v. jugularis interna).

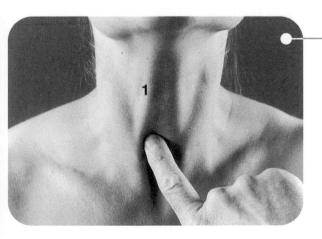

Fig. 1.49 | **The sternothyroid (*m. sternothyroideus*)**

The sternothyroid is a small muscle, located underneath the practitioner's index finger. Push aside the sternohyoid muscle laterally (1) (Figs 1.46 and 1.47) with your index finger to access the sternothyroid. It is not always possible to detect this muscle as such beneath your fingers in all subjects.

Attachments
This is a flattened, elongated muscle, extending from the sternum to the thyroid gland, anterior to the larynx and thyroid.

NERVES AND BLOOD VESSELS

The notable structures that can be detected by palpation are:

- The subclavian artery (*a. subclavia*) (Fig. 1.51).
- The brachial plexus (*plexus brachialis*) (Fig. 1.52).
- The internal carotid artery (*a. carotis interna*). Taking the pulse (Fig. 1.53).

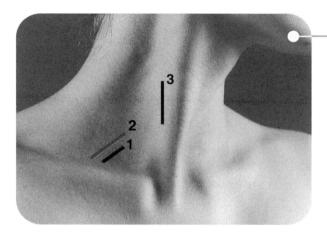

Fig. 1.50

The nerves and blood vessels of the neck

1. The subclavian artery.
2. The brachial plexus.
3. The carotid artery.

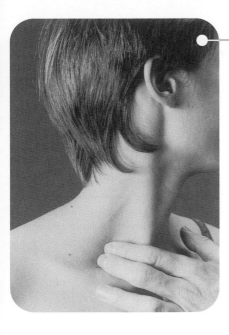

Fig. 1.51 | The subclavian artery (*a. subclavia*)

Begin by locating the clavicular head of the sternocleidomastoid (see Fig. 1.27). Contralateral rotation of the subject's head is needed; ask the subject to turn the head to the opposite side. Place a broad contact with your fingers on the medial third of the clavicle, across the cleido-occipital head of the muscle; beneath your fingers you will detect the pulse of this artery.

Note: The subclavian artery passes just behind the scalenus anterior muscle (Fig. 1.36).

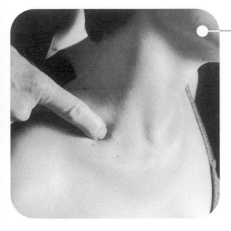

Fig. 1.52 | The brachial plexus (*plexus brachialis*)

The approach is the same as that described above (Fig. 1.51). Through the cleido-occipital head, you will detect a full, cylindrical cord. This is the brachial plexus, indicated here by the practitioner's index finger. Ask the subject to rotate and incline the head to the opposite side; at the same time, extend and externally rotate the subject's arm. This has the effect of stretching the structure and making it more easily perceptible.

Note: The brachial plexus passes between the scalenus anterior (Fig. 1.36) and scalenus medius muscles (Fig. 1.37), together with the subclavian artery.

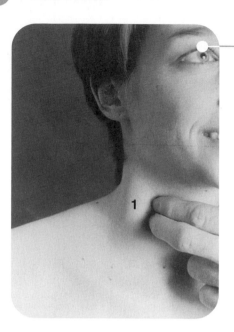

Fig. 1.53 | **The internal carotid artery (*a. carotis interna*)**
Taking the pulse

The carotid pulse can be taken either anteriorly and medially to the sternal head of the sternocleidomastoid (1), as in the adjacent figure, or posteriorly and laterally to it.

Note: The carotid pulse is only ever taken on one side at a time, so as not to arrest cerebral circulation completely. Great care should be taken when applying pressure to the carotid artery, because, if there are any atheromatous plaques present, they could become detached and cause a cerebral embolism. The carotid pulse is extremely useful in an emergency situation, as it can be detected at low blood pressure (around 60 mmHg). This level is just sufficient to keep the brain from hypoxia.

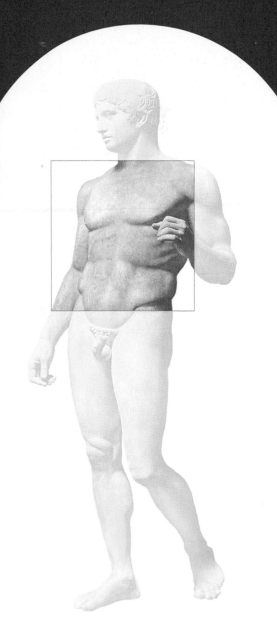

CHAPTER 2

THE TRUNK AND SACRUM

TOPOGRAPHICAL PRESENTATION OF THE TRUNK AND SACRUM

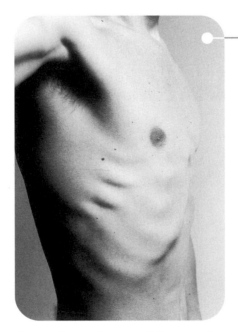

Fig. 2.1

Anterolateral view of the trunk

OSTEOLOGY

THE BONES OF THE THORACIC CAGE

Anterior view

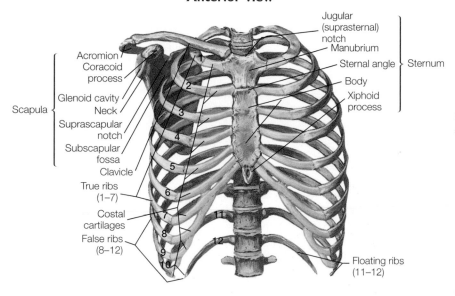

- Jugular (suprasternal) notch
- Manubrium
- Sternal angle
- Body
- Xiphoid process
- Sternum

- Acromion
- Coracoid process
- Glenoid cavity
- Neck
- Suprascapular notch
- Subscapular fossa
- Clavicle
- Scapula

- True ribs (1–7)
- Costal cartilages
- False ribs (8–12)

1
2
3
4
5
6
7
8
9
10
11
12

- Floating ribs (11–12)

Posterior view

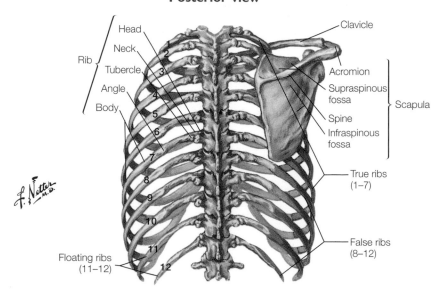

- Clavicle
- Head
- Neck
- Tubercle
- Angle
- Body
- Rib

- Acromion
- Supraspinous fossa
- Spine
- Infraspinous fossa
- Scapula

1
2
3
4
5
6
7
8
9
10
11
12

- True ribs (1–7)
- False ribs (8–12)
- Floating ribs (11–12)

F. Netter M.D.

THE SKELETON OF THE ABDOMEN

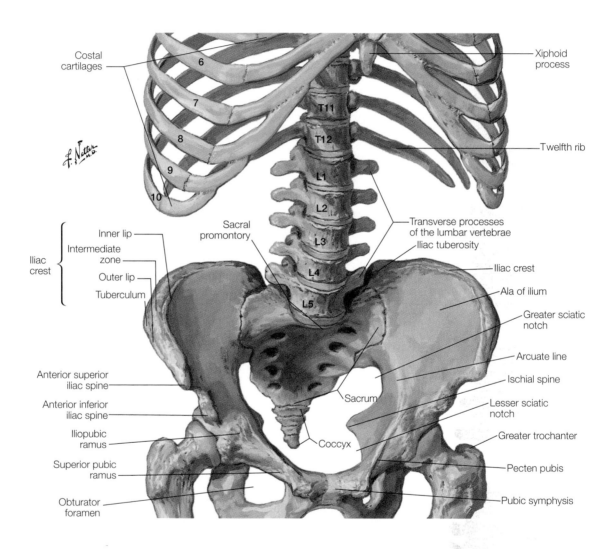

Costal cartilages

6

7

8

9

10

Xiphoid process

T11

T12

Twelfth rib

L1

L2

L3

L4

L5

Iliac crest

Inner lip
Intermediate zone
Outer lip
Tuberculum

Sacral promontory

Transverse processes of the lumbar vertebrae
Iliac tuberosity
Iliac crest
Ala of ilium
Greater sciatic notch
Arcuate line
Ischial spine
Lesser sciatic notch
Greater trochanter

Anterior superior iliac spine

Anterior inferior iliac spine

Iliopubic ramus

Superior pubic ramus

Obturator foramen

Sacrum

Coccyx

Pecten pubis

Pubic symphysis

THE VERTEBRAL COLUMN

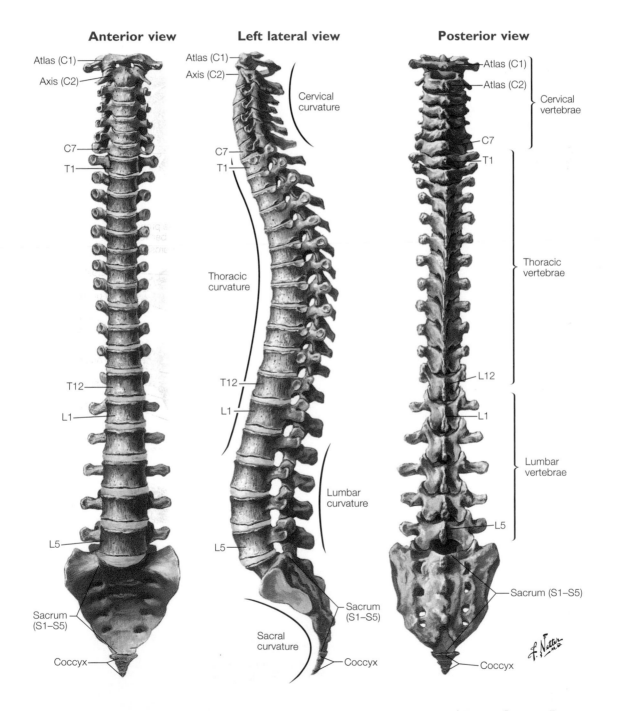

Anterior view

Atlas (C1)
Axis (C2)
C7
T1
T12
L1
L5
Sacrum (S1–S5)
Coccyx

Left lateral view

Atlas (C1)
Axis (C2)
Cervical curvature
C7
T1
Thoracic curvature
T12
L1
Lumbar curvature
L5
Sacrum (S1–S5)
Sacral curvature
Coccyx

Posterior view

Atlas (C1)
Atlas (C2)
Cervical vertebrae
C7
T1
Thoracic vertebrae
L12
L1
Lumbar vertebrae
L5
Sacrum (S1–S5)
Coccyx

THE THORAX

The notable structures that can be detected by palpation are:

- The sternum (*sternum*): general view (Fig. 2.3).
- The manubrium of the sternum (*manubrium sterni*) (Fig. 2.4).
- Jugular (suprasternal) notch (*incisura jugularis*) (Fig. 2.5).
- Sternal angle (*angulus sterni*) (angle of Louis) (Fig. 2.6).
- Body of sternum (*corpus sterni*) (Fig. 2.7).
- Xiphoid process (*processus xiphoideus*) (Fig. 2.8).
- Superior thoracic aperture (thoracic inlet) (*apertura thoracis superior*) (Fig. 2.9).
- First costal cartilage (*cartilago costalis*) (Fig. 2.10).
- First rib: body (*corpus costae*) above the clavicle (*clavicula*) (Fig. 2.11).
- Posterior extremity of the body (shaft) of the first rib (*costa prima*) (Figs 2.12 and 2.13).
- Tubercle of the scalenus anterior muscle (*tuberculum m. scaleni anterioris*) (Lisfranc's tubercle) (Fig. 2.14).
- Anterior extremity of the body (shaft) of the second rib (*costa secunda*) (Fig. 2.15).
- Body of the second rib in the anterior part of the thorax (Fig. 2.16).
- The second rib in the lateral cervical region (posterior triangle of the neck) (Fig. 2.17).
- Posterior extremity of the body of the second rib (*costa secunda*) (Fig. 2.18).
- True ribs (*costae verae*) (see note, Fig. 2.11) (Fig. 2.19).
- False ribs (*costae spuriae*) (Fig. 2.20).
- Inferior thoracic aperture (thoracic outlet) (*apertura thoracis inferior*) (Fig. 2.21).
- Notches of the costal margin (seventh, eighth, ninth, and tenth costal cartilages) (Fig. 2.22).
- Eleventh rib (*costa XI*) (Fig. 2.23): anterior extremity (Fig. 2.24).
- Twelfth rib (*costa XII*) (Fig. 2.25).
- Twelfth rib anterior extremity (Figs 2.26 and 2.27).
- Tenth rib (*costa X*) (Fig. 2.28).
- Angle of rib (*angulus costae*) (Fig. 2.29).

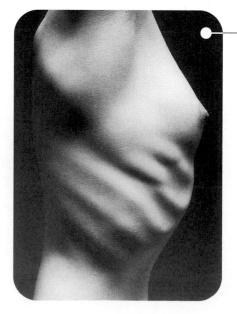

Fig. 2.2 | **Lateral view of the thorax**

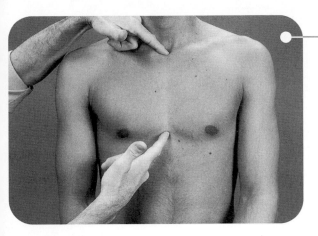

Fig. 2.3 | **The sternum (*sternum*)**
General view

This is a flat, unpaired bone occupying the medial ventral part of the thorax, the area between the practitioner's index fingers in the adjacent figure. It is made up of three parts: the cranial part or manubrium (Fig. 2.4); a middle part, the body of the sternum (or mesosternum) (Fig. 2.7); and a caudal part, the xiphoid process (Fig. 2.8).

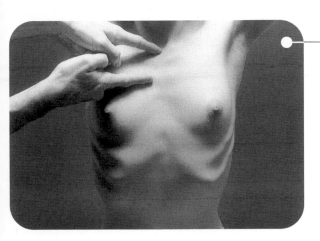

Fig. 2.4 | **The manubrium of the sternum**
(*manubrium sterni*)

The body of the sternum lies in the position indicated in the adjacent figure, and accounts for about one-third of the total length of the sternum. The junction with the body of the sternum is at the level of the second rib.

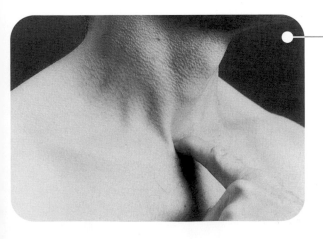

Fig. 2.5 | **Jugular (suprasternal) notch**
(*incisura jugularis*)

This is situated on the base or superior (cranial) border of the sternum, as indicated by the practitioner's index finger. It can be felt beneath the index finger as an upward-facing concave notch.

Note: The two other notches on this segment of the sternum are the clavicular notches, which receive the medial extremity of the clavicles. They are concave in the transverse direction and flat anteriorly and posteriorly, and they face upward and outward.

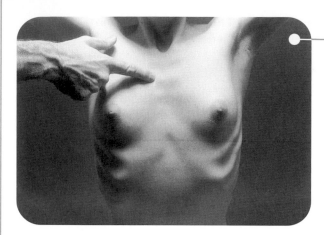

Fig. 2.6 | **The sternal angle (angle of Louis; *angulus sterni*)**

This structure, indicated by the practitioner's index finger, represents the line of union between the manubrium (Fig. 2.4) and body (Fig. 2.7) of the sternum. This junction is at the level of the second rib, and forms the anteriorly raised crest of a dihedral angle.

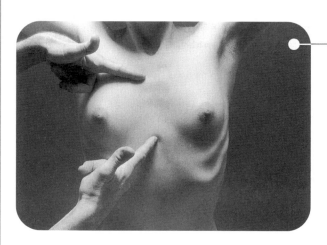

Fig. 2.7 | **The body of the sternum (*corpus sterni*)**

The practitioner's index fingers indicate the general position of this part of the sternum, situated between the sternal angle (Fig. 2.6) and the xiphoid process (Fig. 2.8). When you palpate the anterior part of this structure, you will find three or four transverse crests, which are the vestiges of the fusion of the sternebrae. You will also detect vertical ridges that provide the insertion of the sternochondral parts of the pectoralis major muscles (see also Fig. 3.39).

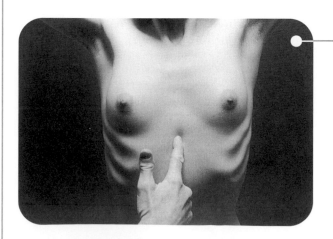

Fig. 2.8 | **The xiphoid process (*processus xiphoideus*)**

This is situated at the caudal extremity of the body of the sternum (Fig. 2.7), aligned as an extension of its posterior surface. Palpation of this structure therefore finds it to be slightly recessed. The tip of the xiphoid process is sometimes forked and may incline forward, backward or to the side. Accessibility is therefore variable between different subjects.

Note: This structure is almost always cartilaginous in adults.

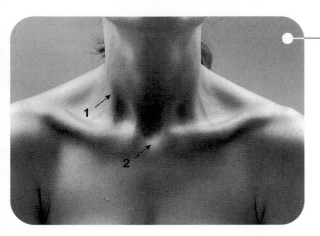

Fig. 2.9 | The superior thoracic aperture (thoracic inlet; *apertura thoracis superior*)

This aperture is elliptical in shape, the transverse diameter being the larger. It is inclined obliquely anteriorly and inferiorly. It is bounded anteriorly by the jugular notch (1) (see also Fig. 2.5), which projects on to the inferior border of the second thoracic vertebra. Laterally it is bounded by the first rib (2) and posteriorly by the superior border of the first thoracic vertebra.

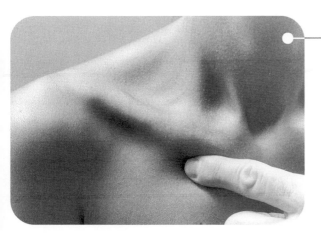

Fig. 2.10 | The first costal cartilage (*cartilago costalis*)

To locate this structure, place your index finger immediately below the clavicle, in contact with the lateral border of the manubrium of the sternum. If this proves difficult, ask the subject to take rapid, repeated in-breaths. This makes it easier to sense the structure beneath your index finger.

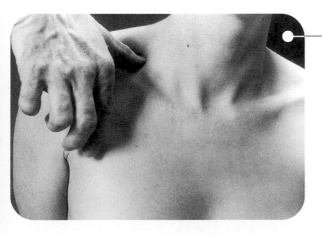

Fig. 2.11 | The first rib: body or shaft (*corpus costae*), above the clavicle (*clavicula*)

Locate a position above and behind the clavicle, where you will find a structure that feels dense. This is the first rib. It can be palpated along almost its entire length.

Note: The first rib is a true rib, i.e. a rib that is attached to the sternum by means of a costal cartilage.

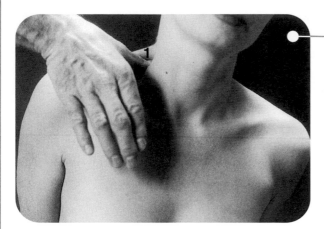

Fig. 2.12   **The posterior extremity of the body (shaft) of the first rib (*costa prima*)**

It is very easy to access the first rib at this point; push back the superior fibers of the trapezius (1) in a posterior direction, as shown here, until you encounter it.

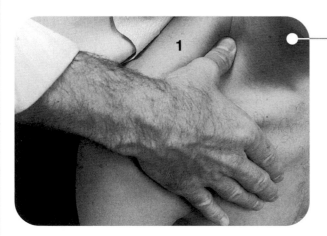

Fig. 2.13   **Close-up of posterior extremity of the body (shaft) of the first rib**

The adjacent figure shows the practitioner's thumb pushing back the superior fibers of the trapezius (1) and resting on the posterior-most part of the cranial surface of the first rib.

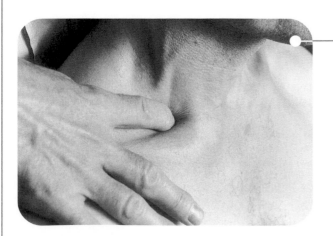

Fig. 2.14   **The tubercle of the scalenus anterior (*tuberculum m. scaleni anterioris*) (Lisfranc's tubercle)**

Beginning from a position above and behind the clavicle, loosen the musculature of the region to facilitate the localization of this structure. The best way to do this is to ask subjects to turn and incline their head to the ipsilateral side. In some subjects, you will feel the tubercle through the thickness of the two clavicular heads of the sternocleidomastoid.

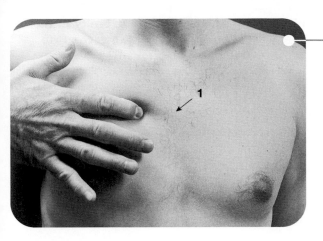

Fig. 2.15 | **The anterior extremity of the body (shaft) of the second rib (*costa secunda*)**

This lies between the first rib and middle ribs, at the lateral extension of the sternal angle (1) (see also Fig. 2.6). In the adjacent figure, the practitioner's index finger is in the second intercostal space, lying in contact with the inferior part of the second rib.

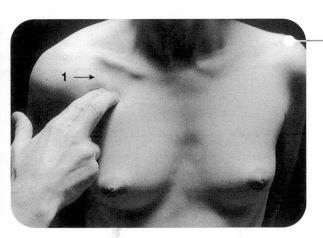

Fig. 2.16 | **The body of the second rib in the anterior part of the thorax**

As indicated in the adjacent figure, the second rib can be followed along its length, in the direction of the coracoid process (1), as far as the point where the rib passes under the clavicle.

Note: The second rib is a true rib (see note to Figure 2.11).

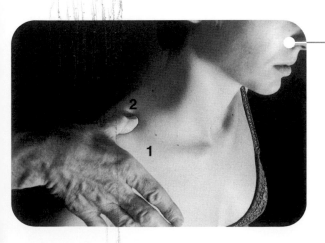

Fig. 2.17 | **The body of the second rib in the lateral cervical region (posterior triangle of the neck)**

In the lateral cervical region, behind the external extremity of the clavicle (1), there is a dense structure that can be felt beneath your fingers when the trapezius (2) is pushed aside posteriorly. This bony structure is the second rib. It is easier to detect if you direct your contact downward and ask the subject to take short, repeated in-breaths using the upper part of the thoracic cage, so mobilizing the second rib.

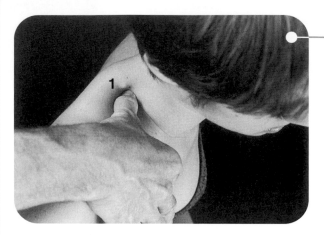

Fig. 2.18 | **The posterior extremity of the body (shaft) of the second rib**

In the adjacent figure, the practitioner is palpating the spinal extremity of the second rib. Push aside the trapezius (1) using a contact positioned posterior and inferior to the first rib (see Fig. 2.12).

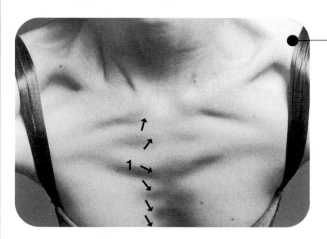

Fig. 2.19 | **The true ribs (*costae verae*)**

The sternal extremity of the true ribs (1) can clearly be seen down as far as the sixth rib in the adjacent figure. The seventh rib can be seen in Figure 2.20 (illustration below). The true ribs can be counted easily, starting from the sternal angle (see Fig. 2.6), which corresponds to the second rib. There are seven true ribs.

(See note to Figure 2.11.)

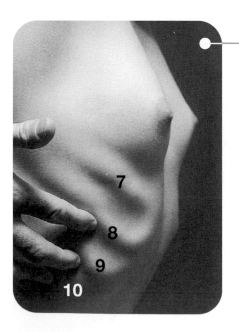

Fig. 2.20 | **The false ribs (*costae spuriae*)**

The three false ribs (8, 9, and 10), indicated by the practitioner's spread fingers in the adjacent figure, have the special feature that they are linked anteriorly by means of their cartilaginous ventral extremity, which extends and unites them to the costal cartilage above. Together with the cartilage of the seventh rib (7), they make up the costal margin (costal arch) (*arcus costalis*).

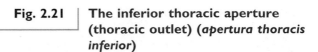

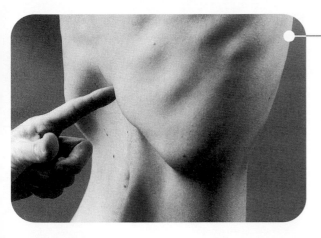

Fig. 2.21 | The inferior thoracic aperture (thoracic outlet) (*apertura thoracis inferior*)

This is an elliptical aperture, whose larger diameter is transverse. It is approximately three times as large as the superior thoracic aperture (Fig. 2.9). It lies on a plane that is inclined downward and posteriorly. Anteriorly (at the front) it is delimited by the xiphoid process (Fig. 2.8), which is in line with the tenth thoracic vertebra, and posteriorly (behind) by the body of the twelfth thoracic vertebra. Laterally it is delimited by the costal margin (seventh, eighth, ninth, and tenth costal cartilages) and floating ribs. (See Figs 2.23–2.27.)

Note: This aperture is filled by the diaphragm (diaphragma).

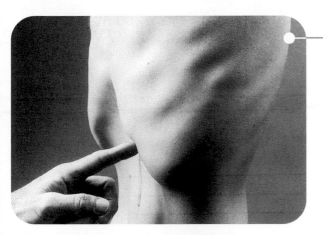

Fig. 2.22 | The notches of the costal margin (seventh, eighth, ninth, and tenth costal cartilages)

As you palpate along the inferior border of the costal margin from the xiphoid process, two notches are evident. The first (indicated on the figure above — Fig. 2.21 — by the practitioner's index finger) corresponds to the junction of the eighth and seventh costal cartilages. There is a second notch (indicated by the practitioner's index finger in the adjacent figure) corresponding to the junction of the tenth and ninth costal cartilages.

Note: These two notches are not always clearly marked.

Fig. 2.23 | The eleventh rib

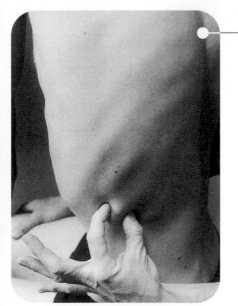

The adjacent figure shows the eleventh rib, held between the practitioner's thumb and index finger. The best approach is to stand behind the subject, placing your two hands on the inferior border of the costal margin (Fig. 2.20). Locate the inferior border of the tenth rib and position your contact here. Now shift your contact to a position level with the anterolateral abdominal wall, toward the iliac crest (*crista iliaca*), feeling for a rib situated immediately below the caudal border of the costal margin, one that has a free ventral (anterior) extremity.

Note: The iliac crest is described in Chapter 8.

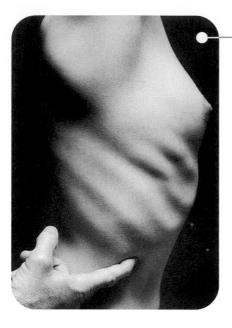

Fig. 2.24 | **The eleventh rib**
Anterior extremity

In the adjacent figure, the practitioner's index finger indicates the ventral (anterior) extremity of the eleventh rib, with a tapered costal cartilage whose end is free. This is termed a floating rib.

Note: This rib has a length of around 20 cm (8 in) and its ventral extremity is usually at some distance from the inferior border of the tenth rib. However, it can be close to it, or even fused with it.

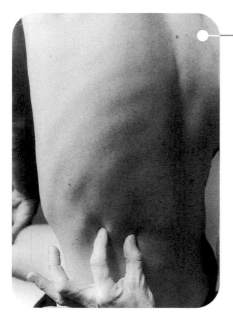

Fig. 2.25 | **The twelfth rib**

The adjacent figure shows the twelfth rib, which the practitioner is grasping between thumb and index finger. Having located the eleventh rib (Figs 2.23 and 2.24), shift your contact down the subject's side in the direction of the iliac crest, at the same time as moving it posteriorly, since the twelfth rib is slightly shorter than the eleventh.

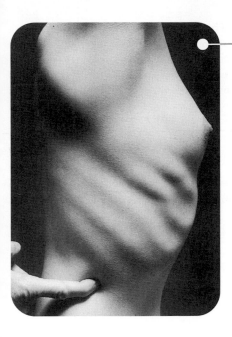

Fig. 2.26 | **The twelfth rib**
Anterior extremity
Lateral view

In the adjacent figure, the practitioner's index finger is positioned on the ventral (anterior) extremity of the twelfth rib. Like the eleventh, it ends in a tapered, free costal cartilage.

Note: The twelfth rib is also floating, and is usually (in about two-thirds of cases) between 10 and 14 cm (4–5¹/₂ in) long. However, it can be very short, measuring 3–6 cm (1¹/₂–2¹/₂ in), in which case it can be confused with the transverse process of a lumbar vertebra.

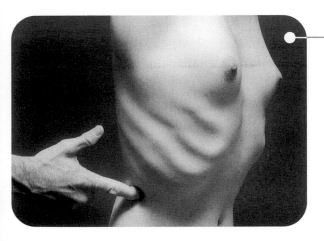

Fig. 2.27 | **The twelfth rib**
Anterior extremity
Anterolateral view

In the adjacent figure, the practitioner's index finger is positioned on the ventral (anterior) extremity of the twelfth rib. This anterolateral view of the thorax shows the relationship between this structure and the eleventh rib (Figs 2.23 and 2.24) and with the costal margin (*arcus costalis*) (Fig. 2.20).

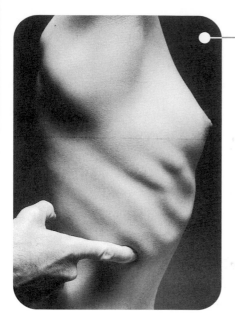

Fig. 2.28 | **The tenth rib**

The ventral (anterior) extremity of the tenth rib may be unattached to the cartilage of the ninth. In that case its anterior extremity remains free. The practitioner's index finger is on that extremity in this figure.

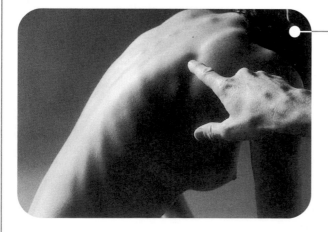

Fig. 2.29 | **The angle of the rib**

This angle represents the first change in direction of the rib on the dorsal part of the thorax. From this point on, it takes a downward, anterior direction.

THE THORACIC AND LUMBAR SPINE

The notable structures that can be detected by palpation are:

- The thoracic spine: all the thoracic vertebrae (*vertebrae thoracicae*) from T1 to T12 (Fig. 2.31).
- The cervicothoracic transition (C6–C7–T1) (Fig. 2.32).
- Vertebrae C6, C7 and T1 (Figs 2.33 and 2.34).
- Visualization of relations between the scapula and spinous processes of the vertebrae (Fig. 2.35).
- Spinous process (*processus spinosus*) of T1 (Fig. 2.36).
- Spinous process of T3 (Fig. 2.37).
- Spinous process of T7 (Fig. 2.38).
- Transverse process (*processus transversus*) of the thoracic vertebrae (Fig. 2.39).
- The lumbar spine: all the lumbar vertebrae (*vertebrae lumbales*) from L1 to L5 (Fig. 2.40).
- Fourth (L4) and fifth (L5) lumbar vertebrae (Figs 2.41 and 2.42).
- Costal process (*processus costiformis; processus costalis*) of the lumbar vertebrae (Fig. 2.43).

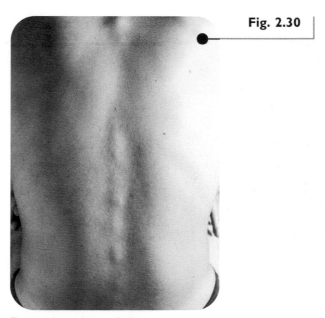

Fig. 2.30

Posterior view of the thoracolumbar spine in the forward flexed position

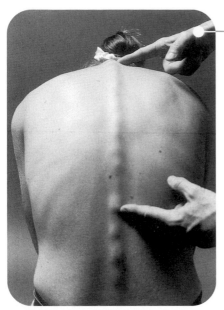

Fig. 2.31 | **The thoracic spine: all the thoracic vertebrae (*vertebrae thoracicae*) from T1 to T12**

The extent of the thoracic spine (all the thoracic vertebrae from T1 to T12) is shown here by the position of the practitioner's two index fingers.

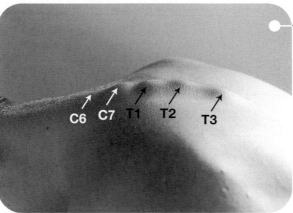

Fig. 2.32 | **The cervicothoracic transition C6–C7–T1**

The adjacent figure clearly shows the spinous processes of the last cervical vertebra, C7, and the first thoracic vertebra, T1, T2, and T3.

Note: The subject is seated, with head bent forward.

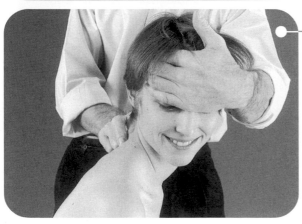

Fig. 2.33 | **Exploration of C6, C7, and T1 — test while rotating the head**

The subject is seated with her head in a neutral position (or slightly bent). The practitioner should stand beside the subject. Place your index, middle, and ring fingers on the spinous processes of the sixth (C6) and seventh (C7) cervical vertebrae and first thoracic vertebra (T1) (Fig. 2.32). Then, with your other hand, take hold of the subject's head and ease it into rotation to the right and then to the left, several times if necessary. You will detect a slight movement at the level of C7; no movement occurs at T1, but there is marked movement at C6.

Note: The slight motion detected when the subject's head is turned can vary; it may be zero when the head is turned to the right, but more marked when turned the other way. That is why it is necessary to test both sides.

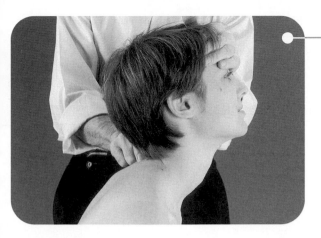

Fig. 2.34 | Exploration of C6, C7 and T1 — test with head extended

The subject is seated with her head in a neutral position (neither flexed nor extended). The practitioner should stand beside the subject. Place the index, middle, and ring fingers of one hand on the spinous processes of the sixth and seventh cervical vertebrae (C6 and C7) and first thoracic vertebra (T1) (Fig. 2.32). Hold the subject's forehead in the palm of your other hand, and ease the head into hyperextension. The spinous process of C6 will "disappear" into the physiological cervical curvature, the spinous process of C7 will be "displaced" (the extent of this varies, depending on the subject), and the spinous process of T1 will remain immobile beneath your fingers.

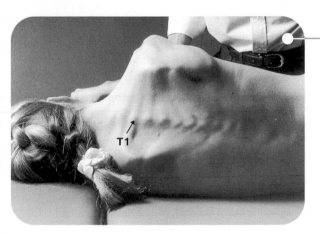

Fig. 2.35 | Visualization of the relationship between the scapula and spinous processes

In the adjacent figure, with the subject in the lateral decubitus position, the craniomedial (superointernal) angle of the scapula is seen to be in line with the spinous process of the first thoracic vertebra, T1. The medial extremity of the spine of the scapula is in line with the spinous process of T3, and the inferior angle of the scapula with the spinous process of T7.

Note: The aim of the above approach should be seen as facilitating initial rapid exploration of the spinous processes. The next stage is to "count" along from C7 (see Figs 2.32–2.34) or from L5 (see Figs 2.41 and 2.42). The positions described here should simply be taken as indicative. Various factors may significantly affect the topographical relationships between the scapula and vertebral column. For example: the position of the scapula on the thoracic cage (and its mobility), the position of the subject on the table, a number of possible dysmorphisms (kyphosis, flat back, scoliosis, etc.)

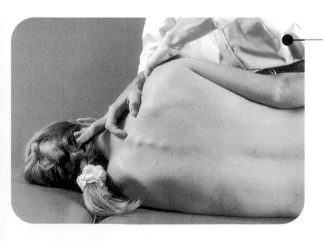

Fig. 2.36 | Exploration of the spinous process (*processus spinosus*) of T1

In the adjacent figure, the practitioner's thumb and index finger demonstrate the relationship (see Fig. 2.35) between the craniomedial (superointernal) angle of the scapula (indicated by the practitioner's thumb) and the spinous process of the first thoracic vertebra (indicated by the practitioner's index finger).

Note: Figures 2.33 and 2.34 show the most reliable method of finding T1.

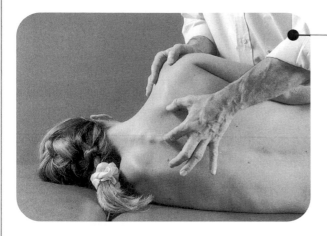

Fig. 2.37 | **Exploration of the spinous process of T3**

In the adjacent figure, the practitioner's thumb and index finger contact demonstrates the relationship (see also Fig. 2.35) between the medial extremity of the spine of the scapula (indicated by the practitioner's thumb) and the spinous process of the third thoracic vertebra (indicated by the practitioner's index finger).

Note: The most reliable method of locating this structure is by counting from vertebra C7 (Figs 2.32–2.34).

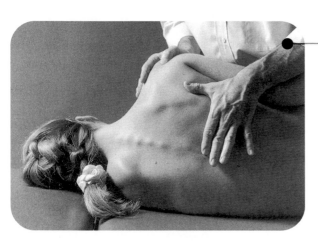

Fig. 2.38 | **Exploration of the spinous process of T7**

In the adjacent figure, the practitioner's thumb and index finger demonstrate the relationship (see also Fig. 2.35) between the inferior angle of the scapula and the spinous process of the seventh thoracic vertebra, T7 (indicated by the practitioner's index finger).

Note: The most reliable method of locating this structure is by counting from vertebra C7 (Figs 2.32–2.34).

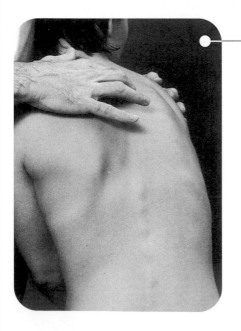

Fig. 2.39 | **The transverse process (*processus transversus*) of the thoracic vertebrae**

The subject is seated, with the practitioner standing alongside. Cradle the anterior surface of the subject's shoulders in the palms of your hands. Search medially to the costal angle and about two finger-widths laterally to the spinous processes. The transverse process is felt as a dense entity, as it is a bony structure. The cradling hold enables the practitioner to induce a rotation of the trunk, which makes it easier to locate the structure. It can be difficult to access in some subjects for reasons of morphology.

Note: The figure shown here demonstrates the method of approach, not the bony structure concerned. Rotation of the trunk makes the costal angle more prominent and easier to distinguish from the transverse process of the vertebra, two finger-widths away from the spinous process.

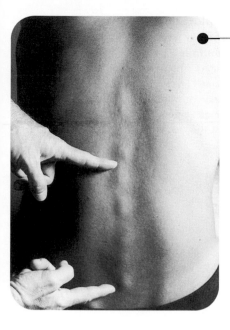

Fig. 2.40 | **The lumbar spine: all the lumbar vertebrae (*vertebrae lumbales*) from L1 to L5**

In the adjacent figure, the practitioner's index fingers indicate the lumbar spine (all the lumbar vertebrae from L1 to L5).

Note: The lumbar spine consists of five lumbar vertebrae. Their number may be increased by one if the first sacral vertebra, S1, appears as a lumbar vertebra, or decreased by one if the last lumbar vertebra, L5, takes the form of a sacral vertebra.

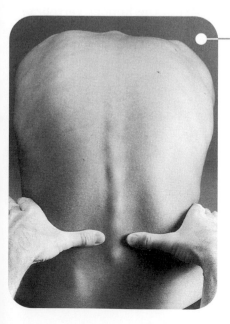

Fig. 2.41 | **Exploration of the fourth (L4) and fifth (L5) lumbar vertebrae**

In the adjacent figure, the practitioner's hands are resting on the iliac crest with the thumbs extended toward the lumbar spine. If you let your thumbs fall naturally, so that they are placed slightly ahead of your palms, they point toward the intervertebral disc (L4–L5, as in the figure here). If your thumbs are placed in the same plane as the palms of your hands, they point toward the spinous processes of the fourth lumbar vertebra, L4.

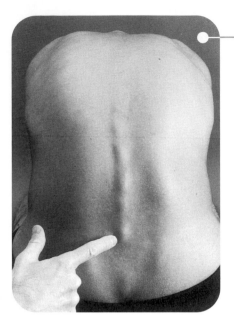

Fig. 2.42 | **Exploration of the fifth (L5) lumbar vertebra (*vertebra lumbalis V*)**

Once you have located L4 (see Fig. 2.41), the spinous process of the vertebra below it can be contacted. This is the fifth lumbar vertebra, indicated in this figure by the practitioner's index finger.

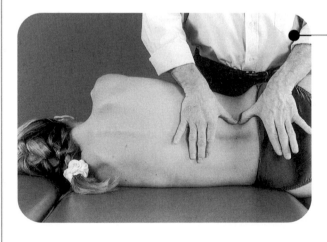

Fig. 2.43 | **The transverse or costal process (*processus costiformis; processus costalis*) of the lumbar vertebrae**

The subject should lie on the contralateral side. Place your thumbs lateral to the erector spinae muscles and direct your contact toward the lumbar spine until you make contact with a dense structure. This is the structure you are looking for.

Notes:
- When examining well-muscled subjects, this density should be localized posteriorly, through the mass of the erector spinae muscles.
- The transverse (costal) process of the first lumbar vertebra is shorter than that of the other lumbar vertebrae. The transverse (costal) process of the fifth lumbar vertebra is longer than that of the other lumbar vertebrae. Exaggerated development of this process may bring about connection and fusion of the fifth lumbar vertebra with the hip bone (coxal bone, pelvic bone; *os coxae*). This has the effect of making L5 a sacral vertebra (see also note to Fig. 2.40).

SACRUM AND COCCYX

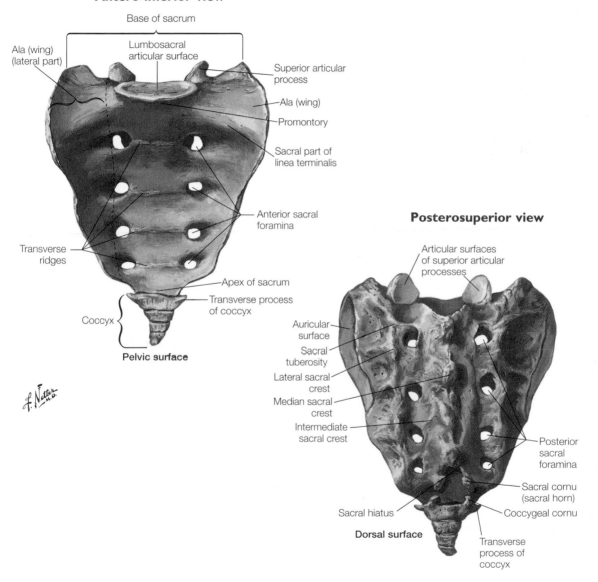

Antero-inferior view

Base of sacrum

Lumbosacral
articular surface

Ala (wing)
(lateral part)

Superior articular
process

Ala (wing)

Promontory

Sacral part of
linea terminalis

Anterior sacral
foramina

Transverse
ridges

Apex of sacrum

Transverse process
of coccyx

Coccyx

Pelvic surface

Posterosuperior view

Articular surfaces
of superior articular
processes

Auricular
surface

Sacral
tuberosity

Lateral sacral
crest

Median sacral
crest

Intermediate
sacral crest

Posterior
sacral
foramina

Sacral cornu
(sacral horn)

Coccygeal cornu

Sacral hiatus

Transverse
process of
coccyx

Dorsal surface

THE SACRUM

The notable structures that can be detected by palpation are:

- Posterolateral visualization of the sacrum (*os sacrum*) (Fig. 2.45).
- The dorsal (posterior) and lateral part of the first sacral vertebra (S1) (*vertebra sacralis I*) (Fig. 2.46).
- The spinous process (*processus spinosus*) of the first sacral vertebra (S1) (*vertebra sacralis I*) (Fig. 2.47).
- The spinous process of the second sacral vertebra (S2) (*vertebra sacralis II*) (Figs 2.48–2.50).
- The median sacral crest (*crista sacralis mediana*) (Fig. 2.51).
- The sacral cornua (sacral horns) (*cornua sacralia*) (Fig. 2.52).
- The sacral hiatus (*hiatus sacralis*) (Fig. 2.53).
- The lateral border of the sacrum (*os sacrum, margo lateralis*): posterolateral view (Fig. 2.54).
- The lateral border of the sacrum: posterior view (Fig. 2.55).

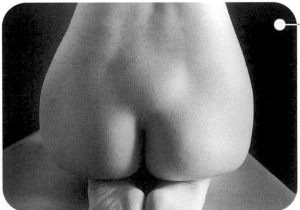

Fig. 2.44

Posterior view of the pelvis (*pelvis*) and sacrum (*os sacrum*)

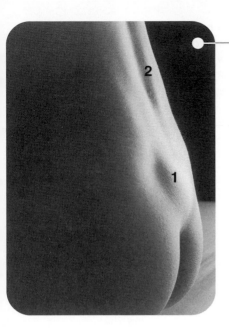

Fig. 2.45 | **Posterolateral visualization of the sacrum**

In the adjacent figure, the position of the sacrum (1) can be seen in relief below the lumbar spine (2).

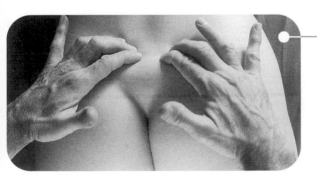

Fig. 2.46 | **The dorsal (posterior) and lateral part of the first sacral vertebra (S1) (*vertebra sacralis I*)**

The subject should lie face down. The practitioner should stand alongside the root of the subject's lower limbs. Begin by placing your hands either side of the lumbar spine, then move them down the lumbar spine, sliding the pressure along until (just below L5) you make contact with a ridge which you will feel beneath your fingers (as shown in the adjacent figure). This is the structure you are seeking.

Note: Beyond L5, the practitioner's hands have naturally come to rest on the sacrum, as its dorsal (or posterior) surface is oriented dorsally and cranially (backward and upward).

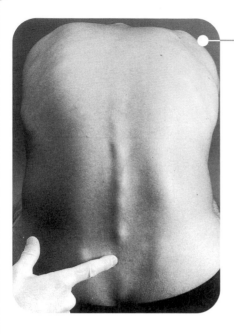

Fig. 2.47 | **The spinous process (*processus spinosus*) of the first sacral vertebra (S1)**

Begin by locating the spinous process of L5 (see Figs 2.41 and 2.42). Then shift your contact caudally to find the first tubercle situated along the median sacral crest. This tubercle is the spinous process of S1.

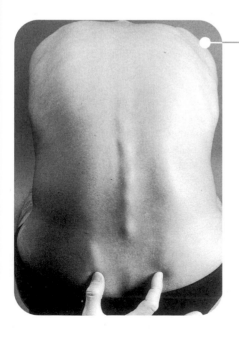

Fig. 2.48 | **The spinous process of the second sacral vertebra (S2) (*vertebra sacralis II*)**
Step 1

In the adjacent figure, the subject is seated, leaning forward. The practitioner's thumb and index finger indicate the posterior superior iliac spine (*spina iliaca posterior superior*) of each of the two hip bones.

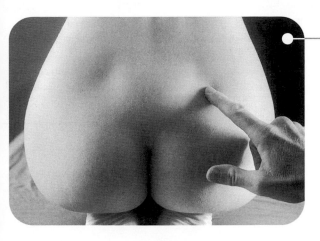

Fig. 2.49 | **The spinous process of the second sacral vertebra (S2) (*vertebra sacralis II*)**
Step 1 (alternative approach)

In the adjacent figure, the practitioner's index finger indicates the depression (which varies in intensity from one subject to another) opposite the sacro-iliac joint (*articulatio sacroiliaca*). This position on the skin corresponds approximately to the posterior superior iliac spine.

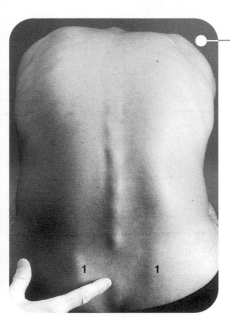

Fig. 2.50 | **The spinous process of the second sacral vertebra (S2)**
Step 2

Once you have located the posterior superior iliac spines (1), which may be clearly visible (as in Fig. 2.48) or not (as in Fig. 2.49), trace a hypothetical horizontal line between the two. The center of this line corresponds to the second tubercle of the median sacral crest. This is the structure you are seeking.

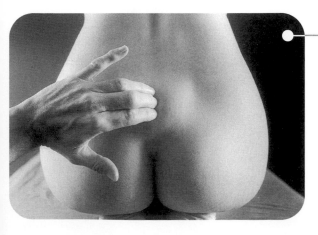

Fig. 2.51 | **The median sacral crest (*crista sacralis mediana*)**

Broad fingertip contact in the middle of the dorsal surface of the sacrum, as shown in this figure, continuous with the spinous processes of the lumbar vertebrae, locates the median sacral crest. You will be better able to sense its anatomical structure if you rub your fingers across it in a transverse direction.

Note: The median sacral crest is made up of three or four tubercles, created by the fusion of the spinous processes of the five sacral vertebrae. A slight depression separates each individual spinous process from the next.

THE TRUNK AND SACRUM

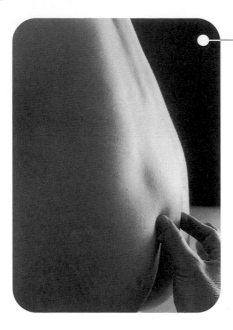

Fig. 2.52 | **The sacral cornua (sacral horns) (*cornua sacralia*)**

These structures can be seen just above the intergluteal cleft, as two small bony columns either side of the depression that constitutes the sacral hiatus (Fig. 2.53), standing out laterally relative to the median sacral crest (Fig. 2.51).

Note: The sacral crest divides in two at its caudal extremity, at the level of the third and fourth posterior sacral foramina, to form two small bony columns. These are the sacral cornua.

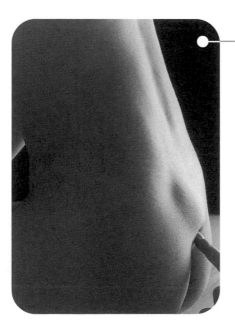

Fig. 2.53 | **The sacral hiatus (*hiatus sacralis*)**

A depression can be seen in the extension of the median sacral crest (Fig. 2.51), just above the intergluteal cleft, as shown here. This depression is formed by the divergence of the sacral cornua (sacral horns) (Fig. 2.52), in a caudal direction from superior (downward from above) and from medial outward. These mark the limits of the sacral hiatus. The top of the sacral hiatus marks the end of the sacral canal (*canalis sacralis*).

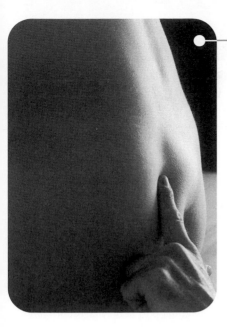

Fig. 2.54 | **The lateral border of the sacrum (os sacrum, margo lateralis) Posterolateral view**

In the adjacent figure, the practitioner's index finger is flat against the lateral border of the sacrum, which can be felt beneath the fingers as a thick, bubbly border.

Note: This border corresponds to the last three sacral vertebrae.

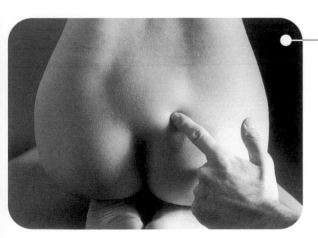

Fig. 2.55 | **The lateral border of the sacrum Posterior view**

The position of this border can be visualized in this view.

Note: Articulatory techniques for the sacro-iliac joint often refer to a fulcrum operating on the "inferolateral angle" of the sacrum. This is not an anatomical term, but refers simply to the most prominent part of the lateral border of the sacrum (indicated here by the practitioner's index finger).

MYOLOGY

THE POSTERIOR MUSCLE GROUP

The notable structures that can be detected by palpation are:

- The trapezius (*m. trapezius*): global visualization (Fig. 2.57).
- The trapezius: superior fibers (Fig. 2.58).
- The trapezius: intermediate fibers (Fig. 2.59).
- The trapezius: inferior fibers (Fig. 2.60).
- The latissimus dorsi (*m. latissimus dorsi*) (Figs 2.61 and 2.62): cranial or superior part at the level of the thoracic vertebral column (posterior) (Fig. 2.63).
- The rhomboid major (*m. rhomboideus major*) (Fig. 2.64).
- The layer of the serratus posterior superior and serratus posterior inferior muscles (*m. serratus posterior superior, m. serratus posterior inferior*) (Fig. 2.65).
- The intermediate aponeurosis of the serratus posterior muscles (Fig. 2.66).
- The erector spinae muscles (*mm. erector spinae*) (Figs 2.67 and 2.68).
- The lumbar part of the iliocostalis lumborum (*m. iliocostalis lumborum, pars lumbalis*) and lumbar part of the longissimus thoracis (*longissimus thoracis, pars lumbalis*) (Fig. 2.69).
- The thoracic part of the iliocostalis lumborum (*m. iliocostalis lumborum, pars thoracis*) (Figs 2.70 and 2.71).
- The quadratus lumborum (*m. quadratus lumborum*) (Fig. 2.72).

Actions

Actions of the quadratus lumborum:

- When its fixed end is inferior: inclines the lumbar spine to the same side.
- It lowers the twelfth vertebra.
- When its fixed end is superior: inclines the pelvis to the same side.

Actions of the serratus posterior superior:

- Raises the upper ribs: an inspiratory muscle.

Actions of the serratus posterior inferior:

- Draws the lower ribs downward: an expiratory muscle.

Actions of the erector spinae muscles:

- All extend the spine.
- The transversospinalis muscles bring about contralateral rotation.
- The longissimus and iliocostalis lumborum muscles bring about lateral flexion and ipsilateral rotation.

Actions of the trapezius, when the fixed end is on the vertebral column:

- The superior fibers move the shoulder upward and inward.
- The middle part draws the scapula inward.
- The inferior fibers draw the medial (vertebral) border of the scapula inward and downward and slightly raise the shoulder.

Actions of the trapezius, when the fixed end is on the shoulder girdle (pectoral girdle):

- The superior fibers bring about ipsilateral flexing and contralateral rotation of the head and neck.
- The two sets of inferior fibers help to elevate the trunk.

Actions of the latissimus dorsi, when the fixed end is inferior:

- It brings about adduction, medial rotation, and posterior movement of the arm.
- It lowers the shoulder and (jointly) laterally flexes the trunk.
- It is an accessory in respiration.
- The latissimus dorsi muscles are also essential "climbing" muscles.

Posterior muscles of the trunk

Left: superficial layer. Right: plane of the rhomboid muscle

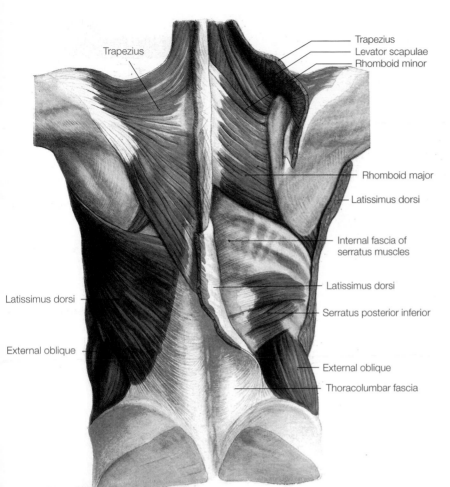

Trapezius

Trapezius
Levator scapulae
Rhomboid minor

Rhomboid major

Latissimus dorsi

Internal fascia of serratus muscles

Latissimus dorsi

Latissimus dorsi

Serratus posterior inferior

External oblique

External oblique

Thoracolumbar fascia

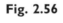

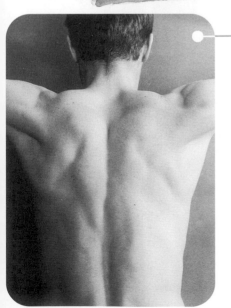

Fig. 2.56 | **Overall view of the posterior muscles of the trunk**

THE TRUNK AND SACRUM

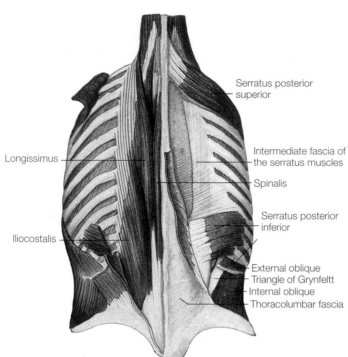

Serratus posterior
superior

Longissimus

Intermediate fascia of
the serratus muscles

Spinalis

Serratus posterior
inferior

Iliocostalis

External oblique
Triangle of Grynfeltt
Internal oblique
Thoracolumbar fascia

Muscles of the posterior region

Left: erector spinae muscles. *Right*: plane of the
serratus posterior muscles.

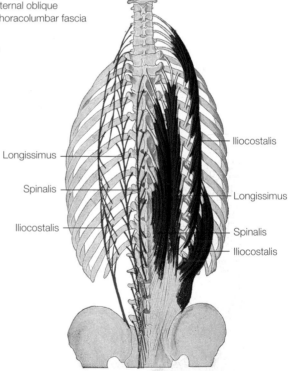

Longissimus

Spinalis

Iliocostalis

Iliocostalis

Longissimus

Spinalis

Iliocostalis

Iliocostalis, longissimus and spinalis muscles

THE POSTEROLATERAL ABDOMINAL WALL

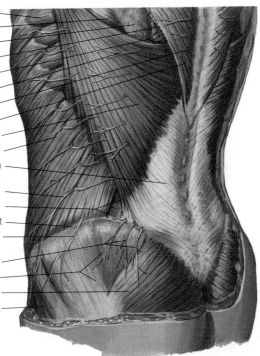

Serratus anterior muscle

Teres major muscle

Infraspinous fascia

Rhomboid major muscle

Auscultatory triangle

Lateral cutaneous branch of dorsal ramus of T7 spinal nerve

Medial cutaneous branch of dorsal ramus of T7 spinal nerve

Trapezius muscle

Latissimus dorsi muscle

External oblique muscle

Thoracolumbar fascia (posterior layer)

Lateral cutaneous branch of subcostal nerve (ventral ramus of T12)

Inferior lumbar triangle (of Petit)

Iliac crest

Lateral cutaneous branch of iliohypogastric nerve (L1)

Superior clunial nerves (lateral cutaneous branches of the dorsal rami of L1, L2, L3 spinal nerves)

Gluteal fascia covering the gluteus medius

Gluteus maximus muscle

Tensor of fascia lata

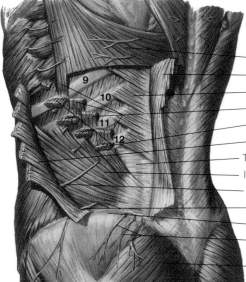

Latissimus dorsi muscle

Latissimus dorsi muscle (*cut and turned back*)

Serratus posterior inferior

Digitations of costal origin of latissimus dorsi muscle

Digitations of costal origin of external oblique muscle

External oblique muscle (*cut and turned back*)

Tendon of origin of transversus abdominis muscle

Internal oblique muscle

Lateral cutaneous branch of subcostal nerve (ventral ramus of T12)

Lateral cutaneous branch of iliohypogastric nerve (L1)

Iliac crest

Superior clunial nerves (lateral cutaneous branches of the dorsal rami of L1, L2, L3 spinal nerves)

Gluteus maximus muscle

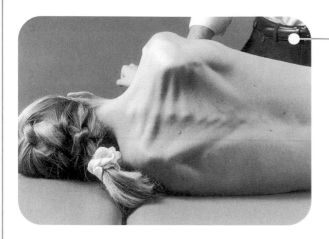

Fig. 2.57 | **The trapezius muscle**
(*m. trapezius*)
Overall visualization and
occipitospinal origin

The adjacent figure shows the topographical location of this muscle. Together with the latissimus dorsi (Figs 2.61–2.63), it constitutes the most superficial layer of the muscles of the back. The intermediate (middle) and inferior fibers of this muscle belong to this region.

Attachments

The origin of this muscle on the cranium is on the exocranial surface of the squama of the occipital bone, on the superior nuchal line (*linea nuchae superior*). At the vertebral column, it arises on the posterior border of the nuchal ligament (*lig. nuchae*) and the top of the spinous processes of C7 to T11 (see also Figs 2.58–2.60).

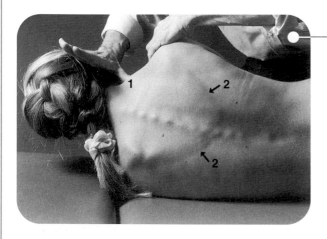

Fig. 2.58 | **The trapezius**
Superior fibers

The subject should lie on one side, facing the practitioner. Place a broad contact, using the palmar surface of one hand, on the lateral part of the subject's head, and place the other hand on the point of the shoulder. Ask the subject to raise this shoulder while flexing the head to the same side. Resist both these movements. The trapezius (1) will appear in the lateral part of the neck.

Attachments to the clavicle

The superior fibers run obliquely downward and laterally, and are inserted on the lateral third of the inferior border of the clavicle and on the adjacent part of the superior surface. The arrows (2) indicate the inferolateral limits of the trapezius. The origins (cranial attachments, and the attachments on the vertebral column) are described above (Fig. 2.57).

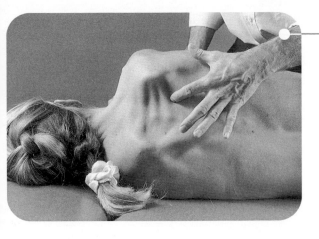

Fig. 2.59 | The trapezius Intermediate fibers

The subject should lie on one side, with both arms positioned to create 90° flexion of the shoulders. Apply resistance to the lateral (external) surface of the arm, above the elbow, as you ask the subject to perform a horizontal abduction of the shoulder. Resist this movement. The intermediate fibers are indicated in this figure by the practitioner's index finger.

Attachments on the scapula and vertebral column
The intermediate (middle) fibers lie transversely, with their insertion on the acromion and the superior side of the posterior border of the spine of the scapula. There is a particularly extensive insertion on the tubercle of the trapezius (see Fig. 3.22). The origin of these fibers on the vertebral column is on the spinous processes of the first five thoracic vertebrae.

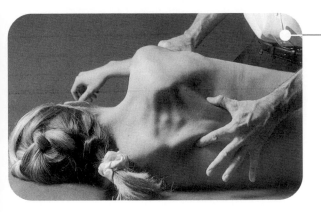

Fig. 2.60 | The trapezius Inferior fibers

In the adjacent figure, the subject is shown lying in the lateral decubitus position, with the shoulder and elbow flexed 90°. Place your hand to resist the lateral surface of the subject's arm, above the elbow, and ask her to abduct the arm horizontally. The practitioner's thumb and index finger contact in this illustration shows the two muscles you are looking for.

Attachments on the scapula and vertebral column
These fibers run obliquely upward and laterally and are inserted on the medial extremity of the spine of the scapula. On the vertebral column, their origin is on the spinous processes of the last six thoracic vertebrae.

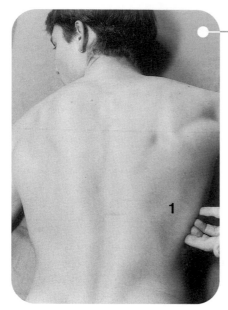

1

Fig. 2.61

The latissimus dorsi (*m. latissimus dorsi*)
Global visualization and topographical location

This muscle, together with the trapezius (Figs 2.57–2.60), makes up the most superficial layer of the muscles of the back. The latissimus dorsi (1) is large and flattened, and is shaped like a triangle with a broad lateral base.

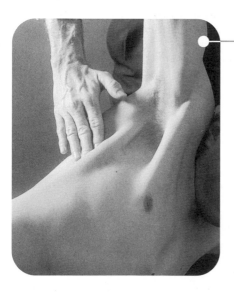

Fig. 2.62 | **The latissimus dorsi**

The adjacent figure shows an anterolateral view of this muscle. The subject is lying on one side, with the arm abducted to 90°. Apply resistance to the internal surface of the arm above the elbow. Ask the subject to perform adduction of the arm, and resist this movement.

Attachments

- The origin is via a tendinous aponeurosis (the thoracolumbar fascia) with attachments to:
    - The spinous processes of T7–L5 and corresponding interspinal ligaments
    - The median sacral crest
    - The outer lip of the iliac crest.
- The latissimus dorsi is also attached at the three or four last ribs and inferior angle of the scapula, by means of muscular digitations.
- The insertion is by means of a flattened tendon passing around the teres major, on the crest of the lesser tubercle of the humerus. (A synovial bursa separates it from the teres major.)

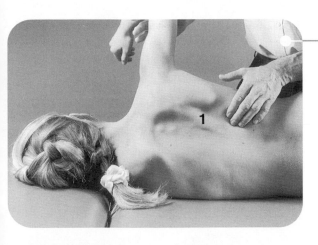

Fig. 2.63 | **The latissimus dorsi**
Cranial or superior part at the
level of the thoracic spine
(posterior)

Figure 2.60 describes the technique for making the inferior fibers of the trapezius (1) more prominent. Begin by locating this muscle, then slide your fingertips underneath the inferior fibers. This will bring them into contact with the most distal part of the latissimus dorsi on the thoracic spine.

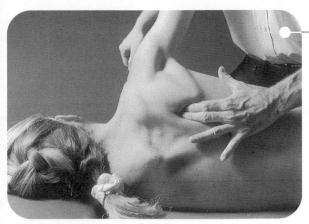

Fig. 2.64 | **The rhomboid major**
(m. rhomboideus major)

Begin by locating the inferior fibers of the trapezius (Fig. 2.60). Then rotate (or swing) the scapula outward sufficiently to free the rhomboid major which is situated here, directly under the trapezius. Palpate between the thoracic spine and the medial border (vertebral border) of the scapula.

Attachment

The rhomboid major arises on the first five thoracic vertebrae and is inserted on the part of the medial border of the scapula below the spine of the scapula.

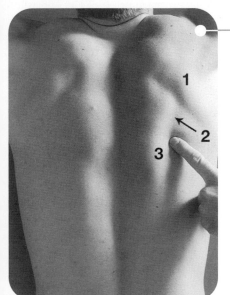

Fig. 2.65 | **The layer of the serratus**
posterior superior and serratus
posterior inferior muscles
(m. serratus posterior superior;
m. serratus posterior inferior)

These are two flattened, quadrilateral muscles, one situated superiorly and one inferiorly, and joined by an intermediate aponeurosis. In the adjacent figure, with the scapula (1) moved aside, the practitioner's index finger indicates the "point of penetration" (inside the posterior angle of the ribs, 2), which is the position you should palpate to approach the layer of the serratus posterior muscles. This is done through the fibers of the latissimus dorsi, by slipping your contact under the trapezius (3).

Attachments

The serratus posterior muscles extend from the line of the spinous processes of C7–L3, to the angle of all the ribs (see Fig. 2.29), slightly laterally to the angle.

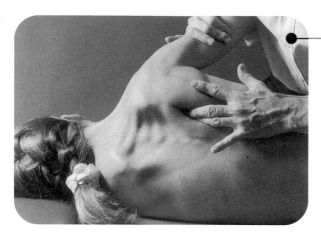

Fig. 2.66 | **The intermediate aponeurosis of the serratus posterior muscles**

Between the serratus posterior superior and serratus posterior inferior muscles, the layer of the serratus posterior muscles consists of a thin intermediate aponeurosis stretched from the vertebral column to the ribs, bounded by the fourth and ninth ribs.

Note: This figure completes the method of approach described in Figure 2.65 (where the subject is lying prone rather than on one side, as here).

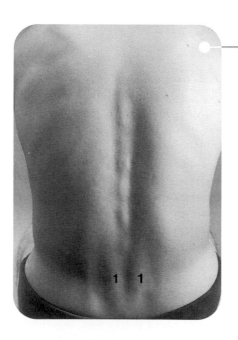

Fig. 2.67 | **The erector spinae muscles (*mm. erector spinae*) (1) Topographical location**

These muscles (1) make up the deep layer of the posterior muscles of the trunk. They are situated on either side of the spinous processes, on the posterior part of the lamina (*lamina arcus vertebrae*) and transverse process (*processus transversus*). They extend from the cervical region to the sacrum, and are composed of closely interwoven muscles (see Fig. 2.68) which completely fill the vertebral grooves.

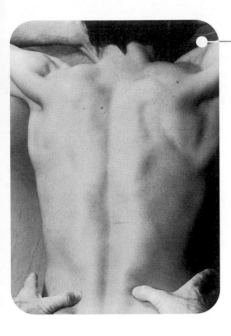

Fig. 2.68 | **The erector spinae muscles Caudal (lower) part**

Subjects should lie face down; then ask them to extend their trunk. A muscular mass will appear in the lumbar region, at the vertebral grooves.

Note: The erector spinae muscles consist of the spinalis muscle of the thorax (m. spinalis), the longissimus thoracis (see note to Fig. 2.69), and the iliocostalis (m. iliocostalis). Caudally, the transversospinalis, spinalis, longissimus, and iliocostalis muscles form an undifferentiated common muscle mass (see 1, on Fig. 2.67).

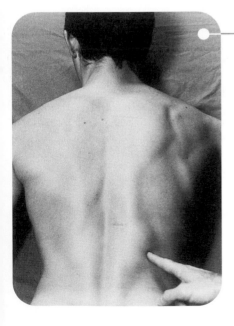

Fig. 2.69 | **The lumbar part of the iliocostalis lumborum (*m. iliocostalis lumborum, pars lumbalis*) and the longissimus thoracis (*m. longissimus thoracis, pars lumbalis*)**

These two muscles are closely interwoven and share the same caudal origin (iliac crest, tuberculum of iliac crest, and sacral crest). Ask the subject to extend the trunk, to make the desired muscles appear more prominently. The muscles to be explored here are indicated by the practitioner's index finger in the illustration. This technique for revealing the muscle mass is the same as that described for Figure 2.68.

Note: The most recently agreed nomenclature does not assign a separate name to the lumbar part of the longissimus muscle; it is a division of the longissimus thoracis. Also, the iliocostalis lumborum has a lumbar and a thoracic part.

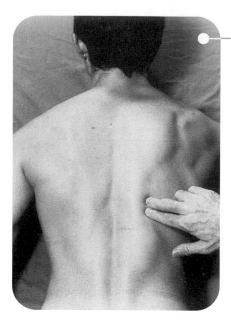

Fig. 2.70 | **The thoracic part of the iliocostalis lumborum (*m. iliocostalis lumborum, pars thoracis*) and the longissimus thoracis (*m. longissimus thoracis*) Topographical location**

The adjacent figure shows the topographical location of these muscles. They are situated at the vertebral grooves, covered by the following muscle layers (listed here in succession from the deep to the superficial layer): the layer of the serratus posterior muscles (Figs 2.65 and 2.66), the layer of the rhomboid major (Fig. 2.64), opposite the scapula, and finally, more superficially, by the trapezius cranially and the latissimus dorsi caudally.

Note: See also the note to Figure 2.69.

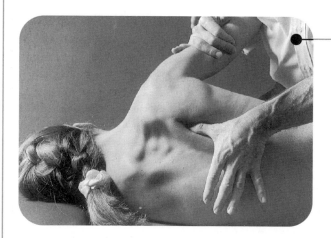

Fig. 2.71 | **The thoracic part of the iliocostalis lumborum and the longissimus thoracis**

Begin by locating the inferior fibers of the trapezius (Fig. 2.60). Then slide your contact (either of two fingers together, or the thumb, as shown in the adjacent figure) in the direction of the thoracic spine. The bundles of fleshy fibers may be seen to roll under your fingers. The fibers belong to the thoracic part of the iliocostalis lumborum on the outside and the longissimus thoracis medially. (See also Fig. 2.70.)

Note: This muscle may be very differently perceived in different subjects.

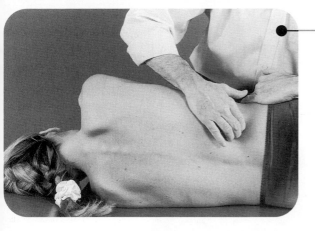

Fig. 2.72 | **The quadratus lumborum (*m. quadratus lumborum*) in the superior lumbar triangle (Grynfeltt's/Lesshaft's triangle) (*trigonum lumbale superius*)**

The subject should lie on one side. Place one hand on the twelfth rib (Figs 2.25–2.27) in the superior lumbar triangle (*trigonum lumbale superius*) (see note below). (This is also variously known as the triangle of Grynfeltt, Lesshaft's space, Grynfeltt–Lesshaft triangle, lumbar tetragon, or superior quadrilateral lumbar space.) The other hand lies on the iliac crest (*crista iliaca*). Ask the subject to draw the iliac crest toward the twelfth rib, and resist this motion. You will sense the contraction of the quadratus lumborum under your cranial hand.

Note: The superior lumbar triangle is formed of aponeuroses and bounded by the following muscles:

- Medially by the erector spinae group
- Below and laterally by the posterior border of the internal oblique muscle of the abdomen
- Above and medially by the serratus posterior superior and serratus posterior inferior muscles
- Above and laterally by the inferior border of the twelfth rib.

This layer of muscles is covered posteriorly by one containing the inferior lumbar triangle (triangle of Petit). This is bounded as follows:

- Below, by the posterior part of the iliac crest
- Laterally and anteriorly, by the posterior border of the external oblique muscle of the abdomen
- Medially, by the lateral border of the latissimus dorsi.

These two spaces, the superior and inferior lumbar triangles, are the two weak points of the posterior abdominal wall.

Attachments

The quadratus lumborum is flattened and quadrilateral in shape, and stretches from the posterior part of the inner lip of the iliac crest to the twelfth rib and lumbar spine. It is situated anterior to the erector spinae muscles, and separated from them by the fascia of the origin of the transversus abdominis.

THE ANTERIOR ABDOMINAL WALL: INTERMEDIATE DISSECTION

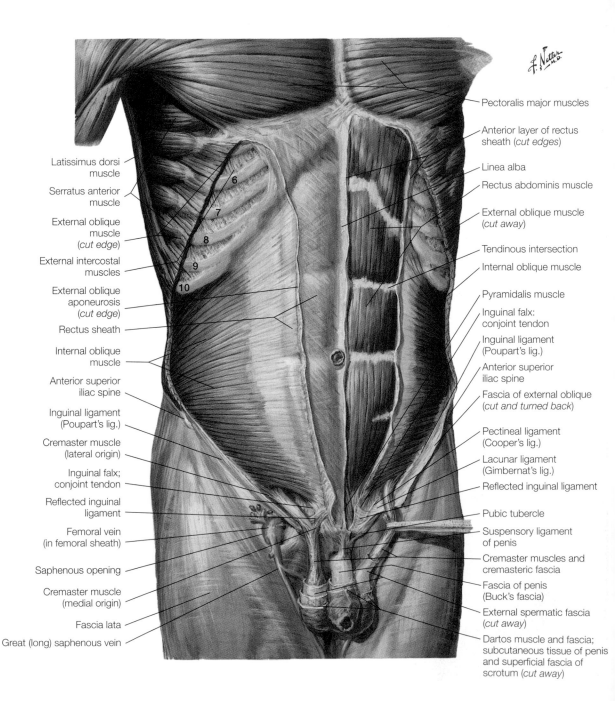

Latissimus dorsi muscle

Serratus anterior muscle

External oblique muscle (*cut edge*)

External intercostal muscles

External oblique aponeurosis (*cut edge*)

Rectus sheath

Internal oblique muscle

Anterior superior iliac spine

Inguinal ligament (Poupart's lig.)

Cremaster muscle (lateral origin)

Inguinal falx; conjoint tendon

Reflected inguinal ligament

Femoral vein (in femoral sheath)

Saphenous opening

Cremaster muscle (medial origin)

Fascia lata

Great (long) saphenous vein

6
7
8
9
10

Pectoralis major muscles

Anterior layer of rectus sheath (*cut edges*)

Linea alba

Rectus abdominis muscle

External oblique muscle (*cut away*)

Tendinous intersection

Internal oblique muscle

Pyramidalis muscle

Inguinal falx: conjoint tendon

Inguinal ligament (Poupart's lig.)

Anterior superior iliac spine

Fascia of external oblique (*cut and turned back*)

Pectineal ligament (Cooper's lig.)

Lacunar ligament (Gimbernat's lig.)

Reflected inguinal ligament

Pubic tubercle

Suspensory ligament of penis

Cremaster muscles and cremasteric fascia

Fascia of penis (Buck's fascia)

External spermatic fascia (*cut away*)

Dartos muscle and fascia; subcutaneous tissue of penis and superficial fascia of scrotum (*cut away*)

THE MUSCLES OF THE ANTEROLATERAL WALL OF THE THORAX AND ABDOMEN

The notable structures that can be detected by palpation are:

- The external intercostal muscles (*mm. intercostales externi*) (Fig. 2.74).
- The external oblique muscle of the abdomen (*m. obliquus externus abdominis*):
    — Costal origins (Figs 2.75, 2.76, 2.80 and 2.81)
    — Costal digitations (Fig. 2.77)
    — Body of the muscle (Figs 2.78 and 2.79).
- The anterolateral muscles of the abdomen (Fig. 2.82).
- The psoas major (greater psoas muscle; *m. psoas major*) (Figs 2.83–2.85).

Actions

The external intercostal muscles:

- These are muscles of respiration.
- They support the thoracic cage by resisting its expansion.

The iliopsoas:

- Flexes and laterally rotates the thigh on the pelvis.
- If the fixed end is the femur, it flexes the trunk and rotates it contralaterally.

The muscles of the anterolateral abdominal wall:

- Contraction of these muscles compresses the abdominal viscera. They are therefore involved in micturition, defecation, vomiting, childbirth, and forced expiration.
- If the fixed end is superior, they bring about retroversion of the pelvis.
- Contraction of the external oblique on one side draws the anterior surface of that half of the thorax toward the opposite side.
- Contraction of the internal oblique on one side draws the anterior surface of the other half of the thorax toward itself.
- If the fixed end is on the thorax, the muscles of the anterolateral abdominal wall bring about retroversion of the pelvis.

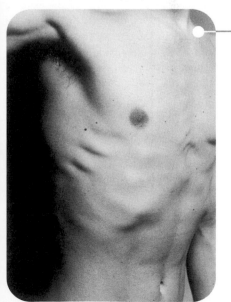

Fig. 2.73 | **Anterolateral view of the thorax and abdomen**

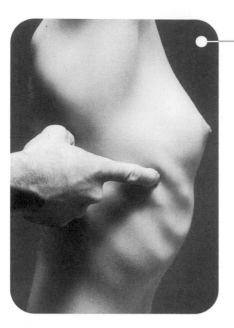

Fig. 2.74 | **The intercostal muscles (*mm. intercostales*)**

Attachments

These muscles lie in each of the intercostal spaces. They consist (working inward from the outside) of the external intercostal muscles (*mm. intercostales externi*), internal (i.e. middle) intercostal muscles (*mm. intercostales interni*), and innermost intercostal muscles (*mm. intercostales intimi*). There are three per space, joining the adjacent borders of the ribs and cartilages. Small muscles are attached to them; these are the levatores costarum and subcostales.

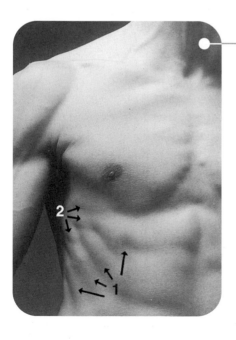

Fig. 2.75 | **The external oblique muscle of the abdomen (*m. obliquus externus abdominis*) Costal attachments: visualization**

The adjacent figure shows the fleshy fibers of the external oblique (1), running in a diagonal direction toward the last seven or eight ribs to insert on the external surface of the ribs. The illustration also shows how this muscle interlinks with the serratus anterior (2). (For a comprehensive view of the attachments of this muscle, see Fig. 2.80.)

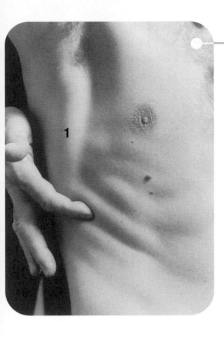

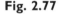

Fig. 2.76 | **The external oblique muscle of the abdomen (*m. obliquus externus abdominis*) and internal oblique muscle of the abdomen (*m. obliquus internus abdominis*)**

The external oblique muscle lies over the internal oblique. (Here, the practitioner's index finger indicates one of the costal digitations of the external oblique.)

1. Latissimus dorsi

Attachments of the internal oblique muscle of the abdomen

This muscle overlies the transversus abdominis, covering it almost completely. It extends from the iliac crest to the last ribs, linea alba, and pubis.

It arises:

- On the three-quarters of the iliac crest anterior to the interstitium and the third external to the inguinal ligament.
- Via a tendinous aponeurosis interwoven with the thoracolumbar fascia, on the quarter posterior to the iliac crest and on the spinous process of L5.

From here, the fibers fan out between the last ribs and the pubis, passing via the linea alba.

- The posterior fibers (running obliquely upward and anteriorly) are inserted on the inferior border and tip of the last four costal cartilages.
- The middle fibers continue by means of a broad tendinous aponeurosis which forms part of the linea alba.
- The inferior fibers attach to the pubic symphysis, pubis, and pecten pubis.

Fig. 2.77 | **Costal digitations of the external oblique muscle of the abdomen Method of approach**

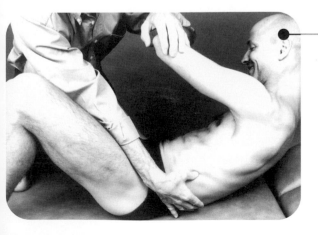

The subject should lie down with shoulder and elbow both flexed at 90°. The practitioner should stand on the other side of the subject. Ask the subject to rise from the table, bringing the flexed elbow across toward the other knee. Resist this action, using your hand on the subject's elbow. The adjacent figure shows this method of approach. The cranial (costal) digitations of this muscle can clearly be seen. They insert on the lateral surface and inferior border of the last seven or eight ribs.

Note: This technique also reveals the body of the external oblique (see Fig. 2.78).

THE TRUNK AND SACRUM

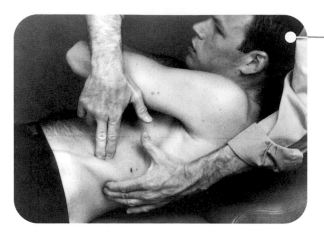

Fig. 2.78 | **The body of the external oblique muscle of the abdomen**
Method of approach

This approach exists in addition to the technique described previously (Fig. 2.77). Simple lateral flexion of the trunk and slight flexion also reveals the body of this muscle. The practitioner should stand at the subject's head. Instruct the subject to flex the trunk to the left, while you watch and control the movement. Resist as necessary with your left forearm, matching your resistance to the force of the lateral flexion. Take hold of the body of the muscle with your fingers.

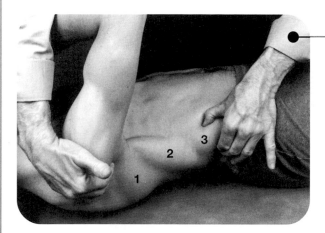

Fig. 2.79 | **The body of the external oblique muscle of the abdomen**
Alternative approach
Relations with the other muscles of the region

Note the relation between the teres major (1), the latissimus dorsi (2), and the body (3) of the external oblique.

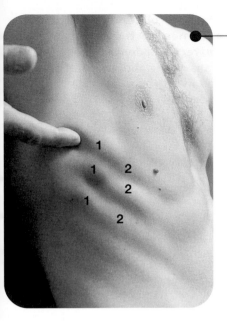

Fig. 2.80 | **The external oblique muscle of the abdomen**
Costal attachments: relations to the serratus anterior

In this figure, the practitioner's index finger indicates the digitations of the serratus anterior (1) and its close relations with the external oblique (2).

The external oblique is a broad, thin muscle, fleshy posteriorly and tendinous anteriorly. It is the most superficial muscle of the anterolateral abdominal wall.

Attachments of the external oblique

- The fibers arise at the thoracic wall (at the external surface and inferior border of the last seven to eight ribs; the last attaches to the cartilage of the twelfth rib). These interdigitate with the inferior fibers of the serratus anterior and with the latissimus dorsi below.
- These fleshy fibers give way to a broad tendinous portion, the aponeurosis of the external oblique, which forms part of the linea alba, and is inserted inferiorly on the pubis and the inguinal ligament.
- The four posterior portions of the external oblique arise on the last two or three ribs and are inserted on the anterior half of the external lip of the iliac crest.

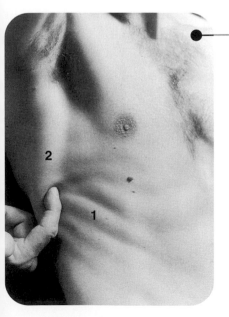

Fig. 2.81 | **The external oblique muscle of the abdomen**
Costal attachments: relations to the latissimus dorsi

In the adjacent figure, the practitioner's index finger rests on one of the digitations of the external oblique (1), and also on the latissimus dorsi (2). This emphasizes the close relation between these two muscles. They are closely interwoven on the lateral surface of the last two or three ribs.

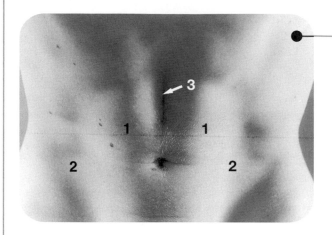

Fig. 2.82 | **The anterolateral muscles of the abdomen: rectus abdominis (*m. rectus abdominis*) and transversus abdominis of the abdomen (*m. transversus abdominis*)**

The two rectus muscles (1) can be visualized in the adjacent figure, separated by the linea alba (3). The bodies (2) of the external oblique, internal oblique, and transversus abdominis can be found to either side of the rectus abdominis muscles. They are listed here in the order they occur, from superficial to deep.

Note: There are five muscles of the anterolateral abdominal wall: rectus abdominis, pyramidalis, transversus abdominis, external oblique, and internal oblique muscles of the abdomen.

Attachments

Rectus abdominis is a long, flattened, thick muscle, stretching the length of the median line in the antero-inferior part of the thorax.

- Its origin is inferiorly, on the anterior surface of the pubis, from the tubercle to the symphysis, and on the anterior surface of the symphysis.
- The muscle is inserted on the external surface and the inferior border of the fifth, eighth, and seventh costal cartilages, via three digitations.

Transversus abdominis is the deepest muscle of the antero-lateral abdominal wall. The middle portion is the muscular body, and the two extremities terminate in a tendinous membrane. Its attachments are:

- On the internal surface of the last six costal cartilages, via six digitations. These are interwoven with the digitations of the diaphragm at ribs 10–12.
- On the tip of the transverse processes of the first four lumbar vertebrae, via an aponeurosis called the thoracolumbar fascia. This extends across the space from the costal to the iliac attachments.
- On the half or two-thirds of the iliac crest anterior to the inner lip, and the third external to the inguinal ligament.

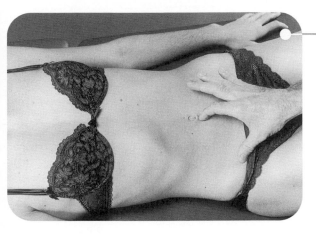

Fig. 2.83 | **The psoas major (greater psoas muscle; *m. psoas major*)**
Method of approach
Step 1

The subject is supine. The practitioner's thumb and index finger mark the anterior superior iliac spine (thumb) and navel (index finger).

Origin and attachment

The iliopsoas is composed of the psoas major and iliacus muscles, which unite at their distal insertion.

The psoas major arises:

- On the lateral surface of vertebral bodies T12–L5, via fibrous arches
- On the adjacent intervertebral discs
- On the inferior border of the transverse processes.

The iliacus arises:

- On the inner lip of the iliac crest
- On the iliac fossa, base of the sacrum, and sacro-iliac joint.

These two muscles have a common insertion on the lesser trochanter of the femur.

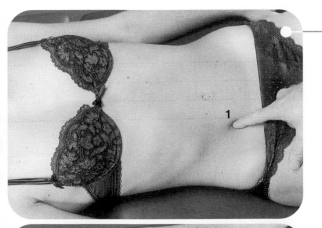

Fig. 2.84 | **The psoas major**
Method of approach
Step 2

Imagine a hypothetical line running between the practitioner's thumb and index finger, as shown in the figure above (Fig. 2.83). Take the middle of this line, placing your index finger broadly against the lateral (external) border of the rectus abdominis (1). (See also Fig. 2.82.)

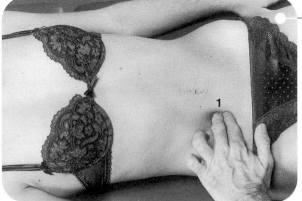

Fig. 2.85 | **The psoas major**
Method of approach
Step 3

Having located the positions described in steps 1 and 2 above (Figs 2.83 and 2.84), you can palpate this muscle by gently penetrating down through the abdominal wall at the lateral border of the rectus abdominis (1). You will detect a fairly significant muscle body beneath your fingers. (It becomes easier to feel if you ask the subject to flex the thigh actively toward the pelvis.)

NERVES AND BLOOD VESSELS

The notable structures that can be detected by palpation are:

• The axillary artery (*a. axillaris*) (Fig. 2.87).
• The abdominal aorta (*pars abdominalis aortae; aorta abdominalis*) (Fig. 2.88).

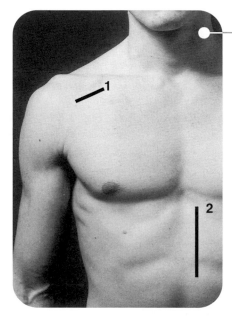

Fig. 2.86

Visualization of the course of the axillary artery (*a. axillaris*) and abdominal aorta (*pars abdominalis aortae; aorta abdominalis*)

1. The axillary artery.
2. The abdominal aorta.

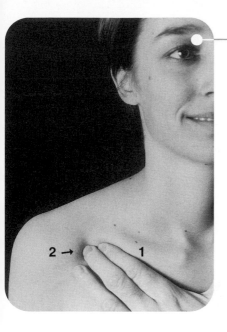

Fig. 2.87 | The axillary artery (*a. axillaris*)

Place the flat of one hand on the anterior surface of the pectoralis major. The practitioner's index finger is resting on the inferior border of the clavicle (1); the ends of the practitioner's fingers press up against the medial surface of the coracoid process (2) (see Fig. 3.28). You will feel the pulse beneath your fingers.

2 →   1

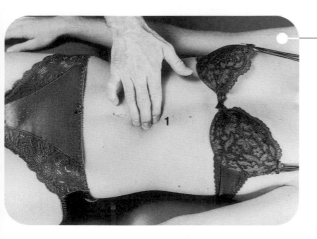

Fig. 2.88 | The abdominal aorta (*pars abdominalis aortae; aorta abdominalis*)

This is the continuation of the thoracic aorta, after it has passed through the diaphragm. It passes anteriorly and to the left of the vertebral column before dividing at the level of disc L4–L5 to form its two terminal branches. To take the pulse of this artery, ask the subject to lie supine with knees bent so as to relax the abdominal tension. Stand to the subject's right side, and place three fingers together just above the navel, one finger-width to the left of the linea alba (1) (see Fig. 2.82). Take great care when penetrating the abdominals.

CHAPTER 3

THE SHOULDER

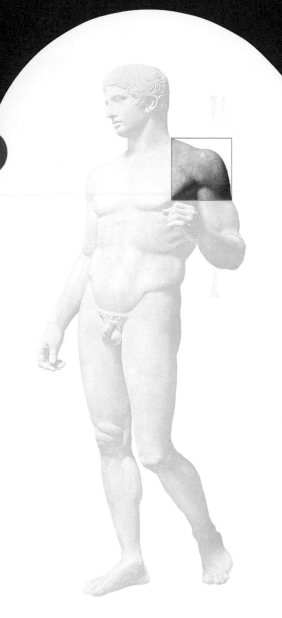

TOPOGRAPHICAL PRESENTATION OF THE SHOULDER

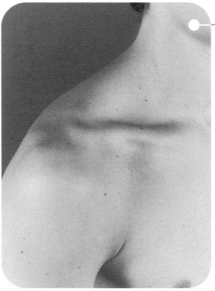

Fig. 3.1

Anterolateral view of the shoulder

OSTEOLOGY

THE CLAVICLE AND STERNOCLAVICULAR JOINT

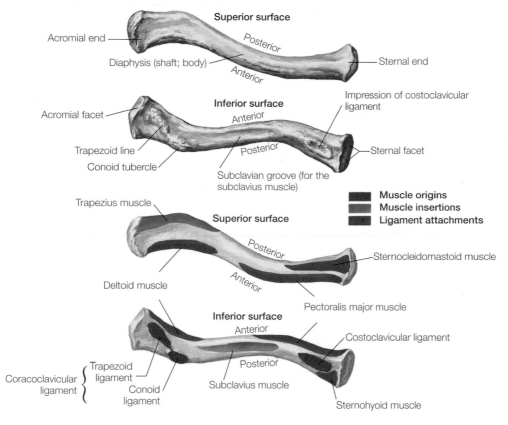

Superior surface

Acromial end

Diaphysis (shaft; body)

Posterior

Anterior

Sternal end

Impression of costoclavicular ligament

Inferior surface

Acromial facet

Anterior

Trapezoid line

Conoid tubercle

Posterior

Subclavian groove (for the subclavius muscle)

Sternal facet

Muscle origins
Muscle insertions
Ligament attachments

Trapezius muscle

Superior surface

Posterior

Anterior

Sternocleidomastoid muscle

Deltoid muscle

Pectoralis major muscle

Inferior surface

Anterior

Coracoclavicular ligament { Trapezoid ligament Conoid ligament

Posterior

Subclavius muscle

Costoclavicular ligament

Sternohyoid muscle

Sternoclavicular joint

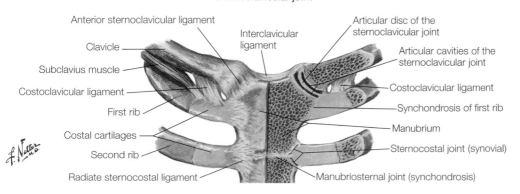

Anterior sternoclavicular ligament

Interclavicular ligament

Articular disc of the sternoclavicular joint

Clavicle

Articular cavities of the sternoclavicular joint

Subclavius muscle

Costoclavicular ligament

First rib

Costal cartilages

Second rib

Radiate sternocostal ligament

Costoclavicular ligament

Synchondrosis of first rib

Manubrium

Sternocostal joint (synovial)

Manubriosternal joint (synchondrosis)

THE HUMERUS AND SCAPULA: ANTERIOR VIEWS

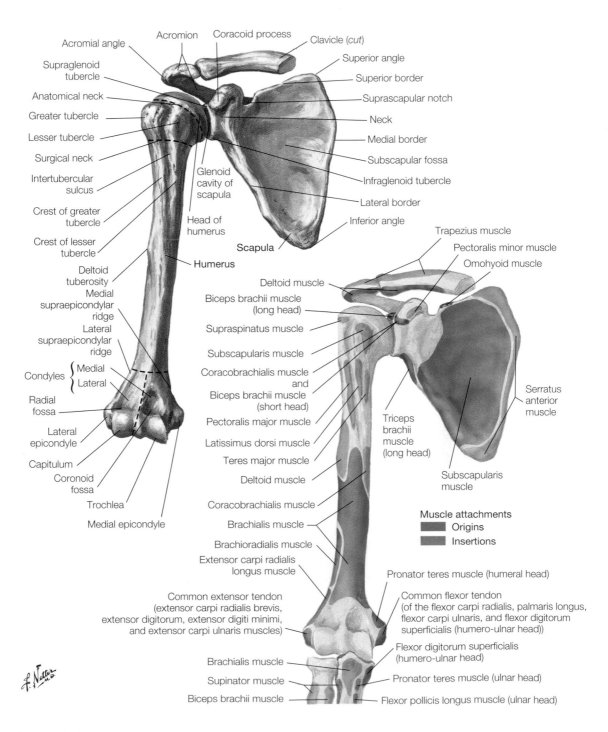

Acromial angle
Acromion
Coracoid process
Clavicle (*cut*)
Supraglenoid tubercle
Anatomical neck
Greater tubercle
Lesser tubercle
Surgical neck
Intertubercular sulcus
Crest of greater tubercle
Crest of lesser tubercle
Deltoid tuberosity
Medial supraepicondylar ridge
Lateral supraepicondylar ridge
Condyles { Medial
Lateral
Radial fossa
Lateral epicondyle
Capitulum
Coronoid fossa
Trochlea
Medial epicondyle

Superior angle
Superior border
Suprascapular notch
Neck
Medial border
Subscapular fossa
Infraglenoid tubercle
Lateral border
Inferior angle

Glenoid cavity of scapula
Head of humerus
Scapula
Humerus

Deltoid muscle
Biceps brachii muscle (long head)
Supraspinatus muscle
Subscapularis muscle
Coracobrachialis muscle and Biceps brachii muscle (short head)
Pectoralis major muscle
Latissimus dorsi muscle
Teres major muscle
Deltoid muscle
Coracobrachialis muscle
Brachialis muscle
Brachioradialis muscle
Extensor carpi radialis longus muscle
Common extensor tendon (extensor carpi radialis brevis, extensor digitorum, extensor digiti minimi, and extensor carpi ulnaris muscles)
Brachialis muscle
Supinator muscle
Biceps brachii muscle

Trapezius muscle
Pectoralis minor muscle
Omohyoid muscle

Serratus anterior muscle

Triceps brachii muscle (long head)

Subscapularis muscle

Muscle attachments
■ Origins
■ Insertions

Pronator teres muscle (humeral head)
Common flexor tendon (of the flexor carpi radialis, palmaris longus, flexor carpi ulnaris, and flexor digitorum superficialis (humero-ulnar head))
Flexor digitorum superficialis (humero-ulnar head)
Pronator teres muscle (ulnar head)
Flexor pollicis longus muscle (ulnar head)

f. Netter M.D.

THE HUMERUS AND SCAPULA: POSTERIOR VIEWS

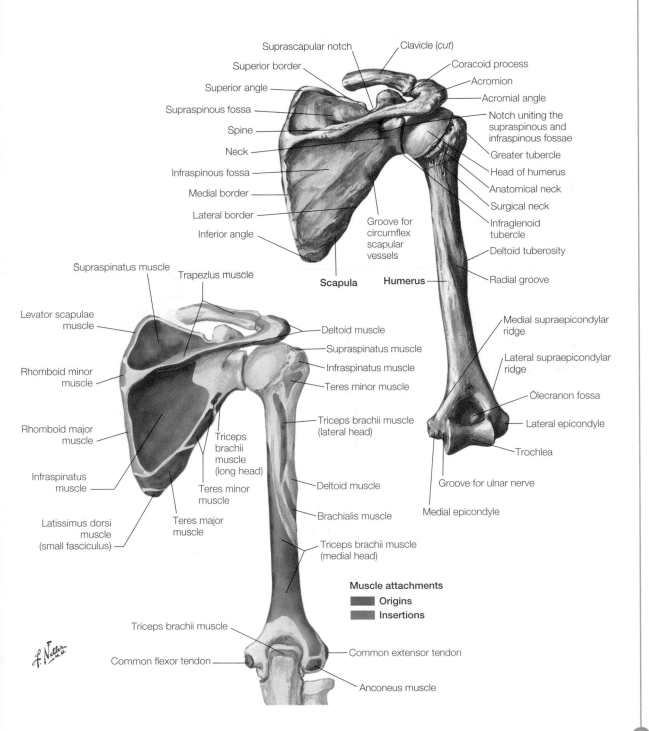

Suprascapular notch

Superior border

Superior angle

Supraspinous fossa

Spine

Neck

Infraspinous fossa

Medial border

Lateral border

Inferior angle

Clavicle (cut)

Coracoid process

Acromion

Acromial angle

Notch uniting the supraspinous and infraspinous fossae

Greater tubercle

Head of humerus

Anatomical neck

Surgical neck

Infraglenoid tubercle

Deltoid tuberosity

Radial groove

Groove for circumflex scapular vessels

Scapula   **Humerus**

Supraspinatus muscle

Trapezius muscle

Levator scapulae muscle

Rhomboid minor muscle

Rhomboid major muscle

Infraspinatus muscle

Latissimus dorsi muscle (small fasciculus)

Teres minor muscle

Teres major muscle

Triceps brachii muscle (long head)

Deltoid muscle

Supraspinatus muscle

Infraspinatus muscle

Teres minor muscle

Triceps brachii muscle (lateral head)

Deltoid muscle

Brachialis muscle

Triceps brachii muscle (medial head)

Medial supraepicondylar ridge

Lateral supraepicondylar ridge

Olecranon fossa

Lateral epicondyle

Trochlea

Groove for ulnar nerve

Medial epicondyle

Muscle attachments

▮ Origins

▮ Insertions

Triceps brachii muscle

Common flexor tendon

Common extensor tendon

Anconeus muscle

THE GLENOHUMERAL JOINT (SHOULDER JOINT)

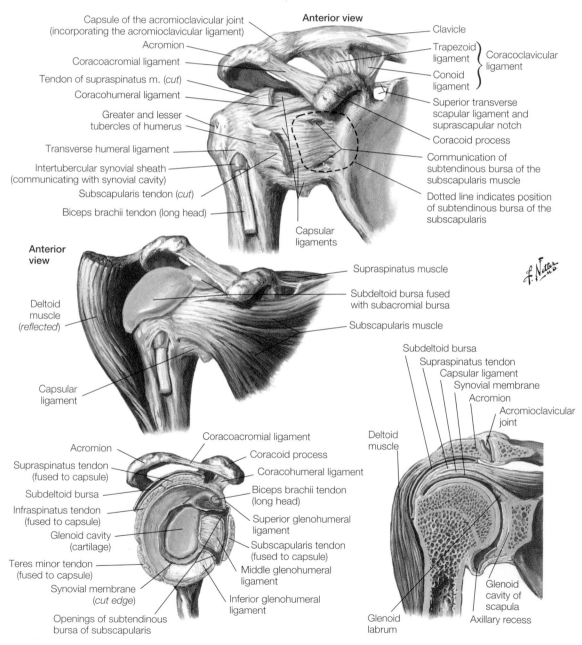

Capsule of the acromioclavicular joint
(incorporating the acromioclavicular ligament)

Acromion

Coracoacromial ligament

Tendon of supraspinatus m. (cut)

Coracohumeral ligament

Greater and lesser
tubercles of humerus

Transverse humeral ligament

Intertubercular synovial sheath
(communicating with synovial cavity)

Subscapularis tendon (cut)

Biceps brachii tendon (long head)

Capsular
ligaments

Anterior view

Clavicle

Trapezoid
ligament

Conoid
ligament

} Coracoclavicular
ligament

Superior transverse
scapular ligament and
suprascapular notch

Coracoid process

Communication of
subtendinous bursa of the
subscapularis muscle

Dotted line indicates position
of subtendinous bursa of the
subscapularis

**Anterior
view**

Deltoid
muscle
(reflected)

Capsular
ligament

Supraspinatus muscle

Subdeltoid bursa fused
with subacromial bursa

Subscapularis muscle

F. Netter M.D.

Coracoacromial ligament

Acromion

Coracoid process

Supraspinatus tendon
(fused to capsule)

Coracohumeral ligament

Subdeltoid bursa

Biceps brachii tendon
(long head)

Infraspinatus tendon
(fused to capsule)

Superior glenohumeral
ligament

Glenoid cavity
(cartilage)

Subscapularis tendon
(fused to capsule)

Teres minor tendon
(fused to capsule)

Middle glenohumeral
ligament

Synovial membrane
(cut edge)

Inferior glenohumeral
ligament

Openings of subtendinous
bursa of subscapularis

Joint opened: lateral view

Deltoid
muscle

Subdeltoid bursa

Supraspinatus tendon

Capsular ligament

Synovial membrane

Acromion

Acromioclavicular
joint

Glenoid
cavity of
scapula

Axillary recess

Glenoid
labrum

Coronal section through joint

THE CLAVICLE (*CLAVICULA*)

The notable structures that can be detected by palpation are:

- The anterolateral concavity (Fig. 3.3).
- The posterolateral convexity (Fig. 3.4).
- The anteromedial convexity (Fig. 3.5).
- The posteromedial concavity (Fig. 3.6).
- The sternal end (*extremitas sternalis*) (Fig. 3.7).
- The acromial end (*extremitas acromialis*) (Fig. 3.8).

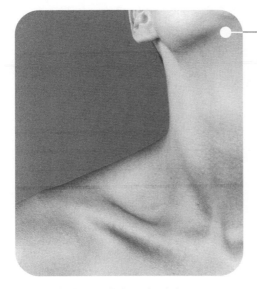

Fig. 3.2

**Overall view of the clavicle
(*clavicula*)**

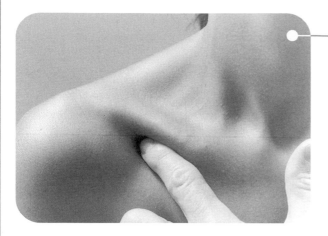

Fig. 3.3 | **The anterolateral concavity of the clavicle (*clavicula*)**

The clavicle is a long bone shaped like an italic letter "S". It runs in a transverse direction between the scapula and the sternum, and forms a key part of the pectoral girdle. The structure provides attachment to the clavicular (anterior) fibers of the deltoid.

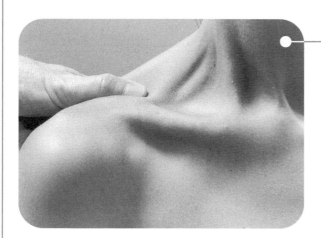

Fig. 3.4 | **The posterolateral convexity of the clavicle**

This part of the clavicle is part of the posterior border. It is convex, with a rough surface that provides attachment to the clavicular fibers of the trapezius. This attachment covers the lateral two-thirds of the posterior border.

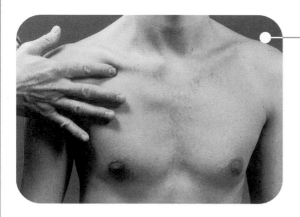

Fig. 3.5 | **The anteromedial convexity of the clavicle**

This convexity occupies the medial two-thirds of the anterior border and provides attachment to the pectoralis major.

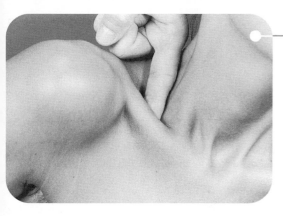

Fig. 3.6 | **The posteromedial concavity of the clavicle**

This concavity occupies the medial two-thirds of the posterior border of the clavicle.

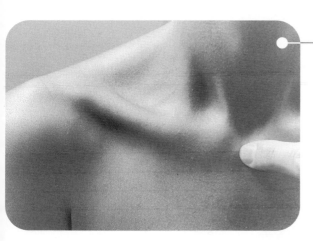

Fig. 3.7 | **The sternal end of the clavicle (*extremitas sternalis claviculae*)**

This extremity of the clavicle broadens into a shape resembling a saddle. It articulates with the sternum and first costal cartilage.

Note: These three structures constitute the sternoclavicular joint (articulatio sternoclavicularis).

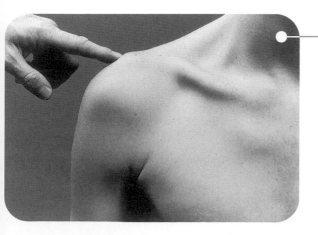

Fig. 3.8 | **The acromial end of the clavicle (*extremitas acromialis claviculae*)**

The acromial end is flattened from top to bottom, and articulates with the acromion by means of a downward, outward, and anterior-facing oval articular surface.

Note: these two structures, the acromion and the acromial end of the clavicle, constitute the acromioclavicular joint (articulatio acromioclavicularis).

THE SCAPULA (*SCAPULA*)

The notable structures that can be detected by palpation are:

- The scapula (*scapula*) (Fig. 3.10).
- The costal (anterior) surface of the scapula (*scapula*) (Figs 3.11 and 3.12).
- The spine of the scapula (*spina scapulae*) and acromion (the lateral extension of this) (Figs 3.13 and 3.14).
- The acromial angle (*angulus acromii*) (Fig. 3.15).
- The postero-inferior border of the acromion inside the acromial angle (*angulus acromii*) (Fig. 3.16).
- The lateral border of the acromion (*acromion*) (Fig. 3.17).
- The tip of the acromion (*acromion*) (Fig. 3.18).
- The medial border of the acromion (*acromion*) (Fig. 3.19).
- The spine of the scapula (*spina scapulae*) (Fig. 3.20).
- The medial extremity of the spine of the scapula (*spina scapulae*) (Fig. 3.21).
- The tubercle for the trapezius (Fig. 3.22).
- The supraspinous fossa (*fossa supraspinata*) (Fig. 3.23).
- The infraspinous fossa (*fossa infraspinata*) (Fig. 3.24).
- The medial (vertebral) border of the scapula (*scapula, margo medialis*) (Fig. 3.25).
- The lateral border of the scapula (*scapula, margo lateralis*) (Fig. 3.26).
- The neck of the scapula (*collum scapulae*) (Fig. 3.27).
- The coracoid process (*processus coracoideus*) (Fig. 3.28).
- The superior border of the scapula (*scapula, margo superior*) (Fig. 3.29).
- The inferior angle of the scapula (*scapula, angulus inferior*) (Fig. 3.30).
- The superior angle of the scapula (*scapula, angulus superior*) (Figs 3.31 and 3.32).

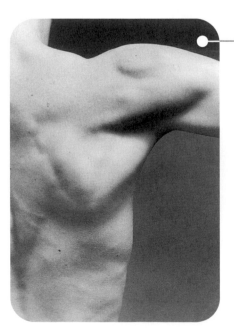

Fig. 3.9 | **Overall view of the scapula**

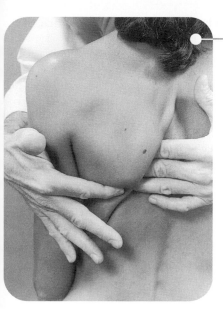

Fig. 3.10 | **The scapula (*scapula*)**
Global approach

The scapula is a flat bone that lies on the posterior surface of the thoracic cage between the second and seventh ribs. It articulates with the clavicle and the humerus.

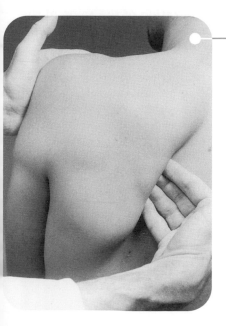

Fig. 3.11 | **The costal (anterior) surface of the scapula**
Spinal approach

The figure alongside shows how this approach from the spinal direction brings the practitioner's contact to the attachments of the serratus anterior muscle, which lie along the medial border of the bone.

Note: There is a ridge along the lateral (axillary) border, linking the neck of the scapula and the inferior angle. It is called the pillar of the scapula.

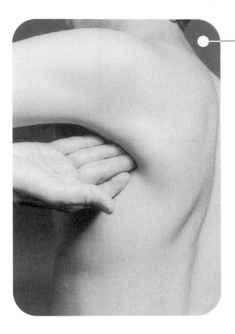

Fig. 3.12 | **The costal (anterior) surface of the scapula**
Lateral or axillary approach

Using this approach, the practitioner's contact is directed toward the subscapularis. This muscle attaches to the anterior surface of the scapula.

Note: There is a ridge along the lateral (axillary) border, linking the neck of the scapula and the inferior angle. It is called the pillar of the scapula.

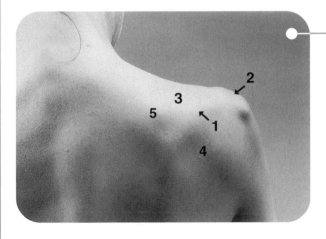

Fig. 3.13 | **Visualization of the spine of the scapula (*spina scapulae*) and acromion (*acromion*)**

The spine of the scapula (1) is a triangular structure with a medial crest. It lies perpendicularly to the surface of the scapula, crossing it at the point where the superior fifth joins the inferior four-fifths of the bone. The anterior border of the scapular spine is therefore, in effect, implanted in the posterior surface of the scapula, separating it into two parts. These are the supraspinous fossa (3) and infraspinous fossa (4). The lateral and posterior borders of the scapular spine broaden laterally to form the acromion (2).

Note: The superior angle of the scapula (5) (see also Fig. 3.31) can also be seen here.

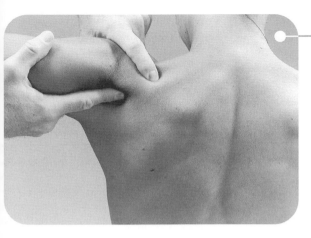

Fig. 3.14 | **The spine of the scapula and acromion**

The figure alongside shows the external extremity of the scapular spine, between the practitioner's two index fingers. It broadens laterally to form what is called the acromion. This is quadrangular, and flattened in the opposite direction to the scapular spine, at right angles to it. It has a superior and an inferior surface, an internal or medial border, an external or lateral border, tip, and acromial angle.

Note: The superior surface seems to be the result of an enlargement of the posterior border of the scapular spine. The inferior surface seems the result of an enlargement of the lateral border of the scapular spine.

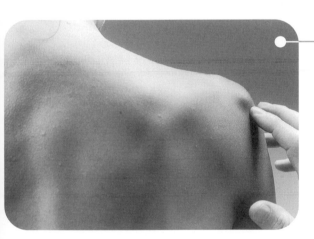

Fig. 3.15 | **The acromial angle (*angulus acromii*)**

This is an anatomical reference point, marking the change in direction of the postero-inferior border of the acromion. It provides attachment to the deltoid.

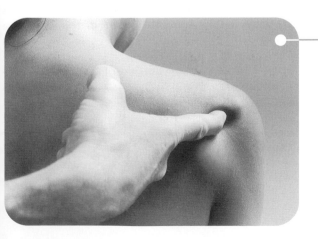

Fig. 3.16 | **The postero-inferior border of the acromion inside the acromial angle**

The practitioner's index finger in the figure alongside indicates this border. It provides attachment to the deltoid.

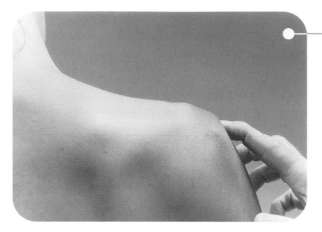

Fig. 3.17 | **The lateral border of the acromion (*acromion*)**

In this figure, the practitioner's index finger indicates this structure. It provides attachment to the deltoid.

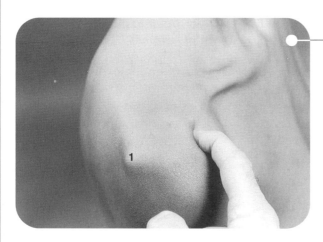

Fig. 3.18 | **The tip of the acromion**

Indicated here by the practitioner's index finger, this lies just lateral and anterior to the acromial end of the clavicle. It provides attachment to the deltoid. The acromial angle (1) can also be seen in this figure.

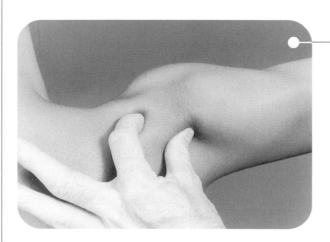

Fig. 3.19 | **The medial border of the acromion**

An upward-facing, inward-facing, oval articular surface occupies the lateral two-thirds of this border. This surface articulates with the acromial end of the clavicle. In this figure, the practitioner's index finger is on this structure, and the thumb in contact with the postero-inferior border of the acromion.

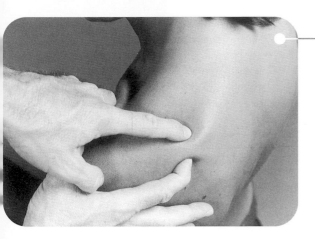

Fig. 3.20 | The spine of the scapula (*spina scapulae*)

This is a triangular osseous structure, implanted in the posterior surface of the scapula and lying transversely across it at the point where the superior quarter joins the inferior three-quarters of that surface.

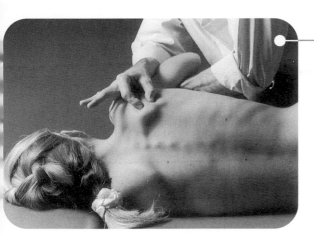

Fig. 3.21 | The medial extremity of the spine of the scapula

The medial extremity of the scapular spine expands into a triangular area which can be seen clearly in this figure beneath the thumb-and-finger contact of the practitioner. It ends at the medial border of the scapula.

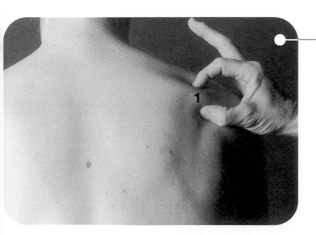

Fig. 3.22 | The tubercle for the trapezius

The middle part of the posterior border of the scapular spine, just beneath the skin, enlarges to form the tubercle for the trapezius muscle (1). This structure can be felt as a bulge beneath your fingers.

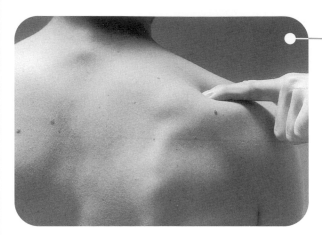

Fig. 3.23 | **The supraspinous fossa (*fossa supraspinata*)**

This lies on the posterior surface of the scapula, above the scapular spine, and provides attachment to the supraspinatus muscle.

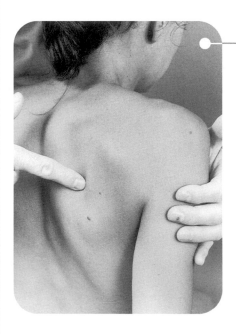

Fig. 3.24 | **The infraspinous fossa (*fossa infraspinata*)**

This lies on the posterior surface of the scapula, below the scapular spine, and provides attachment to the infraspinatus muscle.

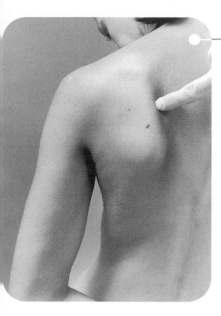

Fig. 3.25 | **The medial (or vertebral) border of the scapula (*scapula, margo medialis*)**

This is the longest of the three borders of the scapula. It has an obtuse angle, the tip of which corresponds to the medial extremity of the scapular spine. Above this angle is the attachment of the levator scapulae muscle. Below the angle are the attachments of the rhomboid minor and rhomboid major muscles.

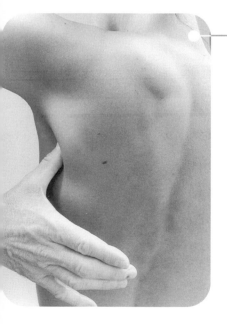

Fig. 3.26 | **The lateral border of the scapula (*scapula, margo lateralis*)**

The lateral border broadens at its upper end, below the glenoid cavity (*cavitas glenoidalis*), creating a tubercle, the infraglenoid tubercle, which provides attachment to the long head of the triceps brachii.

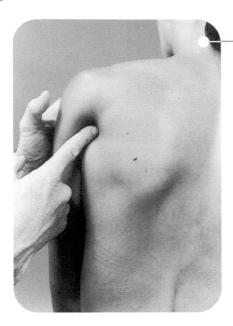

Fig. 3.27 | **The neck of the scapula (*collum scapulae*)**

The neck of the scapula, which supports the glenoid cavity (*cavitas glenoidalis*), forms part of the lateral angle (*angulus lateralis*) of the scapula, along with the glenoid cavity and the coracoid process. There is a groove on the posterior surface of the neck which links the supraspinous and infraspinous processes, laterally to the spine of the scapula.

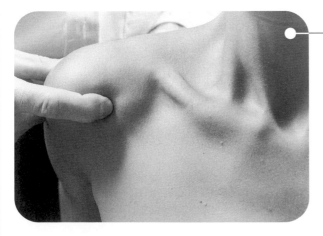

Fig. 3.28 | **The coracoid process (*processus coracoideus*)**

This process can be found just inside the head of the humerus and below the clavicle, as shown in this figure. It is shaped like a semi-flexed finger. The tip and medial border are accessible to palpation.

Muscle attachments
This bony structure provides the insertion of the pectoralis minor muscle (indicated here by the horizontal part of the practitioner's partly flexed finger), the origin of the coracobrachialis muscle, and the origin of the short head of the biceps brachii (both at the tip of the coracoid process).

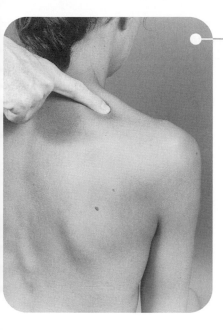

Fig. 3.29 | **The superior border of the scapula (*scapula, margo superior*)**

This short, thin, sharp border terminates laterally in the suprascapular notch (*incisura scapulae*), which provides passage to the suprascapular nerve (*n. suprascapularis*).

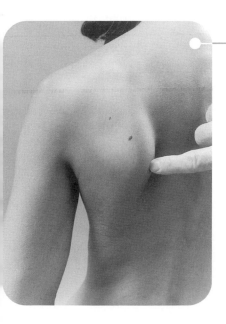

Fig. 3.30 | **The inferior angle of the scapula (*scapula, angulus inferior*)**

The inferior angle is thick, rough, and rounded in shape, and lies at the junction of the medial and lateral borders.

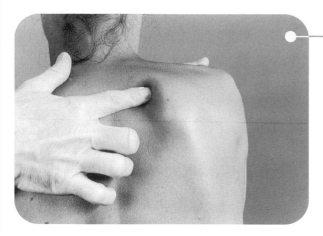

Fig. 3.31 | **The superior angle of the scapula**
(*scapula, angulus superior*)
Dorsal (posterior) approach

With the subject seated, the practitioner takes hold of the shoulder in one hand, pushing it backward and upward so that the medial (vertebral) border of the scapula becomes prominent. The superior angle is indicated by the practitioner's index finger.

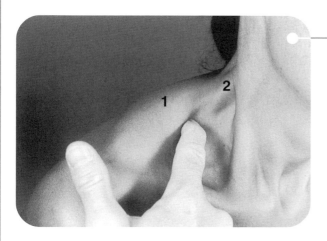

Fig. 3.32 | **The superior angle of the scapula**
(*scapula, angulus superior*)
"Anterior" approach

The subject is seated, and is asked to move the arm backward in such a way that the scapula glides upward and forward over the thoracic cage. The movement of the arm can alternatively be carried out by the practitioner. This movement, active or passive, causes the superior angle to protrude beneath your fingers, in the muscle mass of the trapezius (1). The levator scapulae muscle is indicated by (2). Although the subject is shown seated in the adjacent figure, the contralateral decubitus position is also suitable when seeking this structure.

THE SUPERIOR EXTREMITY OF THE HUMERUS (*HUMERUS*)

The notable structures that can be detected by palpation are:

- The humerus (*humerus*): global contact for the head of the humerus (*caput humeri*) (Fig. 3.34).
- Global approach to three structures belonging to the humerus: lesser tubercle (*tuberculum minus*), intertubercular sulcus (bicipital groove; *sulcus intertubercularis*), and the greater tubercle (*tuberculum majus*) (Figs 3.35 and 3.36).

Fig. 3.33

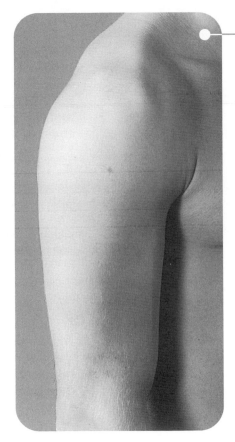

The superior extremity of the humerus (*humerus*)

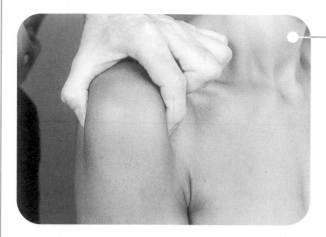

Fig. 3.34 | **The humerus: global contact for the head of the humerus (*caput humeri*)**

The figure here shows a global contact straddling the lateral extremity of the clavicle and the acromion to take hold of the head of the humerus. Ask the subject to rotate the shoulder alternately in internal and external directions. The elbow can be held at an angle of 90°. You will feel the head of the humerus rotating beneath your fingers.

Note: Assuming a starting position in which the subject's elbow is internally rotated, you will clearly detect the greater and lesser tubercles (see also Figs 3.35 and 3.36) as they pass. Between them, the intertubercular sulcus (see also Figs 3.35 and 3.36) can also be clearly detected.

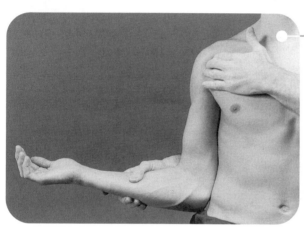

Fig. 3.35 | **Global approach to three structures belonging to the humerus: lesser tubercle (*tuberculum minus*), intertubercular sulcus (bicipital groove; *sulcus intertubercularis*), and the greater tubercle (*tuberculum majus*)**

The subject is seated, with the arm against the body, elbow bent at an angle of 90°, and hand supinated. Using a broad contact with the pads of several fingers, position your contact on the pectoralis major and clavicular part of the deltoid. With your other hand, draw the subject's arm into external rotation. In this position, you will feel the coracoid process beneath your fingers (see Fig. 3.28). Just outside it you can feel the lesser tubercle. If you ease the subject's arm into internal rotation, you will sense laterally, and in this order, the intertubercular sulcus and the greater tubercle beneath your fingers.

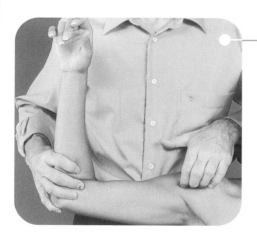

Fig. 3.36 | **Alternative global approach to three structures belonging to the humerus: lesser tubercle, intertubercular sulcus, and the greater tubercle**

The subject is seated, with the shoulder abducted at 90°, and elbow flexed at an angle of 90°. The practitioner should stand behind the subject. Place one hand on the deltopectoral groove, using a broad contact with several fingers together. With your other hand, take hold of the subject's elbow and perform rapid but low-amplitude, alternating movements of internal and external rotation of the shoulder. The dense structure you detect beneath your fingers in the more medial position is the lesser tubercle, and the more lateral one is the greater tubercle. The depression between these two structures is the intertubercular sulcus.

MYOLOGY

THE ANTERIOR MUSCLE GROUP

This group consists of the pectoralis major (greater pectoral muscle; *m. pectoralis major*), pectoralis minor (smaller pectoral muscle; *m. pectoralis minor*), and subclavius (subclavian muscle; *m. subclavius*) muscles.

The notable structures that can be detected by palpation are:

- The clavicular head of the pectoralis major (*m. pectoralis major, pars clavicularis*) (Fig. 3.38).
- The sternocostal head of the pectoralis major (*m. pectoralis major, pars sternocostalis*) (Fig. 3.39).
- The abdominal part of the pectoralis major (*m. pectoralis major, pars abdominalis*) (Fig. 3.40).
- The subclavius (*m. subclavius*) (Fig. 3.41).
- The pectoralis minor (*m. pectoralis minor*) (Fig. 3.42).

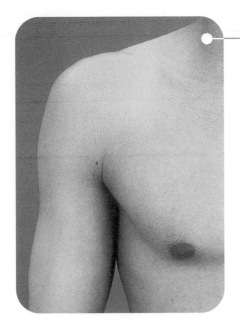

Fig. 3.37

The shoulder: the anterior muscle group

Actions

Actions of the pectoralis major:

- When the fixed end is on the thorax, this muscle is responsible for the adduction and medial rotation of the arm:
  - The clavicular head raises and adducts the arm in the direction of the opposite shoulder.
  - The sternocostal head adducts in the horizontal plane.
  - The abdominal part lowers and adducts the arm toward the opposite hip.
- When the fixed end is on the humerus, it acts as an accessory inspiratory muscle and participates in raising the trunk.

ANTERIOR MUSCLE GROUP: SUPERFICIAL LAYER

Pectoralis major

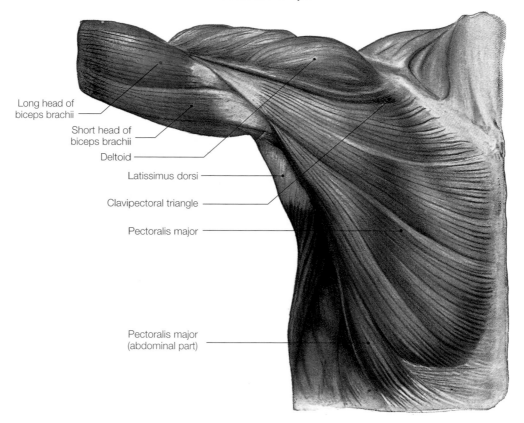

Long head of
biceps brachii

Short head of
biceps brachii

Deltoid

Latissimus dorsi

Clavipectoral triangle

Pectoralis major

Pectoralis major
(abdominal part)

ANTERIOR MUSCLE GROUP: DEEP LAYER

Subclavius and pectoralis minor
Attachments of the pectoralis major

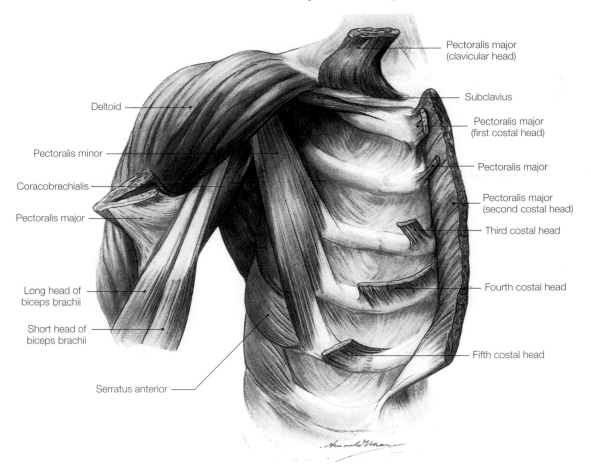

Deltoid

Pectoralis minor

Coracobrachialis

Pectoralis major

Long head of
biceps brachii

Short head of
biceps brachii

Serratus anterior

Pectoralis major
(clavicular head)

Subclavius

Pectoralis major
(first costal head)

Pectoralis major

Pectoralis major
(second costal head)

Third costal head

Fourth costal head

Fifth costal head

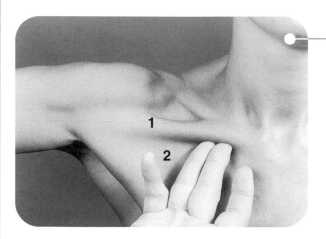

Fig. 3.38 | **The clavicular head of the pectoralis major** (*m. pectoralis major, pars clavicularis*)

Abduct the subject's arm by 90°, with the elbow also bent at an angle of 90° and the forearm directed upward. While offering resistance to the medial part of the arm, ask the subject to perform horizontal adduction of the arm. Contact your two fingers together underneath the subject's clavicle, looking for a groove between the clavicular head (1) and the sternocostal head (2) (Fig. 3.39).

Attachments

- The clavicular head of the pectoralis major arises on the medial two-thirds of the anterior border of the clavicle.
- Insertion: see Figure 3.40.

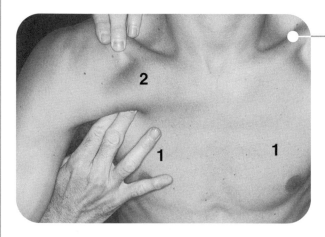

Fig. 3.39 | **The sternocostal head of the pectoralis major** (*m. pectoralis major, pars sternocostalis*)

Abduct the subject's arm by 90°, and provide resistance to the horizontal adduction of the arm. The sternocostal head (1) will appear under the groove that separates it from the clavicular head (2) (see Fig. 3.38).

Attachments

- The sternocostal head of the pectoralis major arises:
    - On the anterior surface of the sternal manubrium
    - On the body of the sternum
    - On the costal cartilages of the second to sixth ribs
    - On the costal (osseous) part of the cartilages of the fifth and sixth ribs.
- Insertion: see Figure 3.40.

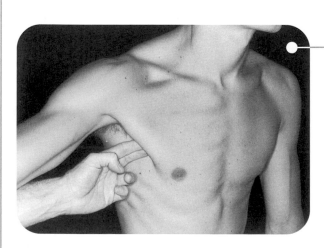

Fig. 3.40 | **The abdominal part of the pectoralis major** (*m. pectoralis major, pars abdominalis*)

Take up a starting position with the subject's arm abducted at an angle of 90°. Resist the adduction of the subject's shoulder by placing resistance against the medial surface of the arm. The muscular head in question forms the inferolateral border of the pectoralis major.

Attachments

- The abdominal part of the pectoralis major arises on the rectus sheath.
- The three heads of the pectoralis major (clavicular and sternocostal heads and abdominal part) terminate in a tendon inserting on the crest of the lesser tubercle of the humerus, lateral to the latissimus dorsi. These are separated by a bursa.

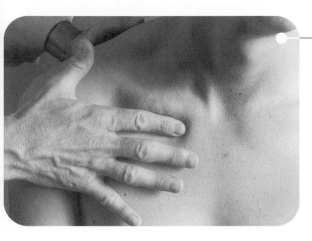

Fig. 3.41 | The subclavius muscle (*m. subclavius*)

The general location of this muscle is indicated here by the practitioner's fingers. The muscle is not easy to detect by palpation.

Note: Acting as an active ligament of the sternocostoclavicular joint, this structure forms a key element in the various movements of the clavicle.

Attachments

The origin of the subclavius is tendinous, and located on the first costal cartilage of the first rib. Its insertion is on the middle part of the inferior surface of the clavicle.

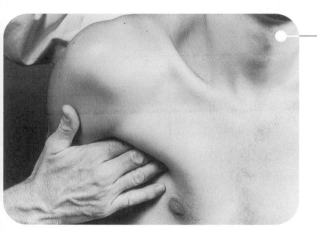

Fig. 3.42 | The pectoralis minor (*m. pectoralis minor*)

The subject is seated or supine. The practitioner should support the subject's arm by cradling the forearm in one hand. The subject's elbow should be bent at 90° and resting on the practitioner's forearm. The aim is to use this supporting hold to ease the subject's shoulder upward and medially so as to slacken the pectoralis major as much as possible. Then, using the pads of the fingers of the other hand and stabilized by the thumb, in the contact shown in the adjacent figure, slide your fingers under the pectoralis major to try to locate a fairly significant cord of muscle. This is the pectoralis minor. It is very easy to detect, even in the relaxed state, but can be made more prominent by calling on the actions of the muscle. To do this, you can either ask the subject to take short, repeated in-breaths, to mobilize the third, fourth, and fifth ribs to which the muscle is attached (in this case the fixed end is on the coracoid process), or, as illustrated here, you can ask the subject to move the shoulder forward. The pectoralis minor is then responsible for performing this action, with its insertion on the coracoid process of the scapula (see Fig. 3.28). In this case, the fixed end of the muscle is costal.

Attachments

The pectoralis minor has a tendinous origin on the third, fourth, and fifth ribs, and its insertion on the medial border of the horizontal portion of the coracoid process.

THE INTERNAL MUSCLE GROUP

This comprises just one muscle, the serratus anterior (*m. serratus anterior*).

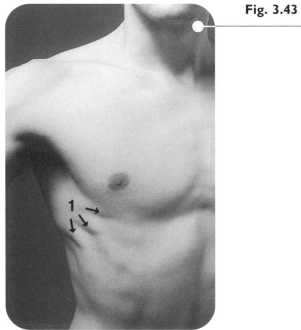

Fig. 3.43

Anterolateral view of the trunk: the internal muscle group of the shoulder

1. The serratus anterior (*m. serratus anterior*).

Actions

The serratus anterior abducts the scapula in relation to the vertebral column, i.e. it moves it laterally across the thorax, at the same time moving it upward and forward.

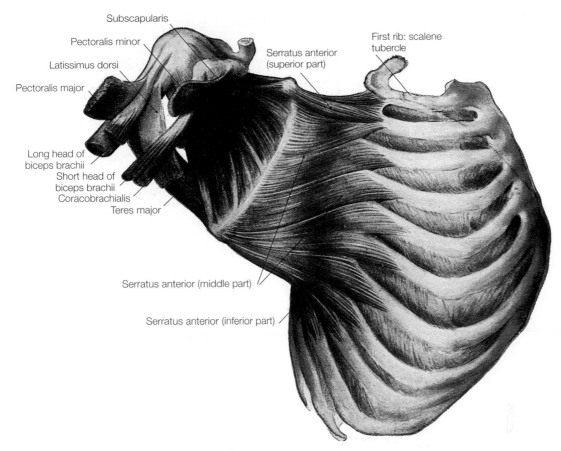

Subscapularis

Pectoralis minor

Latissimus dorsi

Pectoralis major

Long head of
biceps brachii

Short head of
biceps brachii

Coracobrachialis

Teres major

Serratus anterior
(superior part)

First rib: scalene
tubercle

Serratus anterior (middle part)

Serratus anterior (inferior part)

The serratus anterior

The clavicle has been transected and the shoulder turned outward and backward to display the serratus anterior.

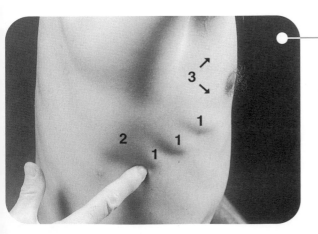

Fig. 3.44 | The serratus anterior (*m. serratus anterior*) — palpation on the ribs

Subjects should be either seated or standing. Ask them to take short, repeated in-breaths so as to make the muscular digitations (1) attached to the ribs appear in between the latissimus dorsi (2) posteriorly and the pectoralis major (3) anteriorly. (See also Figs 2.75 and 2.76.)

Attachments

- The serratus anterior arises on the lateral surfaces of the first six ribs, by means of muscular digitations.
- It is inserted on the superior and inferior angles of the scapula and the medial border of the scapula between these two angles.

THE POSTERIOR MUSCLE GROUP

This group consists of the muscles of the posterior wall of the axilla which are in direct contact with the scapula. Only one of these, the subscapularis, is on the anterior surface of the scapula. The other five lie posterior to the scapula. These are the supraspinatus and infraspinatus muscles, the teres major and minor muscles, and the latissimus dorsi.

The notable structures that can be detected by palpation are:

- The subscapularis (*m. subscapularis*) (Fig. 3.46).
- The supraspinatus (*m. supraspinatus*) (Figs 3.47, 3.54, and 3.55).
- The humeral insertion of the supraspinatus (Fig. 3.48).
- The infraspinatus (*m. infraspinatus*) (Figs 3.49 and 3.56).
- The teres minor (*m. teres minor*) (Figs 3.50 and 3.59).
- The humeral insertions of the infraspinatus (*m. infraspinatus*) and teres minor (*m. teres minor*) muscles (Fig. 3.51).
- The teres major (*m. teres major*) (Figs 3.52, 3.57, and 3.58).
- The latissimus dorsi (*m. latissimus dorsi*) (Figs 3.53 and 3.60).

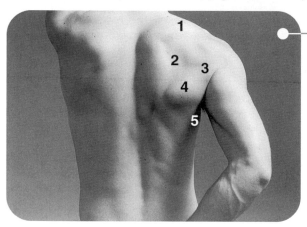

Fig. 3.45 | **The posterior muscle group**

1. The supraspinatus.
2. The infraspinatus.
3. The teres minor.
4. The teres major.
5. The latissimus dorsi.

Note: The position of the subscapularis (m. subscapularis) cannot be seen in this figure. (It lies on the anterior surface of the scapula.)

Actions

Actions of the supraspinatus (*m. supraspinatus*):

- Abduction of the arm.
- Active ligament of the glenohumeral joint (opposes downward luxation of the head of the humerus).
  Actions of the infraspinatus and teres minor muscles:
- Lateral rotation of the arm.
- Supination of the forearm, assisting when this function is required to be performed forcefully.
- Assistance in holding the head of the humerus inside the glenoid cavity.

Actions of the teres major:

- When the fixed end is on the scapula: retropulsion, adduction, and medial rotation of the arm.
- When the fixed end is on the humerus: drawing the angle of the scapula forward and laterally.

Actions of the latissimus dorsi:

- When the fixed end is on the pelvis:
  - The superior fibers provide retropulsion, adduction, and medial rotation of the arm
  - The lateral and inferior fibers incline the trunk and lower the shoulder ipsilaterally
  - The two latissimus dorsi muscles working together extend the vertebral column.
- When the fixed end is on the humerus: ipsilateral closure of the costovertebral space.

Actions of the subscapularis muscle:

- Medial rotation of the arm with a slight adduction component.
- When pronation of the forearm is required to be performed forcefully, the subscapularis assists this function.

The latissimus dorsi

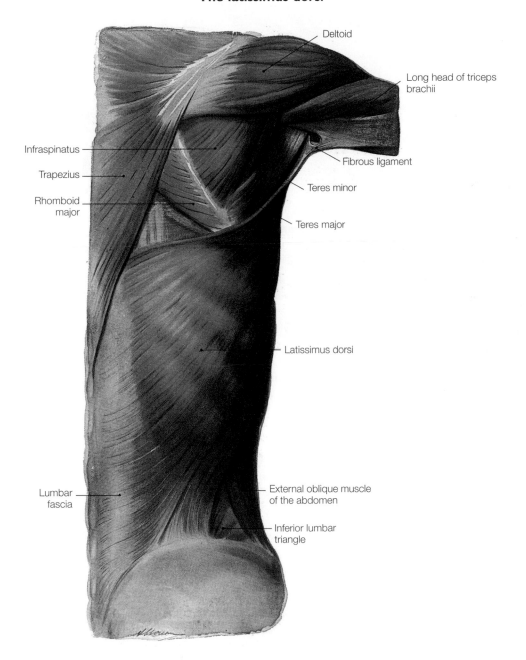

Deltoid

Long head of triceps brachii

Infraspinatus

Trapezius

Rhomboid major

Fibrous ligament

Teres minor

Teres major

Latissimus dorsi

Lumbar fascia

External oblique muscle of the abdomen

Inferior lumbar triangle

The supraspinatus, infraspinatus, teres major, and teres minor muscles

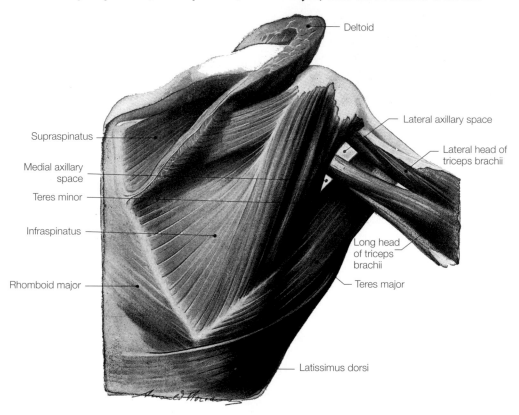

- Deltoid
- Lateral axillary space
- Lateral head of triceps brachii
- Supraspinatus
- Medial axillary space
- Teres minor
- Infraspinatus
- Rhomboid major
- Long head of triceps brachii
- Teres major
- Latissimus dorsi

The subscapularis

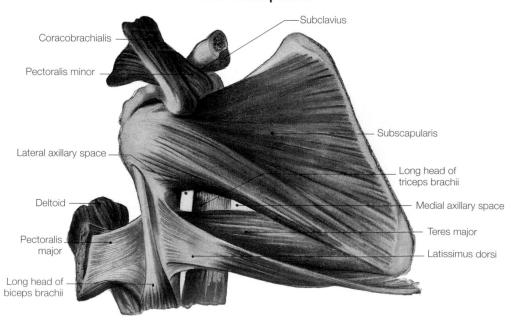

- Coracobrachialis
- Pectoralis minor
- Subclavius
- Subscapularis
- Lateral axillary space
- Long head of triceps brachii
- Deltoid
- Medial axillary space
- Pectoralis major
- Teres major
- Latissimus dorsi
- Long head of biceps brachii

Fig. 3.46 | The subscapularis muscle (*m. subscapularis*)

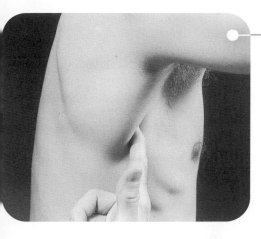

To gain access to this muscle it is necessary to detach the scapula from the thoracic cage, and slide your contact over the anterior surface of the scapula (see Fig. 3.12) between the latissimus dorsi laterally and the pectoralis major medially and anteriorly.

Attachments
- The origin of the subscapularis muscle is on the anterior surface of the scapula:
    — By means of tendinous fibers on the crests
    — By means of muscle fibers between the crests.
- The muscle fibers cross the anterior surface of the scapulohumeral joint, adhering to the capsule.
- The muscle inserts on the lesser tubercle of the humerus.

Note: The neurovascular bundles of the axilla traverse the anterior surface of this muscle. The muscle forms part of what has traditionally been called the rotator cuff.

Fig. 3.47 | The supraspinatus (*m. supraspinatus*)

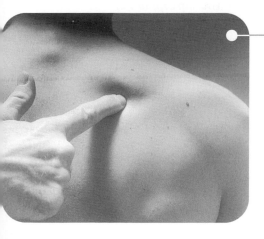

Above the spine of the scapula, the supraspinatus can only be palpated through the trapezius muscle, in the supraspinous fossa. Abduction of the arm makes it possible to detect the muscle beneath your fingers, because this motion brings it into action to stabilize the shoulder.

Attachments
- The origin of the supraspinatus is on the medial two-thirds of the supraspinous fossa and the deep surface of the supraspinous fascia.
- It crosses the superior part of the scapulohumeral joint, adhering to the joint capsule there.
- It is inserted on the superior facet of the greater tubercle of the humerus.

Note: This muscle forms part of what has traditionally been called the rotator cuff.

THE SHOULDER

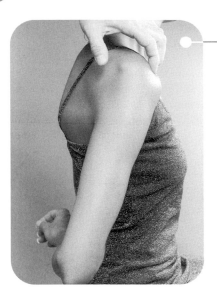

Fig. 3.48 | The humeral insertion of the supraspinatus

Position the subject's arm as shown here. The shoulder should be placed in internal rotation and retropulsion (with the dorsal surface of the hand and the posterior surface of the forearm against the back). The superior facet of the greater tubercle of the humerus, which provides attachment to this tendinous insertion, can be palpated anterior to the tip of the acromion (see Fig. 3.18).

Note: This muscle contributes to the acromioclavicular arch and forms part of what has traditionally been called the rotator cuff.

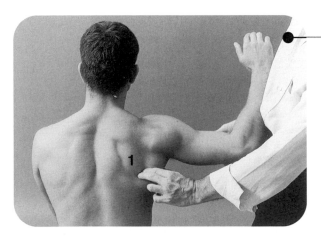

Fig. 3.49 | The infraspinatus muscle (*m. infraspinatus*)

The subject is seated. The practitioner should support the subject's arm (shoulder abducted at 90°, elbow flexed at 90°). From this starting position, ask the subject to rotate the shoulder externally, as shown in the adjacent figure. (This means that the subject should bring the posterior surface of the forearm upward and backward.) The contraction can be detected in the infraspinous fossa of the scapula, where this muscle arises (1).

Attachments

- The origin of the infraspinatus (which is muscular) is on the medial three-quarters of the infraspinous fossa and the deep surface of the infraspinous fascia.
- The muscular fibers adhere to the capsule, crossing the posterosuperior part of the scapulohumeral joint.
- The muscle is inserted on the middle facet of the posterior surface of the greater tubercle of the humerus.

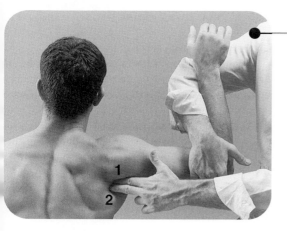

Fig. 3.50 | **The teres minor (*m. teres minor*)**

The subject is seated. The practitioner should hold the subject's arm (shoulder abducted at 90°, elbow flexed at 90°) with a supporting hold. The anterior surface of the subject's forearm should be pronated, resting on the arm of the practitioner. Use a two-finger contact with the pads of the fingers of your other hand on the lateral border of the scapula, between the spinal part of the deltoid (1) above (Fig. 3.55) and the teres major (2) below (Fig. 3.52). Ask the subject to make successive external rotation movements of the shoulder (i.e. to move the hand and forearm backward). This will cause the muscle to contract beneath your fingers.

Attachments

- The origin of the teres minor (which is muscular) is on the infraspinous fossa, along the superior half of the lateral border of the scapula.
- It is inserted by means of a tendon on the inferior facet of the greater tubercle of the humerus.

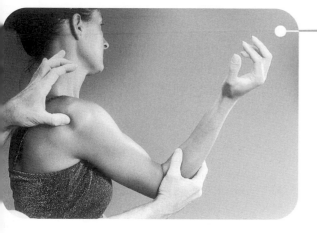

Fig. 3.51 | **The humeral insertions of the infraspinatus and teres minor muscles**

To palpate the tendons of the infraspinatus and teres minor muscles on the humerus, place your thumb as shown in the adjacent figure, below the postero-inferior border of the acromion (Fig. 3.16), in contact with the middle and posterior facets of the greater tubercle of the humerus. In order to do this, you will need to position the subject's arm in antepulsion, adduction, and external rotation.

Note: These two muscles form part of what has traditionally been called the rotator cuff.

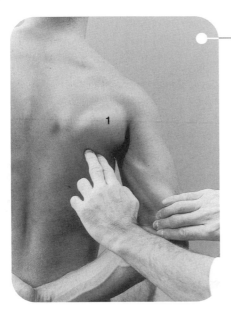

Fig. 3.52 | The teres major (*m. teres major*)

The subject should be lying prone or placed in a sitting position, with the back of the hand and posterior surface of the relevant forearm resting on the sacrum. The practitioner should offer resistance to the medial surface of the subject's arm, and resist retropulsion of the arm. The teres major (here indicated by the practitioner's index finger) creates a raised prominence that is usually clearly marked (1).

Attachments

- The origin of the teres major (which is muscular) is in the infraspinous fossa, along the inferior half of the lateral border of the scapula.
- It inserts by means of a broad tendon on the crest of the lesser tubercle of the humerus, posterior to the latissimus dorsi. A bursa separates these.

Note: The attachment of this muscle is to the inferior third of the lateral quarter of the infraspinous fossa.

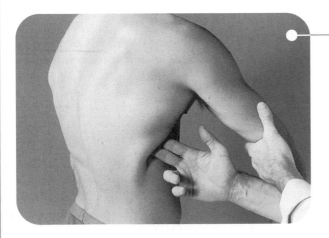

Fig. 3.53 | The latissimus dorsi (*m. latissimus dorsi*)

- Resist the adduction of the subject's arm by positioning your resistance at the internal surface of his or her arm. This causes the muscle to become prominent on the posterolateral part of the thorax (see also Figs 2.61–2.63).

METHOD FOR THE SPECIFIC, SEQUENTIAL EXPLORATION OF THE INDIVIDUAL MUSCLES OF THE POSTERIOR MUSCLE GROUP OF THE SHOULDER

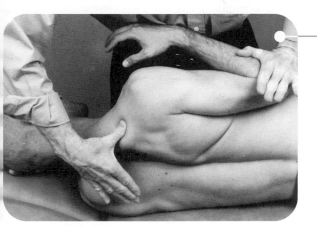

Fig. 3.54 | **The supraspinatus muscle (*m. supraspinatus*) Method of approach**

The subject lies in the left lateral decubitus position, with the right arm resting on the right side of the thorax. The practitioner resists isometric abduction of the subject's right arm; to do this, place your left hand on the subject's elbow. Meanwhile, with your right thumb, palpate the contraction of the supraspinatus above the spine of the scapula.

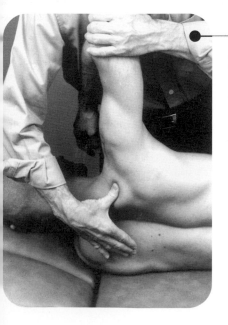

Fig. 3.55 | **The supraspinatus muscle (*m. supraspinatus*) Alternative approach**

The subject lies in the left lateral decubitus position (shoulder at 90°, elbow at 90°), with the right forearm lying against the right half of the practitioner's chest. The practitioner resists isometric abduction of the subject's right arm; place your left hand on the subject's elbow to do so. Meanwhile, with your right thumb, palpate the contraction of the supraspinatus above the spine of the scapula.

THE SHOULDER

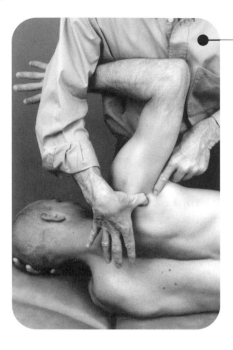

Fig. 3.56 | **The infraspinatus muscle (*m. infraspinatus*) Method of approach**

The subject lies in the left lateral decubitus position (shoulder at 90°, elbow at 90°), with the right forearm lying against the right half of the practitioner's thorax. Ask the subject to perform a lateral rotation of the shoulder, and use the medial surface of your arm to offer isometric resistance.

This will leave both your hands free to take hold of the most lateral part of the body of the infraspinatus between your right thumb and left index finger. This is near the point where the infraspinatus attaches to the middle facet of the greater tubercle of the humerus.

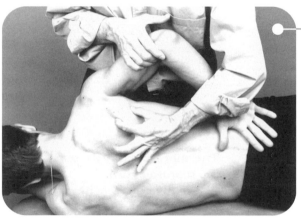

Fig. 3.57 | **The teres major (*m. teres major*) Method of approach**

The subject lies in the left lateral decubitus position. Ask the subject to place the right arm behind the back so that the back of the right hand rests on the sacrum. Place your right hand on the medial surface of the subject's arm (just above the elbow), and resist posterior adduction of the arm. Meanwhile, palpate the teres major between the thumb and index finger of your left hand.

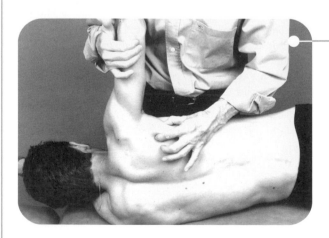

Fig. 3.58 | **The teres major Alternative approach**

The subject lies in the left lateral decubitus position (shoulder at 90°, elbow at 90°), with the right forearm lying against the right half of the practitioner's thorax. Ask the subject to perform medial (internal) rotation of the shoulder, and use the right side of your thorax to offer isometric resistance. Palpate the teres major between the thumb and index finger of your left hand.

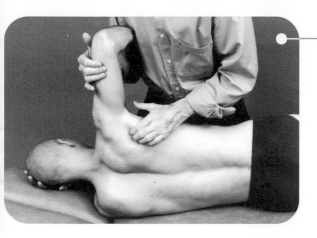

Fig. 3.59 | **The teres minor (*m. teres minor*) Method of approach**

Once you have located the teres major (see Figs 3.57 and 3.58), place the four fingers of your left hand on the muscle's medial (internal) border. Push it aside laterally (outward), and roll the teres minor beneath your fingers against the lateral border of the scapula.

Note: The teres minor is inconstant. When present, it is covered by the muscular mass of the teres major.

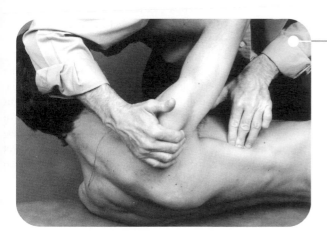

Fig. 3.60 | **The latissimus dorsi (*m. latissimus dorsi*) Method of approach**

The subject is supine. Place the four fingers of your right hand on the inferior part of the subject's shoulder, and resist right lateroflexion of the subject's trunk. Palpate the latissimus dorsi with your left hand.

Note: In the adjacent figure, the practitioner has begun by asking the subject to place the forearm flat against the practitioner's thorax, as a way of disengaging the latissimus dorsi.

THE EXTERNAL MUSCLE GROUP

This group consists of a single muscle, the deltoid (*m. deltoideus*), which lies on the lateral part of the shoulder.

The notable structures that can be detected by palpation are:

- The spinal (posterior) part of the deltoid (*pars spinalis*) (Fig. 3.62).
- The acromial (middle) part of the deltoid (*pars acromialis*) (Fig. 3.63).
- The clavicular (anterior) part of deltoid (*pars clavicularis*) (Fig. 3.64).

The deltoid

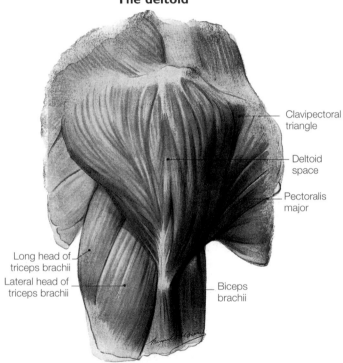

Clavipectoral triangle

Deltoid space

Pectoralis major

Long head of triceps brachii

Lateral head of triceps brachii

Biceps brachii

Actions

- The clavicular part of the deltoid participates in the following actions:
    — Antepulsion (drawing forward) of the arm
    — Direct abduction, together with the acromial part of the deltoid
    — Horizontal anterior adduction, together with the clavicular head of the pectoralis major.
- The acromial part of the deltoid is responsible for abduction of the arm, together with the supraspinatus.
- The spinal part of the deltoid:
    — Posterior horizontal adduction of the arm
    — Retropulsion of the arm, together with the teres major and latissimus dorsi muscles. (Its role in this movement is, however, a specific one; the spinal part of the deltoid operates in a neutral position or in abduction, while the other two muscles perform this motion in adduction.)

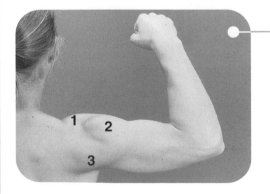

Fig. 3.61 | **Posterior view of the shoulder region**

1. The clavicular (anterior) part of the deltoid.
2. The acromial (middle) part of the deltoid.
3. The spinal (posterior) part of the deltoid.

Fig. 3.62 | **The spinal part of the deltoid (*m. deltoideus*)**

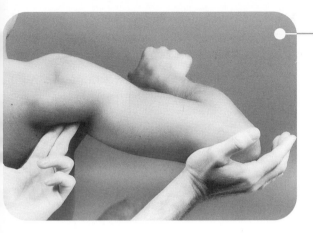

The subject's shoulder is abducted at 90°, with elbow flexed. Position resistance, as shown here, against the posterior, inferior part of the arm just above the elbow. Ask the subject to perform horizontal retropulsion. You will feel or see the body of the muscle on the posterior part of the subject's shoulder. Here it is indicated by the two-finger contact of the practitioner's other hand.

Attachments of the three portions of the deltoid
- The origins of the deltoid are found:
  — By means of a tendinous attachment:
    — On the anterior border and superior surface of the acromial end of the clavicle
    — On the lower border of the spine of the scapula
  — By means of a muscular attachment: on the lateral border of the acromion.
- The deltoid inserts via a tendon on the deltoid tuberosity of the humerus.

Note: The subdeltoid bursa lies between the acromial part of the deltoid and the greater tubercle.

Fig. 3.63 | **The acromial part of the deltoid**

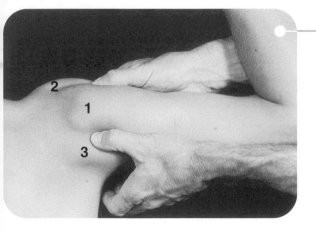

The position of the subject is as in the previous figure (Fig. 3.62). In the adjacent figure, the practitioner's two thumbs indicate the limits of the acromial part (1), which lies between the clavicular (anterior) part (2) and the spinal (posterior) part (3). Ask the subject to perform abduction of the arm, while you resist this movement.

Note: The deltoid covers the scapulohumeral joint, and is separated from it by the subdeltoid bursa (bursa subdeltoidea).

THE SHOULDER

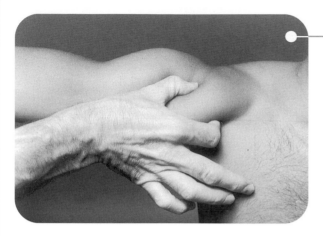

Fig. 3.64 | The clavicular part of the deltoid

The subject's shoulder is still at 90° abduction, with elbow flexed. In the adjacent figure, the practitioner's thumb and index finger indicate the limits of the clavicular part. Ask the subject to perform the action of horizontal antepulsion of the shoulder. Resist this movement.

CHAPTER 4

THE ARM

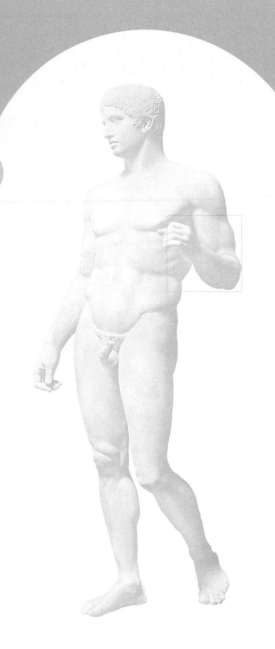

TOPOGRAPHICAL PRESENTATION OF THE ARM

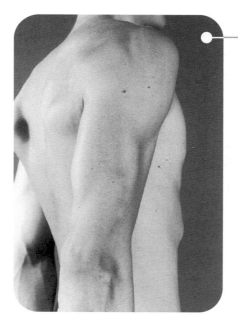

Fig. 4.1

Posterolateral view of the arm region

MYOLOGY

THE ANTERIOR MUSCLE GROUP

This group consists of three muscles: the biceps brachii (*m. biceps brachii*), coracobrachialis (*m. coracobrachialis*), and brachialis (*m. brachialis*). These muscles overlie each other, arranged in two layers: a superficial and a deep layer.

The notable structures that can be detected by palpation are:

- Superficial layer:
  — The body of the long head of the biceps brachii (*m. biceps brachii, caput longum*) (Fig. 4.3)
  — The body of the short head of the biceps brachii (*m. biceps brachii, caput breve*) (Figs 4.4 and 4.5)
  — The tendon of the biceps brachii (*tendo m. bicipitis brachii*) (Fig. 4.6)
  — The bicipital aponeurosis (aponeurosis radiating from the biceps) (*aponeurosis m. bicipitis brachii*) (Fig. 4.7).
- Deep layer:
  — The body of the coracobrachialis (*m. coracobrachialis*) (Fig. 4.8)
  — The brachialis (*m. brachialis*) (Fig. 4.9).

Actions
- The biceps:
  — Flexes and supinates the forearm upon the arm, by the action of the long portion
  — Helps to retain the head of the humerus in the glenoid cavity.
- The coracobrachialis flexes and slightly adducts the arm.
- The brachialis flexes the forearm on the arm.

Fig. 4.2

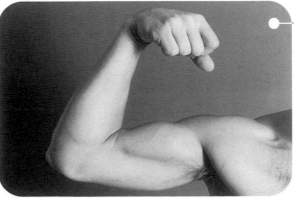

The anterior region of the arm

ANTERIOR MUSCLE GROUP:
SUPERFICIAL LAYER

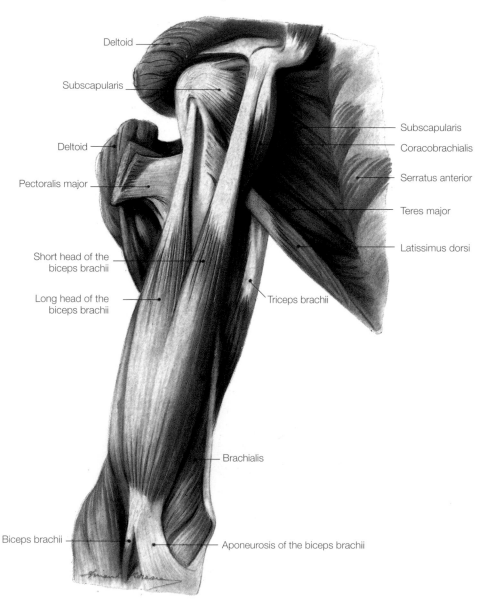

Biceps brachii

Deltoid

Subscapularis

Deltoid

Pectoralis major

Short head of the
biceps brachii

Long head of the
biceps brachii

Subscapularis

Coracobrachialis

Serratus anterior

Teres major

Latissimus dorsi

Triceps brachii

Brachialis

Biceps brachii

Aponeurosis of the biceps brachii

ANTERIOR MUSCLE GROUP: DEEP LAYER

Coracobrachialis and brachialis muscles

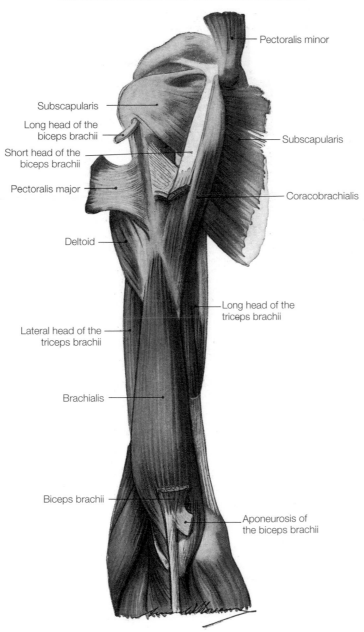

Pectoralis minor

Subscapularis

Long head of the
biceps brachii

Short head of the
biceps brachii

Pectoralis major

Deltoid

Subscapularis

Coracobrachialis

Long head of the
triceps brachii

Lateral head of the
triceps brachii

Brachialis

Biceps brachii

Aponeurosis of
the biceps brachii

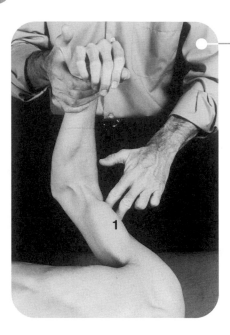

Fig. 4.3 | **The body of the long head of the biceps brachii (*biceps brachii, caput longum*)**

As shown in this figure, the long head (1) can easily be palpated on the anterior surface of the arm, from the elbow region to the point where the muscle disappears behind the deltoid. Ask the subject to contract and relax the muscle repeatedly by raising and lowering the forearm on the arm several times, with the forearm supinated. This makes it easier to see the body of the muscle.

Attachments

The biceps brachii is made up of two parts, the long and short portions.

- The long portion arises on the supraglenoidal tubercle of the scapula, and glenoid labrum.
- The short portion arises on the tip of the coracoid process of the scapula.
- These two portions of the muscle rejoin and are inserted on the posterior surface of the radial tuberosity. The aponeurosis that radiates out from the biceps (Fig. 4.7) leaves the medial tendon level with the elbow and disappears into the antebrachial fascia.

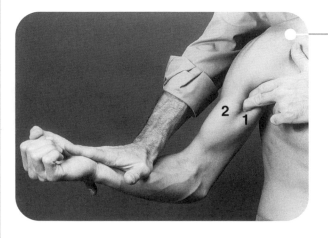

Fig. 4.4 | **The body of the short head of the biceps brachii (*biceps brachii, caput breve*)**

In order to distinguish between the short (1) and long head (2) of the muscle, use one of your hands to resist the subject as he or she flexes the supinated forearm on the arm. Then place two or three fingers of your other hand flat on the proximal third of the anterior surface of the subject's upper arm, with your palm resting on the pectoralis major, as shown. Moving downward and inward in the direction of the subject's elbow, seek a groove separating the two bodies of the long and short heads of the biceps brachii. This is best done by asking the subject to flex the elbow, so as to contract and relax the muscle, a few times in succession.

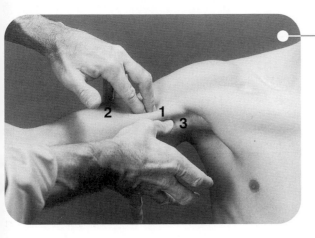

Fig. 4.5 | **The short head of the biceps brachii (*biceps brachii, caput breve*)**

Place the subject's forearm so that it rests between your arm and your thoracic cage, and hold it there. Both your hands need to be free to perform this investigation. In this illustration, the practitioner has isolated the short head (1) of the biceps brachii, separating it from the long head (2) and from the coracobrachialis (3). His right thumb is resting on the coracobrachialis.

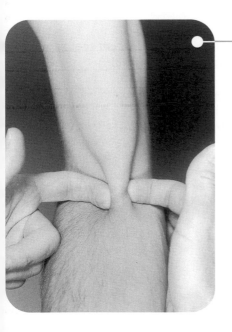

Fig. 4.6 | **The tendon of the biceps brachii (*tendo m. bicipitis brachii*)**

This tendon is very strong and can easily be palpated in the fold of the elbow. If you do need to make the tendon more prominent, ask the subject to flex the supinated forearm, and resist this action.

Note: The attachment of this tendon is to the posterior part of the radial tuberosity.

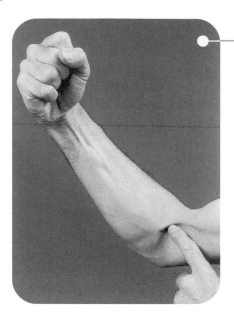

Fig. 4.7 | **The aponeurosis of the biceps brachii (*aponeurosis m. bicipitis brachii*)**

Begin by asking the subject to flex the supinated forearm upon the arm. Then place your index finger on the inside of the subject's elbow against the tendon of the biceps brachii, so that you can detect where the aponeurosis leaves the medial border and anterior surface of this tendon, to disappear into the aponeurosis of the medial epicondylar muscles (forearm flexors).

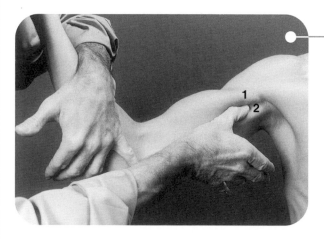

Fig. 4.8 | **The body of the coracobrachialis (*m. coracobrachialis*)**

Place a contact using the pad of your thumb on the medial surface of the subject's upper arm behind the short head (1) of the biceps brachii (see Fig. 4.5). To help you locate the coracobrachialis, the subject should first flex the elbow; then ask him to flex and adduct his shoulder, as shown in this figure, while you resist these movements by placing your other hand against the anterior surface of their forearm. This will throw the biceps into full contraction and make it easier for you to distinguish the biceps from the coracobrachialis, which you are seeking. You will sense a muscular cord (2) tensing beneath your fingers.

Attachment
The coracobrachialis arises via a tendon, fused with that of the short portion of the biceps on the medial side of the tip of the coracoid process of the scapula.

Note: This muscle runs from the coracoid process to the medial surface of the upper arm.

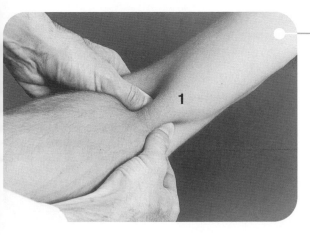

| Fig. 4.9 | **The body of the brachialis (*m. brachialis*) in the inferior third of the upper arm** |

Place a global contact, between thumbs and fingers, on the lateral and medial parts of the upper arm, behind and to either side of the biceps brachii (1). Ask the subject to pronate the forearm and then flex the elbow against resistance.

Origin
- The brachialis arises via muscle fibers:
  — On the inferior half of the medial and lateral surfaces of the humerus
  — On the medial and lateral intermuscular septa.
- It is inserted on to the medial part of the tuberosity of the ulna.

Note: This muscle runs from the humerus to the tuberosity of the ulna.

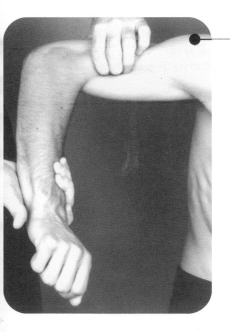

| Fig. 4.10 | **The brachialis muscle (*m. brachialis*) at the arm Alternative approach. Step I** |

It is possible to roll the body of the muscle beneath your fingers against the lateral border of the humerus. To do this, abduct the subject's arm at 90° and position it so that the biceps is pulled downward by gravity. This makes it easier to separate out the brachialis. The subject's elbow should also be bent at 90° so as to relax the biceps and brachialis muscles. Push the biceps brachii aside with your fingers and take hold of as much as possible of the fleshy body of the brachialis.

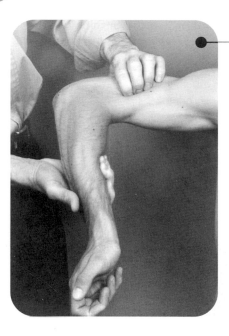

Fig. 4.11 | **The brachialis (*m. brachialis*) at the arm**
Alternative approach. Step 2

With the subject's shoulder and elbow still positioned as described above (Fig. 4.10), roll your fingers on to the brachialis, working backward from anterior until you locate the muscle on the lateral border of the humerus. You will find it quite separate from the biceps, which normally covers it (particularly the anterior part), leaving the lateral and medial parts free.

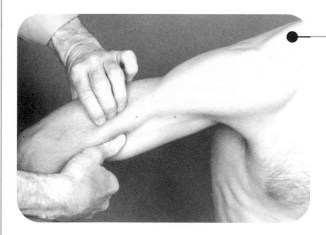

Fig. 4.12 | **The brachialis (*m. brachialis*) at the arm**
Alternative approach

Another way to separate the brachialis from the biceps is to push back the biceps medially. This enables you to take hold of it between the thumb of your right hand and the index, middle, and ring fingers of your left hand (as shown in the figure opposite).

THE POSTERIOR MUSCLE GROUP

This consists of just one muscle, the triceps brachii (*m. triceps brachii*).
The notable structures that can be detected by palpation are:

- The proximal tendon of the long head of the triceps brachii (*m. triceps brachii, caput longum*) (Figs 4.14 and 4.15).
- The body of the long head of the triceps brachii (*m. triceps brachii, caput longum*) (Fig. 4.16).
- The lateral head of the triceps brachii (*m. triceps brachii, caput laterale*) (Fig. 4.17).
- The medial head (deep head) of the triceps brachii (*m. triceps brachii, caput mediale*) (Figs 4.18 and 4.19).
- The distal tendon of the long head of the triceps brachii (*m. triceps brachii, tendo*) (Fig. 4.20).

Actions
- The long head of the triceps brachii extends the forearm on the arm, acting together with the anconeus. (The force of the medial and lateral heads when performing this action is greater than that of the long head.)
- The long head is involved in retropulsion of the arm, and maintains the head of the humerus in the glenoid cavity (for example, during extension of the arm together with extension of the elbow).

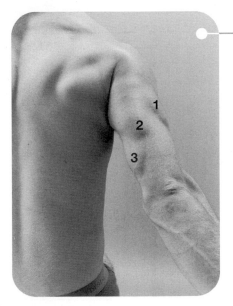

Fig. 4.13

The posterior region of the arm

1. The lateral head of the triceps brachii.
2. The long head of the triceps brachii.
3. The medial head (deep head) of the triceps brachii.

4

The triceps brachii

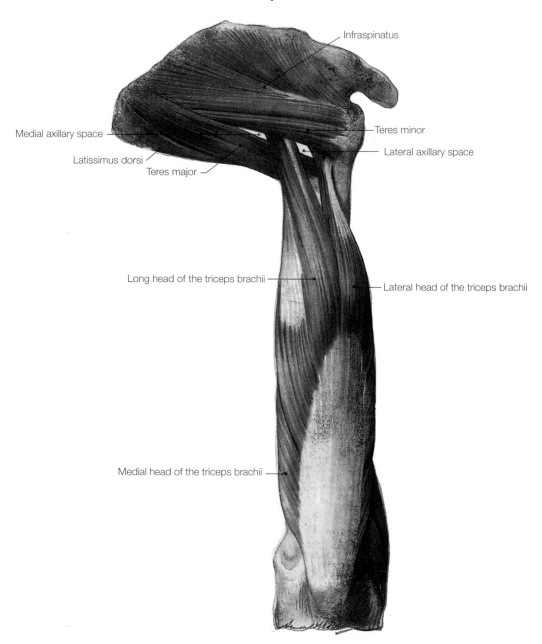

Infraspinatus

Teres minor

Medial axillary space

Lateral axillary space

Latissimus dorsi

Teres major

Long head of the triceps brachii

Lateral head of the triceps brachii

Medial head of the triceps brachii

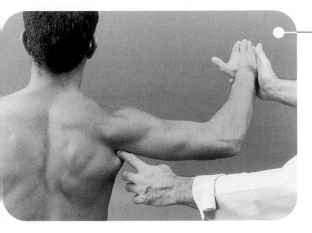

Fig. 4.14 | **The proximal tendon of the long head of the triceps brachii (*triceps brachii, caput longum*)**

The subject is seated. The practitioner should stand beside the subject, on the side of the arm to be examined. Position the subject's arm as shown in the figure opposite, with the subject's elbow abducted at 90° and elbow flexed at 90°. Place your contact on the posterior part of the subject's shoulder using the pad of one or two fingers of your palpating hand as shown, in contact with the spinal part of the deltoid (see Figs 3.61 and 3.62) and lateral to the teres minor (see Fig. 3.50). Ask the subject to extend the forearm on the arm, while you resist this action by placing your other hand on the distal end of the subject's forearm. You will detect the tendon beneath your fingers, on the posterior surface of the subject's shoulder.

Attachments
The triceps brachii consists of three heads: the lateral, medial, and long heads.

- The long head of the triceps arises on the infraglenoid tubercle and glenoid labrum, by means of a tendon.
- The lateral head arises via tendinous fibers:
    — On the lateral part of the posterior surface of the humerus, above the radial groove
    — On the lateral intermuscular septum of the arm.
- The medial head arises via fleshy fibers:
    — On the medial intermuscular septum of the arm
    — On the posterior surface of the shaft of the humerus, below the radial groove.

The three heads converge toward the middle of the posterior surface, on a tendon that is flattened from front to back.

- The fibers of the long head terminate on the superficial part of this tendon.
- The fibers of the lateral head terminate on the deep part and the lateral border of this tendon.
- The fibers of the medial head terminate on the deep part and the medial border of this tendon.

The muscle is inserted:

- By means of a tendon on the posterior part of the superior surface of the olecranon of the ulna.
- By means of muscular fibers from the lateral and medial heads, on the lateral and medial surfaces of the olecranon of the ulna.

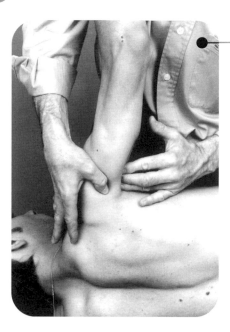

Fig. 4.15 | **The proximal tendon of the long head of the triceps brachii (*triceps brachii, caput longum*) Alternative approach**

The subject lies on the left side, with the right arm abducted at 90° and the forearm resting inside the pit of the practitioner's right arm. Ask the subject to extend the forearm upon the arm. This action enables you to sense the contraction at the tendon and to take hold of the tendon between your fingers.

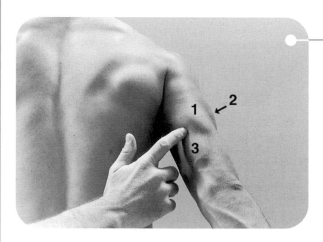

Fig. 4.16 | **The body of the long head of the triceps brachii (*triceps brachii, caput longum*)**

The long head (1) of the triceps brachii should not be confused with the lateral head (2), which lies in front of and laterally to it, or with the medial head (3), which is below the long head and more internally situated. Ask the subject to extend the forearm on the arm against resistance in order to make the body of the long head more prominent, or to palpate it when it is contracted.

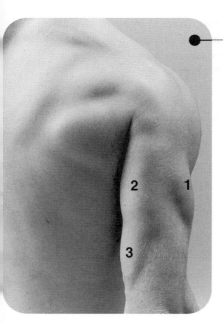

Fig. 4.17 | **The lateral head of the triceps brachii (*triceps brachii, caput laterale*)**

The lateral head (1) is situated on the lateral surface of the arm, lateral and anterior to the long head (2) of the triceps brachii. Extension of the subject's forearm on the arm against resistance will help you to visualize it. The medial head of the triceps brachii (3) is also shown.

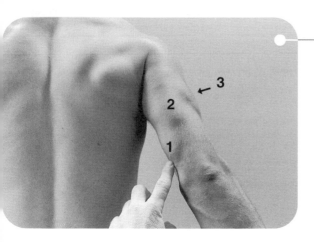

Fig. 4.18 | **The medial head of the triceps brachii (*triceps brachii, caput mediale*) Posterior view**

Ask the subject to extend and flex the forearm repeatedly on his arm against resistance, in order to help you display the medial head (1). It is situated at the distal prolongation of the long head, and is medial to it. The lateral head of the triceps brachii (3) is also shown.

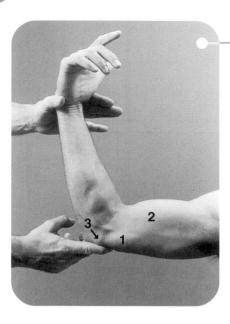

Fig. 4.19 | **The medial head of the triceps brachii (*triceps brachii, caput mediale*) Medial view**

In the figure opposite, the body of the medial head (1) can be seen on the medial part of the arm, behind and medial to the biceps brachii (2) and above the medial epicondyle (3) (see Figs 5.7 and 5.8) Ask the subject to extend the forearm on the arm against resistance to assist you in visualizing and detecting it.

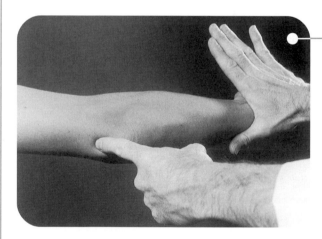

Fig. 4.20 | **The distal tendon of the triceps brachii (*triceps brachii, tendo*)**

The distal tendon is generally flattened from front to back, although it is sometimes found as a full, cylindrical cord that can be perceived on the posterior surface of the elbow, just before its insertion on the superior surface of the olecranon. Ask the subject to extend the forearm on the arm against resistance to help you detect it.

The notable structures that can be detected by palpation are:

- The brachial artery (*a. brachialis*) (Fig. 4.22).
- The median nerve (*n. medianus*) and distal part of the brachial artery (*a. brachialis*) (Fig. 4.23).
- The ulnar nerve (*n. ulnaris*) in the distal part of the arm (Fig. 4.24).
- The radial nerve (*n. radialis*) (Fig. 4.25).

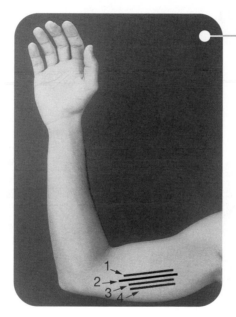

Fig. 4.21

Medial view of the arm

1. The median nerve (*n. medianus*).
2. The brachial artery (*a. brachialis*).
3. The radial nerve (*n. radialis*).
4. The ulnar nerve (*n. ulnaris*).

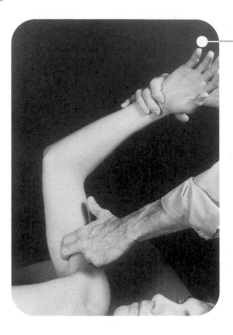

Fig. 4.22 | The brachial artery (*a. brachialis*) (proximal part)

Begin by locating the coracobrachialis (Fig. 4.8). Flexion and adduction of the subject's shoulder (as shown here) will help you to do this. Place a broad contact — with the pads of two or more fingers — behind the body of the muscle. You will be able to detect the pulse of the brachial artery.

Note: Take great care when taking the pulse, as the median nerve passes close to the brachial artery.

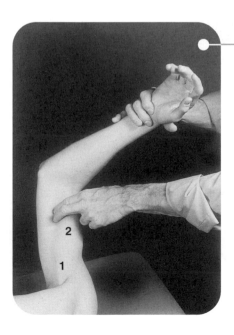

Fig. 4.23 | The median nerve (*n. medianus*) and brachial artery (*a. brachialis*) (distal part)

Begin by locating the body of the coracobrachialis (1) (Fig. 4.8) by flexion and adduction of the subject's shoulder. Place a broad contact — with the pads of two or more fingers — behind the body of this muscle, and draw the whole arm into a position of horizontal abduction. The subject's forearm may be placed in flexion and pronation. You can follow the entire course of the nerve along the anteromedial surface of the arm to the fold of the elbow, pushing aside the biceps brachii (2) laterally to roll the nerve beneath your fingers. It is also possible to follow the brachial artery along the course of the median nerve, on the medial part of the arm. The pulse of this artery can be felt beneath your fingers as far as the fold of the elbow.

Note: Care should be taken when taking the pulse of the brachial artery, as the medial nerve passes close to the brachial artery. (Exceptionally, the nerve lies behind the artery.)

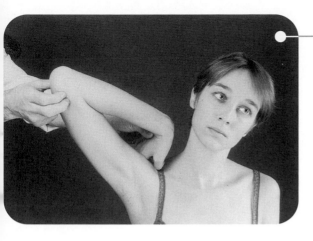

Fig. 4.24 | **The ulnar nerve (*n. ulnaris*) in the distal part of the upper arm**

At the point where the superior third of the arm meets the middle third, the nerve follows a downward, backward, and inward direction. It passes through the medial intermuscular septum of the arm (*septum intermusculare brachii mediale*). From here on, until it reaches the groove between the epicondyle and the olecranon, it is in the posterior compartment of the arm, so that you can roll the nerve beneath your fingers at the contact with the medial head of the triceps brachii (Fig. 4.18). It is easier to perceive this nerve if the subject's arm is placed in maximum antepulsion, as shown here (it may or may not be abducted). The subject's elbow should be flexed to the maximum, forearm pronated, and wrist extended. Take care not to allow the subject to remain in this position for too long, because it is a biomechanical situation in which pressure build-up within the nerve is at its greatest. (See also Figs 5.20 and 5.21).

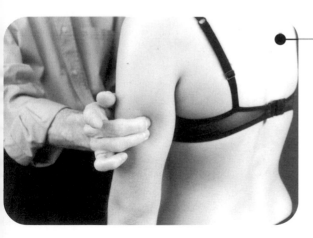

Fig. 4.25 | **The radial nerve (posterior surface of the arm)**

Place one hand below the deltoid tuberosity of the humerus, on the posterior surface of the arm, at the radial groove. The structure to be investigated can be rolled beneath your fingers, through the muscular mass of the triceps brachii.

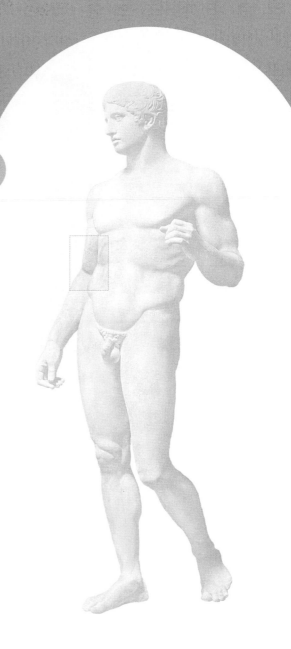

CHAPTER 5

THE ELBOW

TOPOGRAPHICAL PRESENTATION OF THE ELBOW

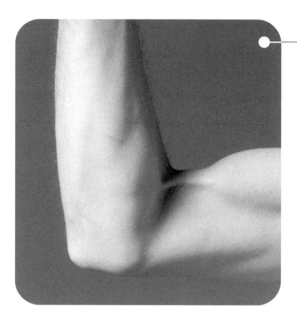

Fig. 5.1

Medial view of the elbow region

OSTEOLOGY

BONES OF THE ELBOW

Distal epiphysis of the humerus, anterior view

Distal epiphysis of the humerus, posterior view

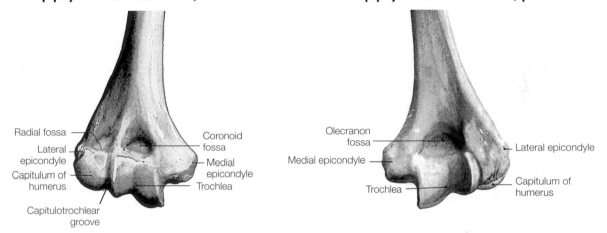

Radial fossa

Lateral epicondyle

Capitulum of humerus

Capitulotrochlear groove

Coronoid fossa

Medial epicondyle

Trochlea

Olecranon fossa

Medial epicondyle

Trochlea

Lateral epicondyle

Capitulum of humerus

Proximal epiphyses of the radius and ulna

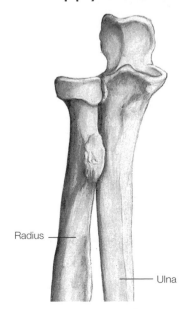

Radius

Ulna

5 THE ELBOW

The notable structures that can be detected by palpation are:

- The humerus (*humerus*):
  - The capitulum of the humerus (*capitulum humeri*) (Fig. 5.3)
  - The lateral epicondyle (*epicondylus lateralis*) (Fig. 5.4)
  - The lateral supraepicondylar ridge (*crista supraepicondylaris lateralis*) (Fig. 5.5)
  - The olecranon fossa (*fossa olecrani*) (Fig. 5.6)
  - The medial epicondyle (*epicondylus medialis*) (Figs 5.7 and 5.8)
  - The medial supraepicondylar ridge (*crista supraepicondylaris medialis*) (Fig. 5.9)
  - The groove for the ulnar nerve (*sulcus nervi ulnaris*) (Fig. 5.10).
- The radius (*radius*):
  - The head of the radius (Fig. 5.11)
  - The neck of the radius (Fig. 5.12)
  - The radial tuberosity (Fig. 5.13).
- The ulna (*ulna*):
  - Visualization of the olecranon (*olecranon*) at the elbow (Fig. 5.14)
  - The superior surface of the olecranon (Fig. 5.15)
  - The medial surface of the olecranon (Fig. 5.16)
  - The lateral surface of the olecranon (Fig. 5.17)
  - The posterior border of the shaft (body) of the ulna (*margo posterior corporis ulnae*) (Fig. 5.18)
  - The coronoid process of the ulna (*processus coronoideus ulnae*) (Fig. 5.19).

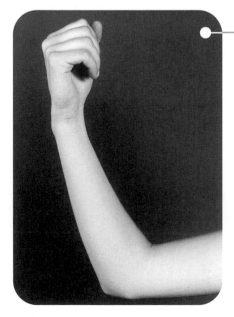

Fig. 5.2

Overall view of the elbow

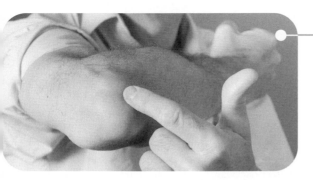

Fig. 5.3 | The capitulum (*capitulum humeri*)

This lies at the distal and lateral extremity of the humerus, and articulates with the articular facet of the radius. In order for you to palpate the full extent of the capitulum, the subject's elbow needs to be fully flexed. This muscular action will also reveal the posterior and inferior parts of this structure. The capitulum will appear smooth beneath your fingers.

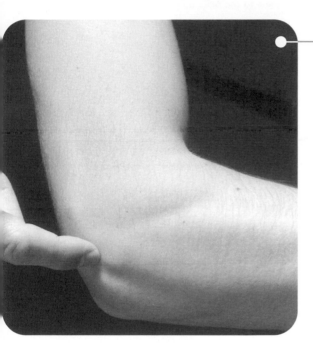

Fig. 5.4 | The lateral epicondyle (*epicondylus lateralis*)

This structure is situated superior and lateral to the capitulum (Fig. 5.3), and inferior to the distal extremity of the lateral supraepicondylar ridge (Fig. 5.5). You can feel its rough surface beneath your fingers. It gives attachment to the lateral epicondylar muscles (forearm extensors) and the radial collateral ligament (*ligamentum collaterale radiale*).

Note: The lateral epicondylar muscles (also called the forearm extensors) are a muscle group consisting of the following: the anconeus, extensor carpi radialis brevis (short radial extensor of the wrist), extensor digitorum, extensor digiti minimi (extensor of the little finger), extensor carpi ulnaris (ulnar extensor of the wrist), and supinator muscles. The attachment of the anconeus is by means of its own tendon on the posterior surface of the lateral epicondyle of the humerus. The origin of the other muscles is by means of a common tendon.

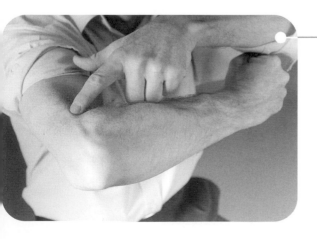

Fig. 5.5 | The lateral supraepicondylar ridge (*crista supraepicondylaris lateralis*)

This can be sensed as a marked, sharp ridge beneath your fingers. It is directly accessible beneath the skin, above the lateral epicondyle (Fig. 5.4), and is considerably more marked than the medial epicondylar ridge.

Note: The proximal continuation of this ridge runs along the lateral border of the humerus (this can be sensed clearly beneath your fingers) as far as the (lateral) deltoid tuberosity (tuberositas deltoidea).

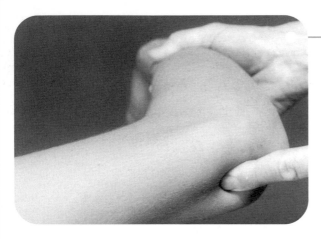

Fig. 5.6 | **The olecranon fossa (*fossa olecrani*)**

This lies at the distal extremity of the posterior surface of the humerus. The fossa receives the proximal extremity of the olecranon when the forearm is extended on the arm. The approach is easier if the subject's elbow is flexed at an angle of 130–140°, so as to relax the tendon of the triceps brachii. Using a contact with the pads of two fingers, supported against the capitulum of the humerus (Fig. 5.3), direct your contact backward, pushing the tendon of the triceps brachii aside medially. The fossa will appear beneath your fingers, superior to the olecranon.

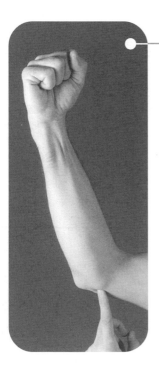

Fig. 5.7 | **The medial epicondyle (*epicondylus medialis*)**

This structure lies above and medial to the trochlea of the humerus, at the distal extremity of the medial border of the shaft of the bone (see also Fig. 5.8).

Note: The anterior surface and tip of the medial epicondyle provide attachment to the medial epicondylar muscles (forearm flexors), i.e. the pronator teres, flexor carpi radialis, palmaris longus, flexor carpi ulnaris, and flexor digitorum superficialis muscles. The posterior surface of the medial epicondyle is smooth, traversed by a vertical groove through which the ulnar nerve passes. The inferior border provides attachment to the ulnar collateral ligament of the elbow joint.

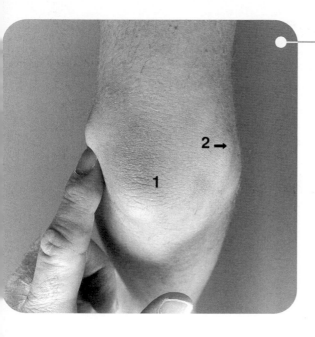

Fig. 5.8 | **Posterior view of the medial epicondyle (*epicondylus medialis*)**

This figure shows the position of the medial epicondyle, indicated by the practitioner's index finger, relative to the olecranon (1) and the lateral epicondyle (2).

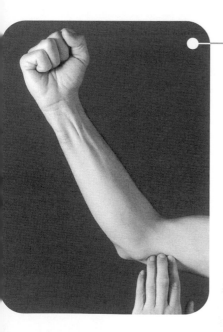

Fig. 5.9 | **The medial supraepicondylar ridge (*crista supraepicondylaris medialis*)**

This ridge is much less marked than the lateral supraepicondylar ridge. It can be found above the medial epicondyle, and is felt beneath your fingers as a blunt ridge which is easy to access.

Note: This ridge approximately follows the medial border of the humerus.

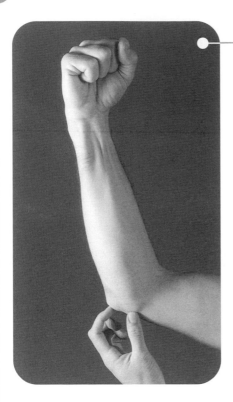

Fig. 5.10 | **The groove for the ulnar nerve (*sulcus nervi ulnaris*)**

This is a vertical groove crossing the posterior surface of the medial epicondyle. In this figure, the practitioner's thumb and finger contact indicates the extent of the groove. The practitioner's thumb rests medially, on the medial epicondyle, while the index finger is on the olecranon.

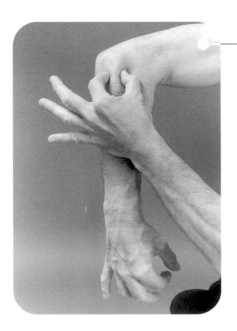

Fig. 5.11 | **The head of the radius (*caput radii*)**

Position your thumb and index finger at the capitulum of the humerus (Fig. 5.3), with the subject's elbow flexed at 90°. Then slide the contact distally, maintaining your contact with the skin. You will sense the joint cavity between the humerus and radius beneath your fingers. You can then take hold of the head of the radius between thumb and index finger. (If you are in any doubt, you can identify the head of the radius by asking the subject to pronate and supinate the forearm, so that the head of the radius rotates beneath your fingers.)

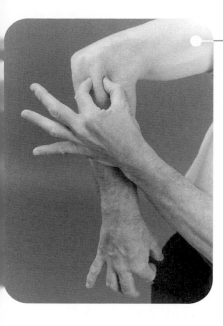

Fig. 5.12 | **The neck of the radius**
(*collum radii*)

Take as your starting point the thumb and index finger contact on the head of the radius, as described above (Fig. 5.11). Descend roughly one finger's width distally, where you will detect a narrowing. This is the desired structure.

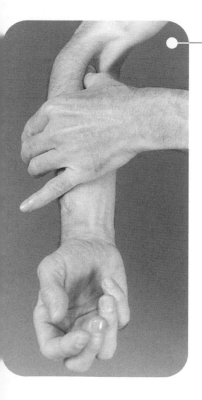

Fig. 5.13 | **The radial tuberosity**
(*tuberositas radii*)

Place your thumb in the base of the lateral groove of the fold of the elbow, as shown here (see note below). Position your thumb against the distal, external extremity of the tendon of the biceps brachii, and you will make contact with the bony structure of the radial tuberosity. Note that supination of the forearm brings the radial tuberosity toward your contact, and pronation moves it away.

Note: The lateral groove of the fold of the elbow runs obliquely downward and inward. It is formed by the lateral part of the biceps brachii medially and anteriorly, laterally by the brachioradialis, and posteriorly by the brachialis. The radial tuberosity is an ovoid structure situated on the antero-internal part of the bone, at the junction of the neck and shaft of the radius. On its posterior surface, it provides attachment to the tendon of the biceps brachii.

Care should be taken when palpating this structure, because there is a bursa between the tendon and the anterior part of the tuberosity.

THE ELBOW

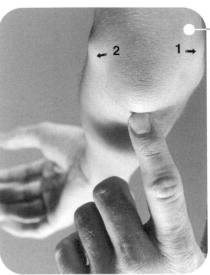

Fig. 5.14 | Visualization of the olecranon (*olecranon*) at the elbow

This is the posterior vertical process of the proximal extremity of the ulna. In the adjacent figure, the practitioner's index finger shows the topographical location of the olecranon relative to the lateral epicondyle (1) and medial epicondyle (2). These three bony structures are among the most important making up the elbow joint.

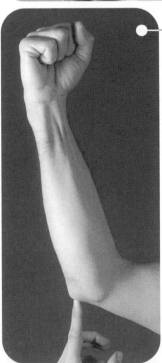

Fig. 5.15 | The superior surface of the olecranon (*olecranon*)

This lies immediately beneath the skin and so presents no difficulties of access, as the adjacent figure demonstrates. A beak-like process extends forward; this rests in the olecranon fossa of the humerus when the forearm is extended at the elbow.

Note: The posterior part gives attachment to the tendon of the triceps brachii.

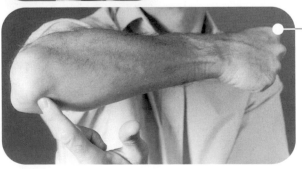

Fig. 5.16 | The medial surface of the olecranon

This surface (indicated by the practitioner's index finger) is important for the reason that it gives insertion to the posterior part of the ulnar collateral ligament of the elbow joint and to the flexor carpi ulnaris.

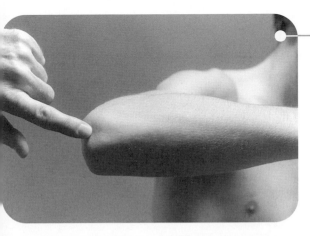

Fig. 5.17 | The lateral surface of the olecranon

The posterior part of the radial collateral ligament of the elbow joint has its attachment here. So too does the anconeus muscle.

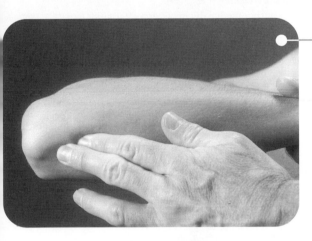

Fig. 5.18 | The posterior border of the shaft (body) of the ulna (*margo posterior corporis ulnae*)

This bony structure is the distal extension of the posterior surface of the olecranon. Examination presents no difficulties.

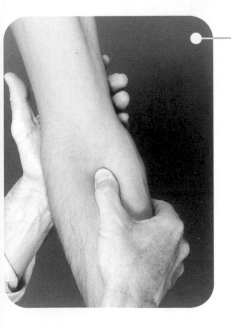

Fig. 5.19 | The coronoid process of the ulna (*processus coronoideus ulnae*)

The subject's elbow should be slightly flexed. Place one hand on the posterior surface of the elbow, at the olecranon (Fig. 5.14), and the other on the medial border of the proximal extremity of the ulna. Position your thumb inside the distal tendon of the biceps brachii (see Fig. 4.6). Grasp the posterior border of the ulna with your other fingers. The practitioner's thumb can be seen here opposite the coronoid process, a bony structure which can only be accessed indirectly, through the mass of muscle: in this case, the anterior group of the muscles of the forearm.

Note: The coronoid process is one of the two processes of the superior extremity of the ulna; the other is the olecranon (Fig. 5.14). These two osseous structures unite to form a hook-shaped articular cavity, the trochlear notch of the ulna.

NERVES AND BLOOD VESSELS

The notable structures that can be detected by palpation are:

- The ulnar nerve (*n. ulnaris*) in the groove for the ulnar nerve (*sulcus nervi ulnaris*) (Fig. 5.21).
- The ulnar nerve (*n. ulnaris*) in the proximal part of the forearm (Fig. 5.22).
- The median nerve (*n. medianus*) in the medial bicipital groove (*sulcus bicipitalis medialis; sulcus bicipitalis ulnaris*) (Fig. 5.23).
- The radial nerve (*n. radialis*) (Figs 5.24 and 5.25).
- The musculocutaneous nerve (*n. musculocutaneus*) (Fig. 5.24).
- The brachial artery (*a. brachialis*) at the medial bicipital groove (*sulcus bicipitalis medialis*) (Fig. 5.26).

Note: The nerves can be palpated by one of the following means: scratching the location with your fingernail; rolling it beneath the pads of your fingers; or visualizing them by inducing a state of tension in them (according to region).

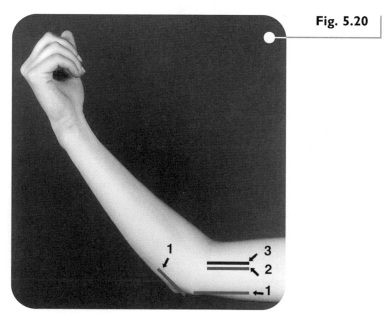

Fig. 5.20

Visualization of the course of the main nerves and blood vessels of the medial part of the elbow

1. Ulnar nerve (*n. ulnaris*).
2. Median nerve (*n. medianus*).
3. The brachial artery (*a. brachialis*).

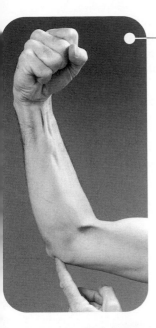

Fig. 5.21 | **The ulnar nerve (*n. ulnaris*) in the groove for the ulnar nerve (*sulcus nervi ulnaris*)**

Examination presents no difficulty. Simply place your index finger in the groove for the ulnar nerve (Fig. 5.10) to contact the structure concerned. The nerve can be sensed beneath your fingers as a full, cylindrical cord. Great care is needed in the approach to the nerve. It lies in the groove for the ulnar nerve (see Fig. 5.20) and then enters beneath the arch that unites the humeral head and ulnar head of the flexor carpi ulnaris muscle.

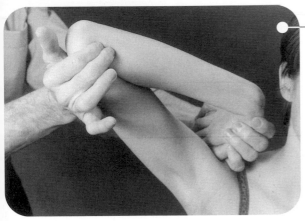

Fig. 5.22 | **The ulnar nerve (*n. ulnaris*) in the proximal part of the forearm**

Beyond the groove for the ulnar nerve (Fig. 5.21), it is still possible to palpate the ulnar nerve in the proximal part of the forearm (see also Fig. 5.20). To do this, ease the subject's arm into flexion with his or her forearm pronated and hand extended. The nerve can be palpated in the "antebrachial" extension of the groove for the ulnar nerve of the medial epicondyle. It can be felt beneath your fingers as a full, cylindrical cord in the proximal third of the forearm.

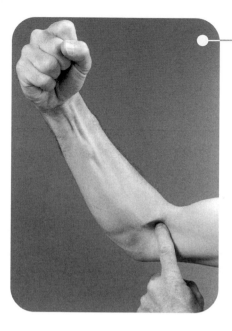

Fig. 5.23 The median nerve (*n. medianus*) in the medial bicipital groove (*sulcus bicipitalis medialis; sulcus bicipitalis ulnaris*)

The contact required to locate this nerve uses the pad of your first two fingertips, inside the tendon of the biceps brachii. As shown in the photograph, it is fairly simple to locate it in this position. You will sense a full, cylindrical cord that can be rolled beneath the pads of your index and middle fingers. This is the median nerve.

Note: The brachial artery lies outside the median nerve.

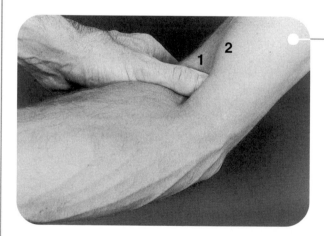

Fig. 5.24 The radial nerve (*n. radialis*) and musculocutaneous nerve (*n. musculocutaneus*) Method of approach

The musculocutaneous nerve is the one that lies closest to the tendon of the biceps. It continues as the lateral cutaneous nerve of the forearm, which in turn divides into an anterior and a posterior branch. It is more superficial than the radial nerve, which lies deeper and more laterally in the lateral bicipital groove.

These two nerves are accessible to palpation, either by rolling them under the pads of your fingers, or by scratching with the nail of your thumb or index finger.

(1) Brachioradialis muscle; (2) biceps brachii muscle.

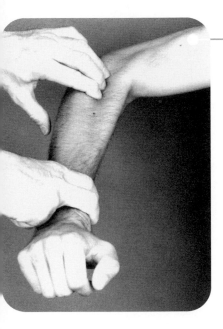

Fig. 5.25 | **The radial nerve (*n. radialis*) at the neck of the radius and posterior surface of the forearm Method of approach**

The motor deep branch of this nerve can be palpated at the neck of the radius; it can also be palpated inferiorly, on the posterior surface of the forearm. To do this, you should first locate the bodies of two muscles, the extensor carpi radialis brevis and the extensor digitorum (see anatomical plate, p. 173). Place a broad contact in between these two muscles, and roll the radial nerve beneath the pads of your fingers, pushing aside the extensor digitorum as you do so.

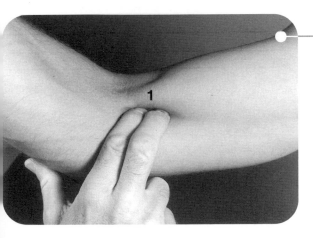

Fig. 5.26 | **The brachial artery (*a. brachialis*) at the medial bicipital groove (*sulcus bicipitalis medialis*)**

Place a two-finger contact in the fold of the elbow, medial and posterior to the tendon of the biceps brachii (1). Here you can clearly detect the pulse of the brachial artery. Note that the median nerve lies medially to it.

CHAPTER 6

THE FOREARM

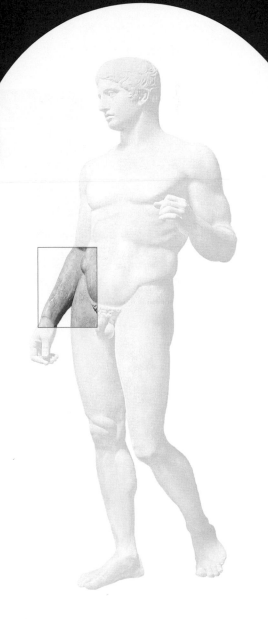

TOPOGRAPHICAL PRESENTATION OF THE FOREARM

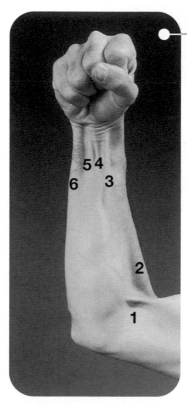

Fig. 6.1

Medial view of the forearm region

1. The aponeurosis radiating from the biceps brachii.
2. The brachioradialis.
3. The flexor carpi radialis.
4. The palmaris longus.
5. The flexor digitorum superficialis (tendon to the fourth finger).
6. The flexor carpi ulnaris.

MYOLOGY

ATTACHMENTS OF THE MUSCLES OF THE FOREARM

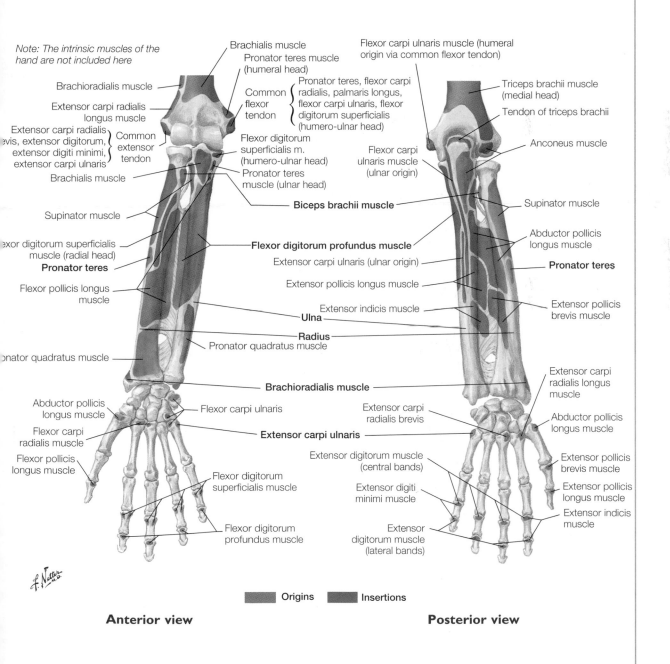

Note: The intrinsic muscles of the hand are not included here

Brachialis muscle
Brachioradialis muscle
Extensor carpi radialis longus muscle
Extensor carpi radialis brevis, extensor digitorum, extensor digiti minimi, extensor carpi ulnaris
Common extensor tendon
Brachialis muscle
Supinator muscle
Flexor digitorum superficialis muscle (radial head)
Pronator teres
Flexor pollicis longus muscle
Pronator quadratus muscle
Abductor pollicis longus muscle
Flexor carpi radialis muscle
Flexor pollicis longus muscle

Pronator teres muscle (humeral head)
Common flexor tendon
Pronator teres, flexor carpi radialis, palmaris longus, flexor carpi ulnaris, flexor digitorum superficialis (humero-ulnar head)
Flexor digitorum superficialis m. (humero-ulnar head)
Pronator teres muscle (ulnar head)
Biceps brachii muscle
Flexor digitorum profundus muscle
Extensor carpi ulnaris (ulnar origin)
Extensor pollicis longus muscle
Extensor indicis muscle
Ulna
Radius
Pronator quadratus muscle
Brachioradialis muscle
Flexor carpi ulnaris
Extensor carpi ulnaris
Flexor digitorum superficialis muscle
Flexor digitorum profundus muscle

Flexor carpi ulnaris muscle (humeral origin via common flexor tendon)
Triceps brachii muscle (medial head)
Tendon of triceps brachii
Anconeus muscle
Flexor carpi ulnaris muscle (ulnar origin)
Supinator muscle
Abductor pollicis longus muscle
Pronator teres
Extensor pollicis brevis muscle
Extensor carpi radialis longus muscle
Abductor pollicis longus muscle
Extensor pollicis brevis muscle
Extensor pollicis longus muscle
Extensor indicis muscle

Extensor carpi radialis brevis
Extensor digitorum muscle (central bands)
Extensor digiti minimi muscle
Extensor digitorum muscle (lateral bands)

Origins   Insertions

Anterior view   **Posterior view**

THE LATERAL MUSCLE GROUP

This group consists of four muscles, arranged in two layers.

- Superficial layer. There are three muscles in this layer. Working across medially, these are:
    - The brachioradialis
    - The extensor carpi radialis longus
    - The extensor carpi radialis brevis.
- Deep layer. This consists of a single muscle, the supinator.

The notable structures that can be detected by palpation are:

- The proximal part of the brachioradialis (*m. brachioradialis*) (Fig. 6.3).
- The body of the brachioradialis (Fig. 6.4).
- The insertion of the brachioradialis (Fig. 6.5).
- The origin of the extensor carpi radialis longus (long radial extensor m. of wrist) (*m. extensor carpi radialis longus*) (Fig. 6.6).
- The body of the extensor carpi radialis longus (Figs 6.7 and 6.8).
- The tendon of the extensor carpi radialis longus (Figs 6.9–6.12).
- The extensor carpi radialis brevis (short radial extensor m. of wrist) (*m. extensor carpi radialis brevis*) (Figs 6.13–6.15).
- The insertion of the extensor carpi radialis brevis (Fig. 6.16).
- The supinator (*m. supinator*) (Fig. 6.17).

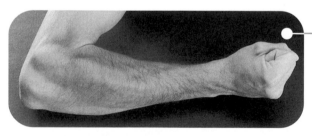

Fig. 6.2

View of the lateral muscle group

Actions
- The brachioradialis flexes the forearm on the arm in the neutral position (neither pronated nor supinated).
- The extensor carpi radialis longus extends and abducts the forearm on the arm (inclines it radially).
- The extensor carpi radialis brevis extends the wrist on the forearm. It also helps to incline it radially when the forearm is semi-pronated.
- The supinator (together with the biceps) helps to supinate the forearm on the arm (assisted, where the impulse to supinate the forearm is strong, by the adductors and lateral rotator muscles of the shoulder, which work together to bring about this action).

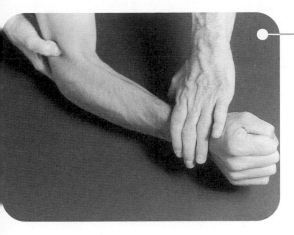

Fig. 6.3 | **The proximal part of the brachioradialis (*m. brachioradialis*)**

With the subject's arm in a neutral position, neither pronated nor supinated, apply resistance on the inferior third of the radius, and ask the subject to flex the forearm on the arm. You will sense the contraction on the distal part of the lateral border of the humerus.

Attachments
- The brachioradialis arises:
  — On the inferior third of the lateral border of the humerus, by means of tendinous fibers
  — On the lateral intermuscular septum of the arm, by means of fleshy fibers.
- It is inserted on the lateral surface of the base of the radial styloid process.

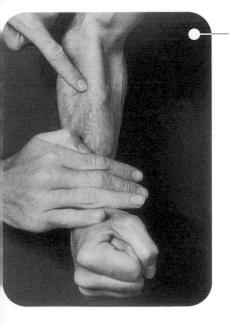

Fig. 6.4 | **The body of the brachioradialis**

Apply the same resistance and request the same action as that described above. The body of the muscle becomes prominent, appearing clearly, as shown in the adjacent figure.

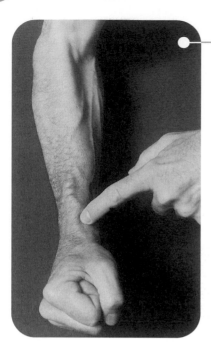

Fig. 6.5 | **The insertion of the brachioradialis**

The muscle is inserted at the base of the radial styloid process, by means of a flat tendon. This attachment is indicated here by the practitioner's index finger.

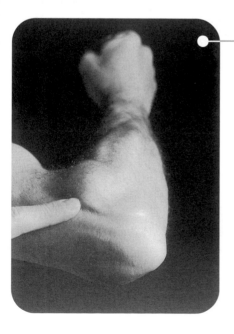

Fig. 6.6 | **The origin of the extensor carpi radialis longus (long radial extensor m. of wrist) (*m. extensor carpi radialis longus*)**

The subject's elbow should be flexed. Ask him to extend the wrist and incline it radially. You will see the muscle contract on the lateral border of the humerus, approximately three finger-widths below the attachment of the brachioradialis.

Attachments
- The extensor carpi radialis longus arises on the lateral supraepicondylar ridge and at the lateral intermuscular septum of the arm.
- It is inserted on the lateral tubercle of the base of the second metacarpal.

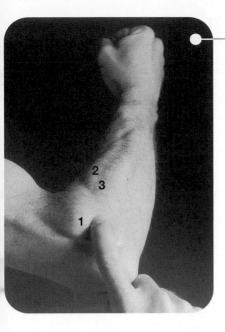

Fig. 6.7 | The body of the extensor carpi radialis longus at the elbow

In many subjects, the body of this muscle appears clearly on the external surface of the elbow if you ask them to extend the wrist and incline it toward the radius. In other subjects, you may find that the contraction of the muscle appears on the lateral surface of the elbow, outside the proximal part of the brachioradialis muscle (Fig. 6.3) (at the fold of the elbow).

1. Body of extensor carpi radialis longus.
2. Extensor carpi radialis brevis.
3. Extensor digitorum.

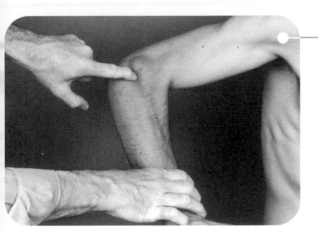

Fig. 6.8 | The extensor carpi radialis longus at the forearm

The figure alongside shows the body of this muscle from another angle. It becomes visible when contracted, and tends to appear as a short, fairly voluminous muscle in males (depending on profession and type or degree of physical activity) and more elongated in females.

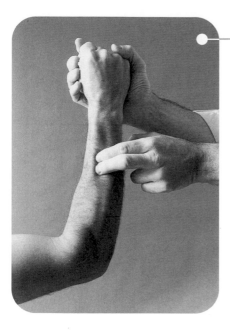

Fig. 6.9 | **The tendon of the extensor carpi radialis longus**

In the middle third of the forearm, the body of the muscle gives way to a tendon, located on the anterolateral part of the body of the extensor carpi radialis brevis. The two tendons can be distinguished in the more distal region by using a broad two-finger contact and "rolling" the tendons on the shaft of the radius.

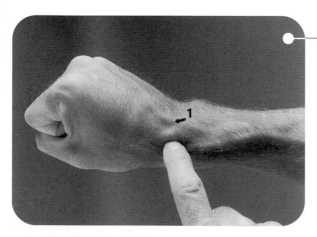

Fig. 6.10 | **To display the tendon of the extensor carpi radialis longus at the wrist**

This tendon is inserted on the lateral part of the dorsal surface of the base of the second metacarpal, and becomes clearly visible in some subjects (as in the adjacent figure) on the outer side of the tendon of the extensor carpi radialis brevis (1) (Fig. 6.16), if the subject is requested to clench the fist.

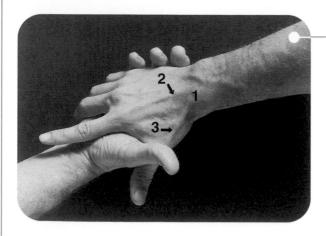

Fig. 6.11 | **Distal palpation of the tendon of the extensor carpi radialis longus Alternative approach. Step 1**

A triangle with a proximal apex (1) and distal base can clearly be seen in the adjacent figure. The two tendons belonging to the extensor carpi radialis longus and extensor carpi radialis brevis can be palpated in this angle. The triangle has a distal base (the first commissure); its ulnar side is formed by the tendon of the extensor digitorum going to the second finger (2) and its radial side by the tendon of the extensor pollicis longus (3).

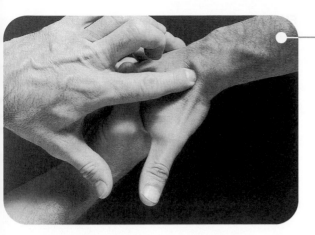

Fig. 6.12 | **Distal palpation of the tendon of the extensor carpi radialis longus Alternative approach. Step 2**

Contact the ulnar border of the tendon of the extensor pollicis longus with one finger and ease the tendon aside radially, feeling for the tendon of the extensor carpi radialis longus (see also Fig. 7.77).

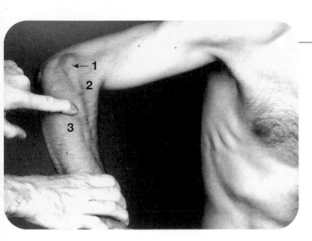

Fig. 6.13 | **The extensor carpi radialis brevis (short radial extensor m. of wrist) (*m. extensor carpi radialis brevis*) in the forearm**

This figure shows the body of the extensor carpi radialis brevis, from another angle. It is indicated by the practitioner's index finger. You can also see the course of the muscle and how it relates to other muscles of the forearm.

1. Extensor carpi radialis longus.
2. Brachioradialis.
3. Extensor digitorum.

Attachments
- The extensor carpi radialis brevis arises on the anterior surface of the lateral epicondyle of the humerus (via the common tendon of the epicondylar muscles).
- It is inserted on the dorsal and lateral base of the third metacarpal.

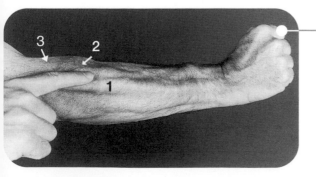

Fig. 6.14 | **The topographical relations of the extensor carpi radialis brevis**

The muscle body indicated here by the practitioner's index finger is situated radially to the extensor digitorum (1). At this level it runs along the tendon of the extensor carpi radialis longus (2) (not visible in this photograph), which lies laterally to it. The brachioradialis (3) (Fig. 6.4) is also on its lateral side.

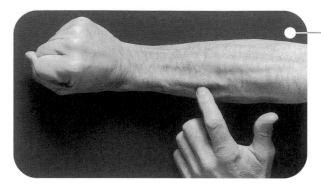

Fig. 6.15 · **The extensor carpi radialis brevis in the inferior third of the forearm**

At this level the tendon (indicated by the practitioner's index finger), along with that of the extensor carpi radialis longus, passes in front of the abductor pollicis longus (Fig. 6.37). More distally they also pass in front of the extensor pollicis brevis (Fig. 6.39).

See anatomical plate page 173.

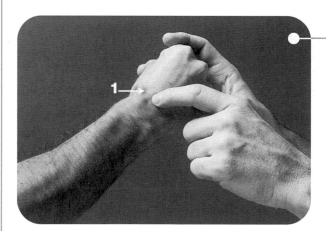

Fig. 6.16 · **The insertion of the extensor carpi radialis brevis**

This tendon can be seen in the adjacent figure, indicated by the practitioner's index finger. It is situated medially to the tendon of the extensor carpi radialis longus (1) (see also Fig. 6.10).

Note: The tendon of this muscle is attached on the posterior process of the base of the third metacarpal (see also Fig. 7.77).

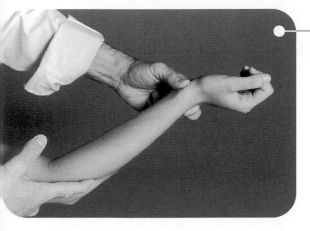

Fig. 6.17 | The supinator muscle (*m. supinator*)

The subject's elbow should be flexed and almost completely supinated. (This muscle is the only one that is effective when the arm is almost fully supinated.) Using your index and middle fingers, place your contact below the head of the radius, opposite the neck of the radius, where some fibers of the supinator muscle are attached (on the anterior, posterior, and lateral surfaces). Wedge your index and middle fingers against the inferior edge of the head of the radius, and ask the subject to supinate the forearm actively, using repeated, short, rapid movements, to enable you to sense the contraction of the muscle fibers beneath your fingers.

Attachments
The supinator has two heads, one superficial and one deep.

- Origins. Taking the muscle as a whole, it arises:
    — On the inferior part of the lateral epicondyle of the humerus
    — On the middle portion of the radial collateral ligament
    — On the supinator ridge of the ulna
    — On the supinator fossa of the ulna.
- Insertions:
    — On the superior part of the oblique line of the anterior border of the radius (superficial portion)
    — On the anterior, lateral, and posterior surfaces of the neck of the radius (deep portion).

THE POSTERIOR MUSCLE GROUP

This group consists of eight muscles, arranged as follows:

- Superficial layer. Working across medially, the muscles of this layer are:
    — The extensor digitorum
    — Extensor digiti minimi
    — Extensor carpi ulnaris
    — Anconeus.
- Deep layer. Working downward from superior to inferior, the muscles of this layer are:
    — The abductor pollicis longus
    — Abductor pollicis brevis
    — Extensor pollicis longus
    — Extensor indicis.

The notable structures that can be detected by palpation are:

- The extensor digitorum (*m. extensor digitorum*) (Figs 6.19–6.22):
    — Tendons on the back of the hand (Figs 6.23 and 6.26)
    — Insertions at the phalanges (Fig. 6.24)
    — Tendon to the second finger and extension of apo-neurosis (Figs 6.26, 6.27, and 6.32).
- The extensor indicis (index extensor m.) (*m. extensor indicis*) (Figs 6.25 and 6.26).
- The extensor digiti minimi (extensor m. of the little finger) (*m. extensor digiti minimi*):
    — Origin (Fig. 6.28)
    — Body of muscle (Fig. 6.29)
    — Tendon (Figs 6.30–6.32).
- The extensor carpi ulnaris (ulnar extensor of the wrist) (*m. extensor carpi ulnaris*) (Figs 6.33–6.35).
- The anconeus (*m. anconeus*) (Fig. 6.36).
- The abductor pollicis longus (long abductor muscle of the thumb) (*m. abductor pollicis longus*):
    — Body of muscle (Fig. 6.37)
    — Tendon (Fig. 6.38).
- The extensor pollicis brevis (short extensor muscle of the thumb) (*m. extensor pollicis brevis*):
    — Body of muscle (Fig. 6.39)

    — Tendon at the wrist (Fig. 6.40)
    — Insertion (Fig. 6.41).
- The extensor pollicis longus (long extensor m. of the thumb) (*m. extensor pollicis longus*) (Figs 6.42–6.44).

Actions

- The anconeus extends the forearm on the arm.
- The extensor carpi ulnaris extends and adducts the wrist (inclines it to the ulnar side).
- As regards the extensor digitorum:
    — It extends the three phalanges of the last four fingers; the action is much more marked for the extension of the proximal (first) phalanx:
        — The extensor indicis and extensor digiti minimi assist in the extension action of the index and little fingers
        — The lumbricals and the dorsal and palmar inter-osseous muscles assist in the extension of the second and third phalanges
    — It helps in the extension of the wrist on the forearm.

The extensor indicis and extensor digiti minimi also assist in the extension of the wrist.

- The abductor pollicis longus:
    — Draws the first metacarpal anteriorly when the thumb is abducted
    — Initiates the opposition of the thumb together with the most lateral muscles of the thumb
    — Assists in flexing the wrist.
- The extensor pollicis brevis:
    — Extends the proximal phalanx on the first metacar-pal, and abducts the first metacarpal. (This is essen-tially the muscle that abducts the thumb.)
    — Assists in the radial inclination of the thumb.
- The extensor pollicis longus:
    — Extends the middle phalanx on the proximal one
    — Extends the proximal phalanx on the first metacarpal
    — It then draws the first metacarpal posterior to the plane of metacarpals.

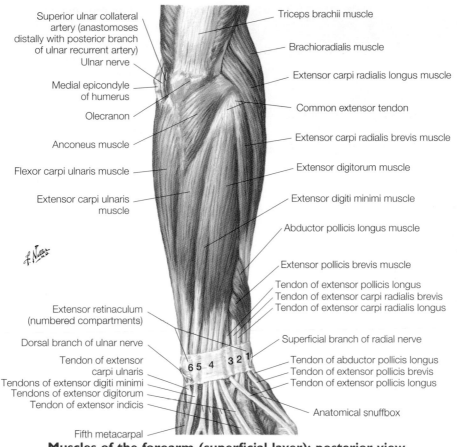

Superior ulnar collateral artery (anastomoses distally with posterior branch of ulnar recurrent artery)

Ulnar nerve

Medial epicondyle of humerus

Olecranon

Anconeus muscle

Flexor carpi ulnaris muscle

Extensor carpi ulnaris muscle

Extensor retinaculum (numbered compartments)

Dorsal branch of ulnar nerve

Tendon of extensor carpi ulnaris

Tendons of extensor digiti minimi

Tendons of extensor digitorum

Tendon of extensor indicis

Fifth metacarpal

Triceps brachii muscle

Brachioradialis muscle

Extensor carpi radialis longus muscle

Common extensor tendon

Extensor carpi radialis brevis muscle

Extensor digitorum muscle

Extensor digiti minimi muscle

Abductor pollicis longus muscle

Extensor pollicis brevis muscle

Tendon of extensor pollicis longus
Tendon of extensor carpi radialis brevis
Tendon of extensor carpi radialis longus

Superficial branch of radial nerve

Tendon of abductor pollicis longus
Tendon of extensor pollicis brevis
Tendon of extensor pollicis longus

Anatomical snuffbox

6 5 4 3 2 1

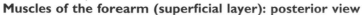

Muscles of the forearm (superficial layer): posterior view

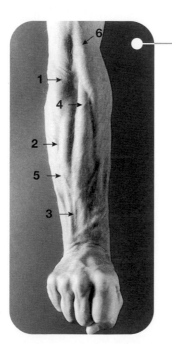

Fig. 6.18 | **Posterior view of the forearm**

1. Anconeus.
2. Extensor carpi ulnaris.
3. Extensor digiti minimi.
4. Extensor digitorum.
5. Flexor carpi ulnaris.
6. Extensor carpi radialis longus.

THE FOREARM

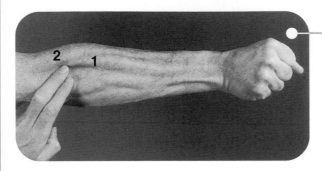

Fig. 6.19 | **The extensor digitorum (*m. extensor digitorum*), proximal part**

This muscle (1) is situated posteriorly and medially to the extensor carpi radialis longus (2) (Fig. 6.7). It can be revealed by asking the subject to make a fist and then repeatedly open it and extend the fingers.

Attachments

- Origins:
  — These are on the lateral epicondyle, via the common tendon of origin of the epicondylar muscles (forearm extensors).
- Insertions:
  — At the first phalanx, each tendon of the extensor digitorum receives the tendinous expansion of the lumbricals and of the interossei on its lateral and medial borders.
  — Each tendon is inserted on the three phalanges as follows:
    — At the metacarpophalangeal joint, each tendon has a fibrous expansion that is inserted at the base of the first phalanx.
    — Each tendon then subdivides into three slips at the proximal phalanx.
    — A middle slip is attached to the posterior surface of the superior extremity of the middle phalanx.
    — Two lateral slips unite on the dorsal surface of the middle phalanx, and are inserted on the superior extremity of the posterior surface of the distal phalanx.

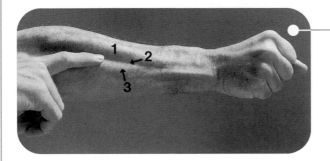

Fig. 6.20 | **The extensor digitorum on the forearm**

This muscle (1) is situated centrally on the posterior surface of the forearm. It runs down behind the supinator and the four muscles of the deep layer of the posterior region of the forearm. It is bounded by the extensor digiti minimi (2) (not visible on this photograph) (see also Fig. 6.29) medially, and by the extensor carpi ulnaris (3) (see Fig. 6.34). Ask the subject to perform the same muscular action as that described above.

Note: At this level the body of the muscle is made up of four portions.

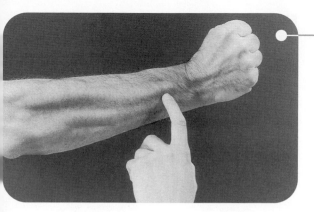

Fig. 6.21 | The extensor digitorum, distal part

On the distal part of the posterior surface of the forearm, the muscle consists of a group of four tendons, issuing from the four portions of the muscle described above.

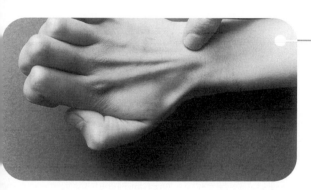

Fig. 6.22 | The extensor digitorum at the wrist

At this level the four tendons of the extensor digitorum and the tendon of the extensor indicis come together and pass through an osteofibrous sheath, part of the extensor retinaculum, which holds them against the posterior surface of the radius before they pass on to the dorsal surface of the hand.

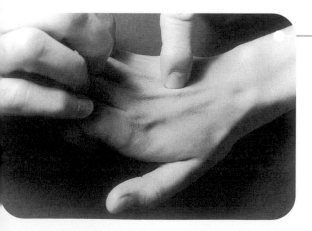

Fig. 6.23 | The tendons of the extensor digitorum on the back of the hand

Extend the subject's hand, applying resistance on the posterior surface of the first phalanges, as shown in the adjacent figure. This will make the tendons appear on the back of the subject's hand.

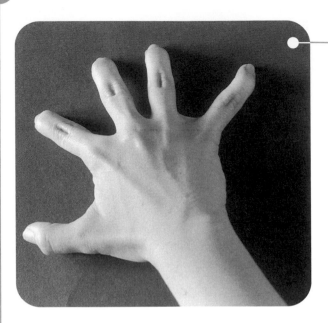

Fig. 6.24 | The insertions of the extensor digitorum at the phalanges

Each tendon is inserted at the respective base of each of the three phalanges of the four fingers on which the tendons operate.

Note: The photograph in the adjacent figure shows extensor digitorum tendons that are each divided into two at the level of the phalanges. This is an exceptional case, and not the usual rule.

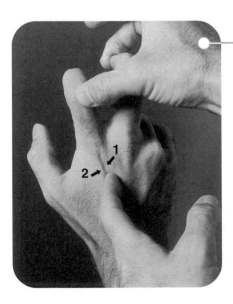

Fig. 6.25 | The extensor indicis (index extensor m.) (*m. extensor indicis*) on the back of the hand

This muscle extends from the ulna to the index finger. On the dorsal surface of the wrist and hand, the tendon of the extensor indicis (1) lies by the ulnar border of the tendon of the extensor digitorum going to the index finger (2). In most cases it unites with this tendon at the metacarpophalangeal joint.

Attachments
- The extensor indicis arises:
    — On the inferior third of the posterior surface of the ulna
    — On the interosseous membrane of the forearm.
- It is inserted at the metacarpophalangeal joint of the index finger, where it fuses with the tendon of the extensor digitorum going to the index finger.

Note: In the figure shown here, the practitioner's index finger points between the two tendons described above.

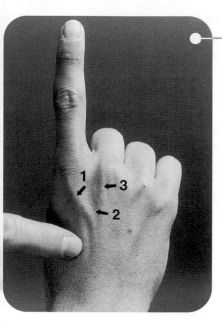

Fig. 6.26 | **The topographical relations of the tendon of the extensor indicis (*m. extensor indicis*) and the tendons of the extensor digitorum**

Subjects' metacarpophalangeal joints should be flexed to begin with. Ask them to extend the second finger. The tendon of the extensor digitorum (1) going to the second finger passes over the tendon of the extensor indicis (indicated here by the practitioner). It is drawn across by an expansion of the aponeurosis (2) which links it to the tendon of the extensor digitorum going to the middle finger (3). This has the effect of drawing the tendon of the extensor digitorum going to the second finger to the ulnar border of the tendon of the extensor indicis.

Note: The italic S-shaped tendon (1) seen on the back of the hand when performing the action described here is the tendon of the extensor digitorum going to the second finger.

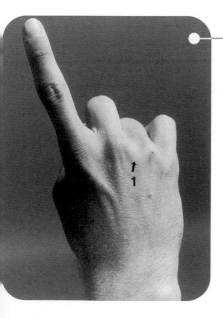

Fig. 6.27 | **The tendon of the extensor digitorum belonging to the second finger, and the expansions of the aponeurosis (1)**

On the back of the hand, the tendons of the extensor digitorum are interlinked by fibrous slips (1). These may be transverse or oblique (see also Figs 6.26 and 6.32).

THE FOREARM

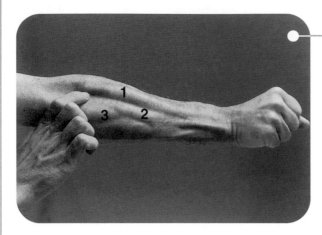

Fig. 6.28

The extensor digiti minimi (extensor m. of the little finger) (*m. extensor digiti minimi*): origin

This muscle arises on the lateral epicondyle of the humerus, inside the origin of the extensor digitorum (1).

1. Extensor digitorum.
2. Extensor carpi ulnaris.
3. Anconeus.

In the adjacent figure, the practitioner's index finger indicates the location of the extensor digiti minimi in the groove between the extensor digitorum (1) and the extensor carpi ulnaris (2).

Attachments
- The extensor digiti minimi arises:
    — On the lateral epicondyle of the humerus
    — On the antebrachial fascia.
- Distally, it fuses with the tendon of the extensor digitorum belonging to the fifth finger near the fifth metacarpal (this varies from one individual to another).

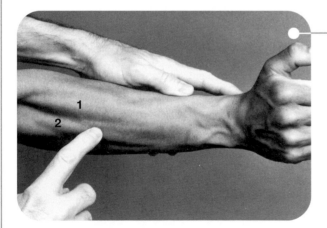

Fig. 6.29

The body of the extensor digiti minimi

This is a very long, slender muscle situated in the depression between the bodies of the extensor digitorum (1) and the extensor carpi ulnaris (2). It is indicated here by the practitioner's index finger. To sense the contraction of this muscle, place a broad contact (using two or three fingers) in the depression described above. Then ask the subject to extend the little finger repeatedly.

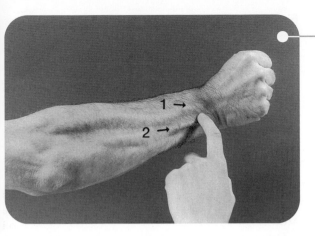

Fig. 6.30 | **The tendon of the extensor digiti minimi**

In order to locate this tendon, place your contact (using your index finger, or two or three fingers) medial to the tendon of the extensor digitorum (1), and lateral to the tendon of the extensor carpi ulnaris (2). You will feel it beneath your fingers. This can be facilitated by asking the subject to extend the proximal phalanx of the fifth finger repeatedly while the other two remain flexed.

Note: The tendon passes behind the head of the ulna and wrist joint in a separate sheath.

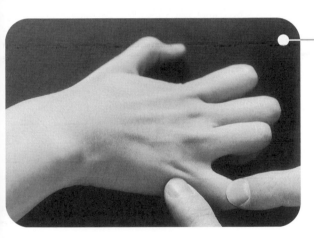

Fig. 6.31 | **The tendon of the extensor digiti minimi on the back of the hand**

Occasionally, the tendon of the extensor digiti minimi is sometimes divided in two, as seen here. This can be displayed by asking the subject to hyperextend the metacarpophalangeal joint of the fifth finger, while you resist this action.

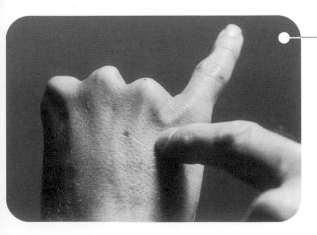

Fig. 6.32 | **The extension of the aponeurosis of the extensor digitorum on the tendon of the extensor digiti minimi**

The tendons of the extensor digitorum belonging to the fourth finger and of the extensor digiti minimi are normally connected with each other. This connection is indicated here by the practitioner's index finger.

Note: There are similar connections between the tendons of the other fingers.

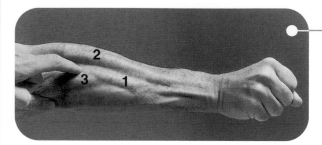

Fig. 6.33 | The origin of the extensor carpi ulnaris (ulnar extensor of the wrist) (*m. extensor carpi ulnaris*)

The practitioner's index finger in the adjacent figure indicates the proximal part of this muscle (1). Begin by locating the extensor digitorum (2). Then position your contact inside that muscle and ask the subject to extend the wrist repeatedly, inclining it to the ulnar side at the same time. You can then detect the extensor carpi ulnaris beneath your fingers. It can help you find the best point of contact if you also locate the anconeus (3).

Attachments
- The extensor carpi ulnaris arises via the common tendon of the lateral epicondylar muscles:
    — On the lateral epicondyle of the humerus
    — On the superior two-thirds of the lateral side of the posterior border of the ulna
    — On the deep surface of the antebrachial fascia.
- It is inserted on the posteromedial tubercle of the base of the fifth metacarpal.

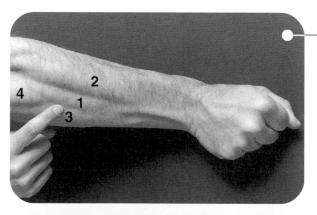

Fig. 6.34 | The body of the extensor carpi ulnaris

In the adjacent figure, the practitioner's index finger indicates the body of the extensor carpi ulnaris (1) between those of the extensor digitorum (2) (laterally) and the flexor carpi ulnaris (3) (medially). The anconeus (4) lies medially and superior to it.

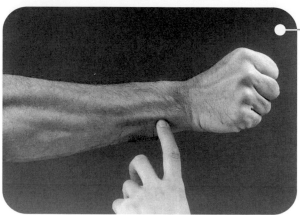

Fig. 6.35 | The extensor carpi ulnaris: distal part

The tendon of the extensor carpi ulnaris (indicated here by the practitioner's index finger) passes behind the distal extremity of the ulna, in an osteofibrous sheath. It is inserted on the medial tubercle of the fifth metacarpal.

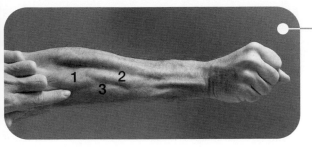

Fig. 6.36 | **The anconeus muscle (*m. anconeus*)**

It is easier to palpate this muscle if you begin with a three-finger contact resting against the lateral border of the olecranon. Then slide your fingers down toward the inferior and lateral part of the forearm, maintaining contact with the skin. You will feel the contour of this muscle beneath your fingers. Ask the subject to contract the muscles repeatedly to extend the forearm on the arm. This will make the body of the muscle more prominent.

In the adjacent figure, the practitioner's index finger indicates the anconeus (1) between the bodies of the extensor carpi ulnaris (2) (laterally) and the flexor carpi ulnaris (3) (medially).

Attachments

- The anconeus arises via a tendon on the posterior surface of the lateral epicondyle of the humerus.
- It is inserted on the lateral, posterior surface of the olecranon and on the superior quarter of the posterior border of the ulna.

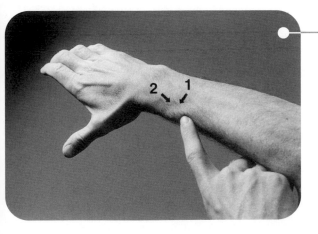

Fig. 6.37 | **The body of the abductor pollicis longus (long abductor muscle of the thumb) (*m. abductor pollicis longus*)**

The body of this muscle can be palpated on the posterior surface of the radius. It is shown in the figure alongside, indicated by the practitioner's index finger, at the point where it passes over the lateral surface of the radius. Ask the subject to abduct the thumb repeatedly as shown, extending it away from the other fingers to enable you to detect the contraction of the muscle.

Attachments

- The abductor pollicis longus arises:
    - On the posterior surface of the ulna
    - On the interosseous membrane of the forearm
    - On the medial part of the posterior surface of the radius.
- It is inserted on the lateral tubercle of the base of the first metacarpal.

Note: There is an oblique groove (1) separating the abductor pollicis longus and extensor pollicis brevis (2).

THE FOREARM

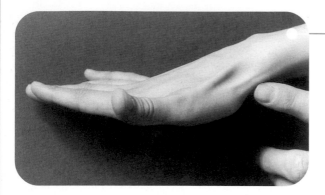

Fig. 6.38 | **The tendon of the abductor pollicis longus**

Ask the subject to abduct the thumb as shown, extending it away from the other fingers, to enable you to detect this tendon. It is indicated here by the practitioner's index finger. The tendon is inserted on the lateral tubercle of the base of the first metacarpal.

Note: It is not always easy to distinguish the tendon of the abductor pollicis longus clearly from that of the abductor pollicis brevis (Fig. 6.40). The two are often found running closely alongside each other in such a way that they seem to be a single tendon. It helps to remember that the tendon of the abductor pollicis longus lies farther anteriorly.

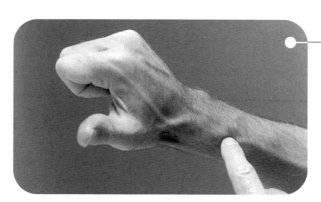

Fig. 6.39 | **The body of the extensor pollicis brevis (short extensor muscle of the thumb) (*m. extensor pollicis brevis*)**

This muscle lies on the posterior surface of the forearm, below the abductor pollicis longus. Both turn around the lateral surface of the radius. A point to remember in identifying these two muscles is that the abductor pollicis brevis occupies the more distal position. An oblique groove (Fig. 6.37) can be palpated between the bodies of the two muscles on the posterolateral part of the radius; the abductor pollicis brevis will be found inferior to this groove. Ask the subject to abduct the thumb repeatedly, extending it away from the other fingers, to help you sense the muscle contraction.

Attachments
- The abductor pollicis brevis arises:
    — On the medial third of the posterior surface of the radius
    — On the interosseous membrane of the forearm.
- It is inserted on the dorsal surface of the first phalanx of the thumb.

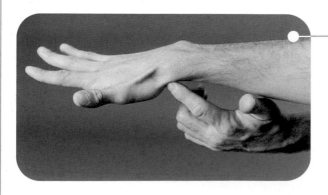

Fig. 6.40 | **The tendon of the extensor pollicis brevis at the wrist**

It is often difficult to distinguish the tendon of this muscle from that of the abductor pollicis longus (Fig. 6.38) at this level, as the two run closely side by side. To make the tendon apparent at the external part of the wrist, ask the subject first to extend all the fingers, and then abduct the thumb away from the other fingers. When trying to identify this tendon, remember that it occupies a dorsal position relative to that of the abductor pollicis longus.

Note: This tendon marks the anterolateral extent of the anatomical snuffbox (see note to Fig. 6.43).

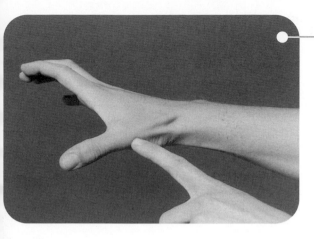

Fig. 6.41 | **The insertion of the extensor pollicis brevis**

The tendon indicated here by the practitioner's index finger runs along the dorsal surface of the first metacarpal, and is inserted on the dorsal part of the base of the first phalanx.

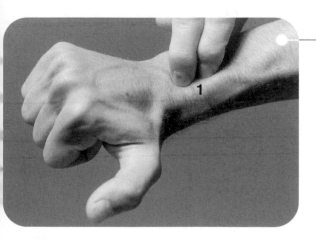

Fig. 6.42 | **The extensor pollicis longus (long extensor m. of the thumb) (*m. extensor pollicis longus*) on the posterior surface of the radius**

Place a two-finger contact on the posterior surface of the radius, medial to the body of the extensor pollicis brevis (1) (Fig. 6.39). Ask the subject to extend the thumb back beyond the plane of the hand, and you will feel the tendon of the extensor pollicis longus becoming taut beneath your fingers.

Attachments

- The extensor pollicis longus arises:
    - On the medial third of the posterior surface of the ulna
    - On the interosseous membrane of the forearm.
- It is inserted on the dorsal surface of the base of the second phalanx of the thumb.

Note: The body of the extensor pollicis longus runs down the posterior surface of the forearm in an oblique outward and downward direction; it runs under and closely against the extensor pollicis brevis.

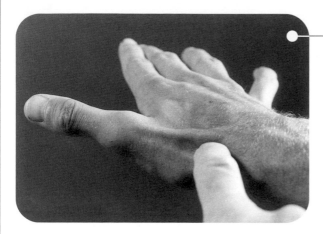

Fig. 6.43 | **The tendon of the extensor pollicis longus at the wrist**

This tendon can be made more prominent by asking the subject to perform the same action as that described in Figure 6.42. This tendon marks the posterolateral extent of the anatomical snuffbox at the wrist. The anterolateral boundary of this feature is marked by the tendon of the extensor pollicis brevis.

Note: The anatomical snuffbox is a triangular depression which appears on the posterolateral aspect of the wrist when the extensor muscles of the thumb contract. The floor of this depression is formed by the scaphoid bone.

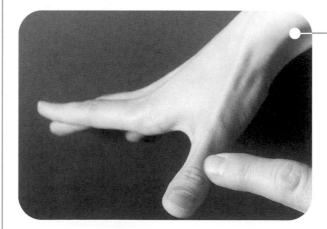

Fig. 6.44 | **The insertion of the extensor pollicis longus**

The tendon runs along the dorsal surface of the first metacarpal and proximal phalanx, and is inserted on the dorsal part of the base of the distal phalanx, shown here by the practitioner's index finger.

THE ANTERIOR MUSCLE GROUP

This group consists of eight muscles, arranged in four layers as follows:

- The first layer of the anterior compartment consists (working medially) of the pronator teres, flexor carpi radialis, palmaris longus, and flexor carpi ulnaris muscles.
- The second layer contains the flexor digitorum superficialis.
- The third layer consists of the flexor digitorum profundus medially and the flexor pollicis longus laterally.
- The fourth layer contains the pronator quadratus muscle.

The notable structures that can be detected by palpation are:

- The medial epicondylar muscles (forearm flexors) (Fig. 6.46); the common tendon of origin (*caput commune musculorum flexorum*) (Fig. 6.47).
- The pronator teres (*m. pronator teres*) (Figs 6.48 and 6.49).
- The flexor carpi radialis (*m. flexor carpi radialis*):
  — Body (Fig. 6.50)
  — Tendons (Figs 6.51 and 6.52).
- The palmaris longus (*m. palmaris longus*) (Figs 6.53 and 6.54).
- The flexor carpi ulnaris (*m. flexor carpi ulnaris*) (Figs 6.55–6.57).
- The flexor digitorum superficialis (*m. flexor digitorum superficialis*):
  — Superficial layer, tendon to the fourth finger (Fig. 6.58)
  — Superficial layer, tendon to the third finger (Fig. 6.59)
  — Deep layer of tendons for the fifth finger and index finger (Fig. 6.60)
  — Distal body of muscle (Fig. 6.61)
  — Tendons in the palm of the hand (Fig. 6.62).
- The flexor pollicis longus (*m. flexor pollicis longus*) (Figs 6.63 and 6.64).

Actions

The flexor pollicis longus:

- Flexes the distal phalanx of the thumb on the proximal one.

- Helps flex the proximal (first) phalanx of the thumb on the first metacarpal.
- Helps oppose the thumb to the other fingers, and in the various grasping actions of the hand.

The flexor digitorum profundus:

- Acts on the last four fingers to:
  — Flex the distal (third) phalanges on the middle (second) ones
  — Help flex the middle phalanges on the proximal (first) ones
  — Help flex the proximal phalanges on the metacarpals.
- Helps to flex the wrist.
- Helps oppose the thumb to the other fingers, and in the various grasping actions of the hand.

The flexor digitorum superficialis:

- Acts on the first four fingers to:
  — Flex the middle phalanges on the proximal ones
  — Help flex the proximal phalanges on the metacarpals.
- Helps oppose the thumb to the other fingers, and in the various grasping actions of the hand.

The flexor carpi ulnaris:

- Helps flex the wrist on the forearm and incline it on the ulnar side.

The flexor carpi radialis:

- Flexes the wrist and abducts it (inclines it on the radial side).
- Assists pronation of the forearm on the arm.

The pronator teres:

- Pronates and flexes the forearm on the arm. (In normal use, pronation is usually associated with abduction and medial rotation of the shoulder.)

The pronator quadratus:

- Pronates and flexes the forearm on the arm.
  The palmaris longus:
- Flexes the wrist on the forearm.

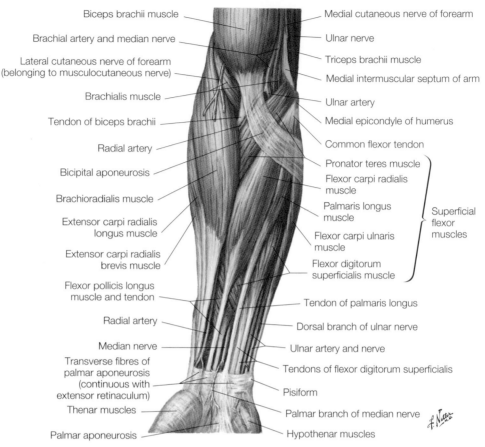

Biceps brachii muscle

Brachial artery and median nerve

Lateral cutaneous nerve of forearm
(belonging to musculocutaneous nerve)

Brachialis muscle

Tendon of biceps brachii

Radial artery

Bicipital aponeurosis

Brachioradialis muscle

Extensor carpi radialis
longus muscle

Extensor carpi radialis
brevis muscle

Flexor pollicis longus
muscle and tendon

Radial artery

Median nerve

Transverse fibres of
palmar aponeurosis
(continuous with
extensor retinaculum)

Thenar muscles

Palmar aponeurosis

Medial cutaneous nerve of forearm

Ulnar nerve

Triceps brachii muscle

Medial intermuscular septum of arm

Ulnar artery

Medial epicondyle of humerus

Common flexor tendon

Pronator teres muscle

Flexor carpi radialis
muscle

Palmaris longus
muscle

Flexor carpi ulnaris
muscle

Flexor digitorum
superficialis muscle

Tendon of palmaris longus

Dorsal branch of ulnar nerve

Ulnar artery and nerve

Tendons of flexor digitorum superficialis

Pisiform

Palmar branch of median nerve

Hypothenar muscles

Superficial
flexor
muscles

Muscles of the forearm (superficial layer): anterior view

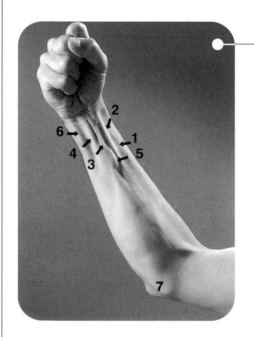

Fig. 6.45 | **Anterior view of the forearm**

1. Flexor pollicis longus (*m. flexor pollicis longus*).
2. Flexor carpi radialis (*m. flexor carpi radialis*).
3. Palmaris longus (*m. palmaris longus*).

Flexor digitorum superficialis (*m. flexor digitorum superficialis*):

4. Tendon to the fourth finger.
5. Body of muscle.
6. Flexor carpi ulnaris (*m. flexor carpi ulnaris*).
7. Common tendon of origin of the medial epicondylar muscles (forearm flexors).

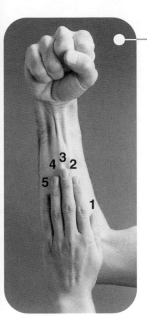

Fig. 6.46 | **The medial epicondylar muscles (forearm flexors)**

The subject's elbow should be flexed, with the wrist in a neutral position or slightly flexed. The fist should be clenched in a neutral position, neither pronated nor supinated. Place your hand, fingers together, against the medial part of the elbow, with your thenar eminence resting on the medial epicondyle. The position of the practitioner's hand as shown here is as follows:

1. Thumb corresponding to the direction of the pronator teres muscle.
2. Index finger in line with the flexor carpi radialis.
3. Middle finger in line with the palmaris longus.
4. Ring finger in line with the flexor digitorum superficialis (tendon going to the fourth finger).
5. Little finger in line with the flexor carpi ulnaris.

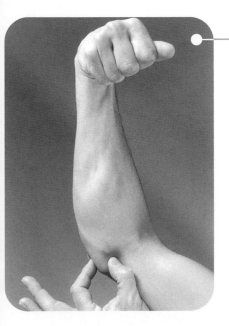

Fig. 6.47 | **The common tendon of origin of the medial epicondylar muscles (forearm flexors) (*caput commune musculorum flexorum*)**

Place a thumb-and-finger contact on the subject's medial epicondyle, and ask him to flex his wrist at the same time as inclining it to the ulnar side. You will feel the common tendon contracting beneath your fingers.

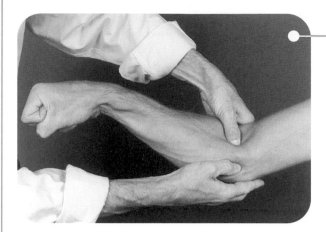

Fig. 6.48 | The body of the pronator teres (*m. pronator teres*)

Position your contact just inside the tendon of the biceps brachii (see Fig. 4.6). Then ask the subject to pronate the forearm with fist clenched. You will sense the body of this muscle tensing beneath your fingers.

Attachments
The pronator teres consists of two heads: the humeral and the ulnar head.

- The humeral head arises on the medial epicondyle of the humerus and on the antebrachial fascia.
- The ulnar head arises on the coronoid process of the ulna.
- The two heads join and the muscle is inserted via a short tendon on the middle third of the lateral surface of the radius.

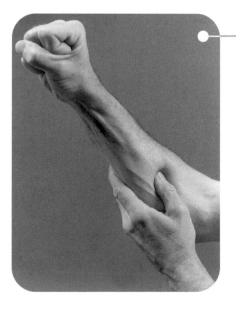

Fig. 6.49 | The distal part of the pronator teres

Once you have located the body of the muscle (Fig. 6.48), follow it along its oblique course, downward and outward to its insertion on the middle third of the lateral surface of the radius. Ask the subject to pronate the forearm with fist clenched. This will help you locate the muscle.

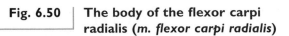
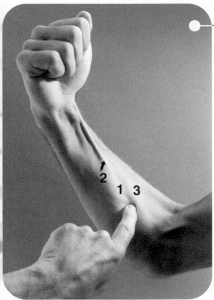

Fig. 6.50 | **The body of the flexor carpi radialis (*m. flexor carpi radialis*)**

Ask the subject to flex the wrist, at the same time inclining it radially. You will detect the body of the muscle (1) in continuity with the tendon (2) and medial to the pronator teres (3) (Fig. 6.49).

Attachments
- The flexor carpi radialis arises via a tendon on the anterior surface of the medial epicondyle of the humerus and of the antebrachial fascia.
- It crosses the lateral part of the carpal tunnel and is inserted on the palmar base of the second metacarpal.

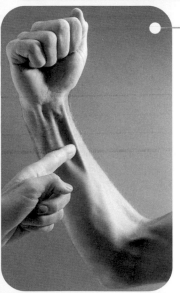

Fig. 6.51 | **The tendon of the flexor carpi radialis**

Ask the subject to perform the same action as that described above. The tendon of the flexor carpi radialis is the most lateral of the tendons that can be seen in the inferior third of the anterior surface of the forearm.

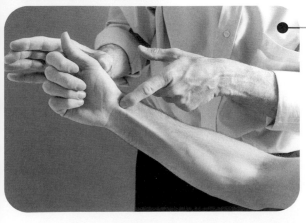

Fig. 6.52 | **The distal tendon of the flexor carpi radialis**

Ask the subject to flex the wrist slightly, at the same time inclining it to the radial side. In the adjacent figure the practitioner is resisting the radial inclination.

Note: The tendon is inserted on the anterior surface of the base of the second metacarpal, and sometimes also that of the third metacarpal.

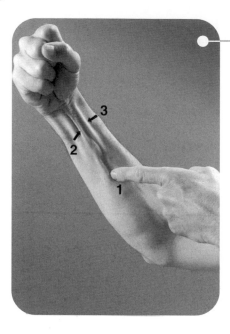

Fig. 6.53 | **The body of the palmaris longus (*m. palmaris longus*)**

Ask the subject to flex the wrist. You will detect the body of the muscle (1) in continuity with the tendon (2) and medial to the flexor carpi radialis (3), as shown here by the practitioner's index finger. This muscle is inconstant.

Attachments
- The palmaris longus arises on the anterior surface of the medial epicondyle of the humerus and on the antebrachial fascia.
- It is inserted via a tendon at the wrist:
  — Median fibers: on the flexor retinaculum and middle palmar fascia
  — Lateral fibers: on the thenar eminence
  — Medial fibers: on the hypothenar eminence.

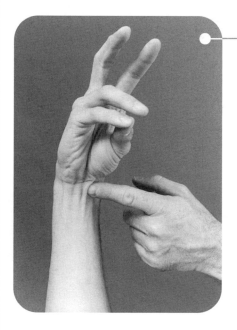

Fig. 6.54 | **The tendon of the palmaris longus**

Ask the subject to oppose the thumb to the little finger. This will make the tendon of the palmaris longus more prominent. It is a long tendon occupying approximately the inferior two-thirds of the anterior surface of the forearm.

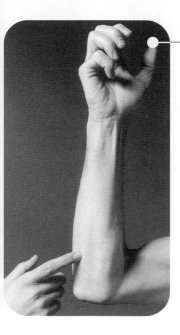

Fig. 6.55 | **The proximal part of the flexor carpi ulnaris (*m. flexor carpi ulnaris*)**

Ask the subject to flex the wrist and incline it on the ulnar side. You will detect the body of the muscle close to the ulna, medial to the palmaris longus.

Note: It is very difficult to distinguish the bodies of the medial epicondylar muscles (forearm flexors) on the proximal part of the forearm.

Attachments
- The flexor carpi ulnaris arises by two heads:
  — One on the medial epicondyle of the humerus (humeral head)
  — One on the medial border of the olecranon and the superior two-thirds of the posterior border of the ulna (ulnar head).
- The tendon is inserted on the anterior surface of the pisiform bone, by means of expansions on the hook of the hamate.

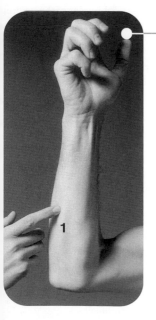

Fig. 6.56 | **The flexor carpi ulnaris**

The two heads of this muscle (described above) unite into a single muscle body (1) running down the medial surface of the forearm to the distal tendon (see Fig. 6.57).

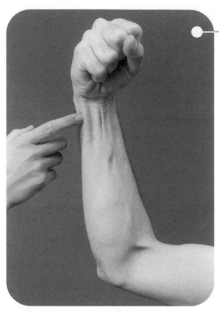

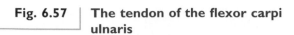

Fig. 6.57 | **The tendon of the flexor carpi ulnaris**

This tendon is the most medial of the tendons visible on the anterior surface of the forearm. The action required to make the tendon more prominent is the same as that described for Figure 6.55.

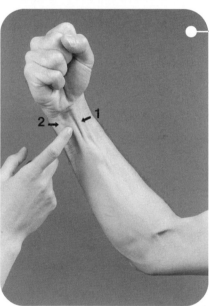

Fig. 6.58 | **The flexor digitorum superficialis (*m. flexor digitorum superficialis*) Superficial layer, tendon to the fourth finger**

In the adjacent figure, the practitioner's index finger indicates the tendon going to the fourth finger. It lies medial to (on the ulnar side of) the tendon of the palmaris longus (1). The practitioner's index finger is against the radial border of the tendon of the flexor carpi ulnaris (2). Ask the subject to clench the fist and flex the wrist quickly and repeatedly. (See also Fig. 7.66.)

Note: The tendons to the fourth finger and to the third finger belong to the anterior (superficial) layer of the flexor digitorum superficialis.

Attachments

The flexor digitorum superficialis consists of two heads: the humero-ulnar and the radial head.

- The humero-ulnar head arises from the medial epicondyle of the humerus and on the coronoid process of the ulna.
- The radial head arises from the superior half of the anterior border of the radius.

Muscle fibers arise from a muscular arch between these two heads, and are arranged in two layers:

- A superficial humero-ulnar layer (or head) runs to the third and fourth fingers.
- A deep radial layer (or head), which sometimes has two bellies, runs to the second and fifth fingers.

The four tendons from the body of the muscle pass through the carpal tunnel and are inserted on the palmar surface of the middle phalanx.

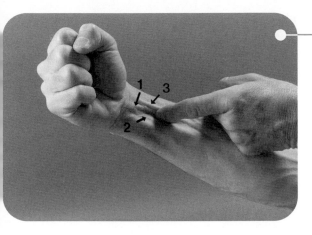

Fig. 6.59 | **The flexor digitorum superficialis Superficial layer, tendon to the third finger**

The adjacent figure shows the practitioner's index finger pushing aside the tendon of the palmaris longus (1) laterally (to the radial side) to contact the tendon of the flexor digitorum to the third finger (2). This lies on the radial border of the tendon of the flexor superficialis going to the fourth finger. Ask the subject to oppose thumb and middle finger (this action is not shown here) and to flex the wrist briefly and repeatedly. This will display the tendon more clearly beneath your fingers. Another method is to ask the subject to clench the fist and flex the wrist briefly and repeatedly, at the same time inclining it slightly to the ulnar side. (See also Fig. 7.67.) The tendon of the flexor carpi radialis (3) is also shown.

Note: This tendon and the one to the fourth finger belong to the anterior (superficial) layer of the flexor digitorum superficialis.

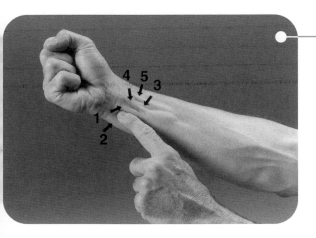

Fig. 6.60 | **The flexor digitorum superficialis Deep layer, tendons to the fifth finger and index finger**

— The tendon to the fifth finger. In the adjacent figure, the practitioner's index finger rests on the ulnar border of the tendon going to the fourth finger (1) in order to make contact with the tendon to the fifth finger. This lies between the tendon of the flexor carpi ulnaris (2) medially (on the ulnar side) and the tendon to the fourth finger (1) (already mentioned above) laterally (on the radial side). Ask the subject to oppose thumb and fifth finger while slightly flexing the wrist. This will display the tightening of the tendon more clearly. (See also Fig. 7.68.)

— The tendon to the index finger. In the adjacent figure, the tendon to the index finger (3) can also be seen between the tendon of the palmaris longus (4) medially and the tendon of the flexor carpi radialis (5) laterally. Ask the subject to oppose thumb and second finger while slightly flexing the wrist, to display this tendon more clearly. (See also Fig. 7.69.)

Note: The tendons described above belong to the posterior (deep) layer of the flexor digitorum superficialis.

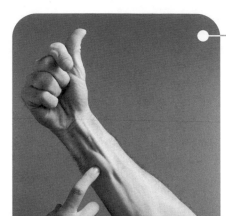

Fig. 6.61 | The distal body of the flexor digitorum superficialis

In the adjacent figure, the practitioner's index finger indicates one belly of the deep (posterior) layer of the flexor digitorum superficialis. This layer contains the tendons to the index and little fingers. The superficial (anterior) layer contains the tendons to the ring finger and middle finger. This belly of the muscle can be displayed more clearly if you ask the subject to clench the fist firmly and at the same time flex the wrist slightly, and to flex the index finger briefly and repeatedly.

Note: This muscle layer cannot be accessed in all subjects.

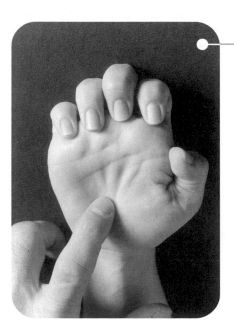

Fig. 6.62 | The tendons of the flexor digitorum superficialis in the palm of the hand

The tendons are clearly visible on the palm of the subject's hand in the adjacent figure. Ask the subject to hyperextend the metacarpophalangeal joints and at the same time to flex the middle and distal (second and third) phalanges. Even if the tendons cannot be detected visually as they can here, they are clearly evident to palpation.

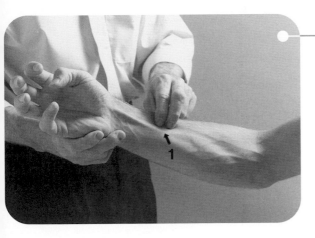

Fig. 6.63 | **The body of the flexor pollicis longus (*m. flexor pollicis longus*)**

Place your contact, using one or two fingers, lateral to the flexor carpi radialis (1) (Fig. 6.51). Ask the subject to execute repeated contractions of the distal phalanx of the thumb on the proximal one. You can feel the contraction beneath your fingers.

Attachments

- The flexor pollicis longus arises on the superior three-quarters of the anterior surface of the radius and on the interosseous membrane of the forearm.
- It is inserted on the palmar surface of the base of the distal phalanx of the thumb.

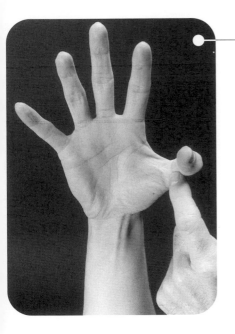

Fig. 6.64 | **The tendon of the flexor pollicis longus (*m. flexor pollicis longus*)**

This tendon can be clearly detected on the palmar surface of the proximal phalanx of the thumb if you ask the subject to flex the distal phalanx on the first quickly and repeatedly.

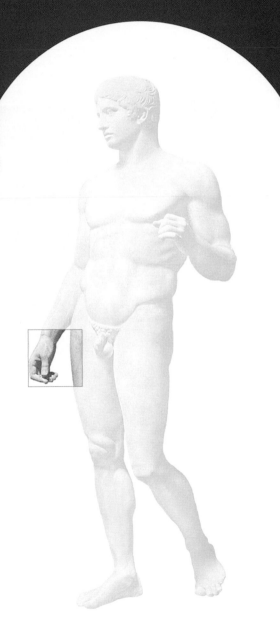

CHAPTER 7

THE WRIST
AND HAND

TOPOGRAPHICAL PRESENTATION OF THE WRIST AND HAND

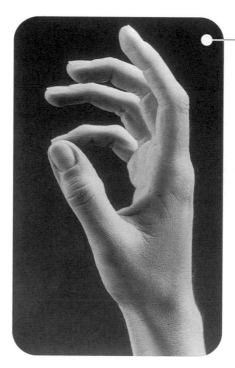

Fig. 7.1

Overall presentation of the hand

OSTEOLOGY

BONES OF THE WRIST JOINT AND HAND AND CARPAL BONES

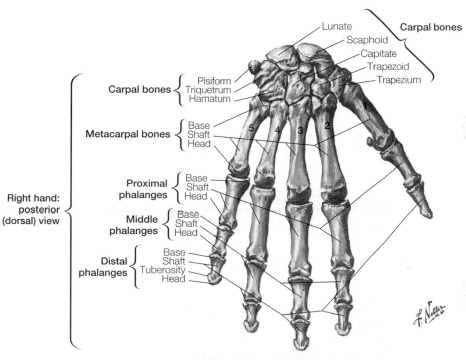

Carpal bones

Lunate
Scaphoid
Capitate
Trapezoid
Trapezium

Carpal bones {
Pisiform
Triquetrum
Hamatum

Metacarpal bones {
Base
Shaft
Head

Right hand: posterior (dorsal) view

Proximal phalanges {
Base
Shaft
Head

Middle phalanges {
Base
Shaft
Head

Distal phalanges {
Base
Shaft
Tuberosity
Head

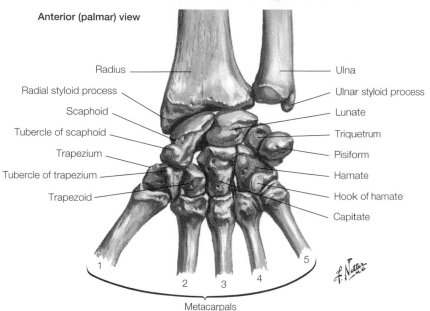

Anterior (palmar) view

Radius
Radial styloid process
Scaphoid
Tubercle of scaphoid
Trapezium
Tubercle of trapezium
Trapezoid

Ulna
Ulnar styloid process
Lunate
Triquetrum
Pisiform
Hamate
Hook of hamate
Capitate

Metacarpals

THE INFERIOR EXTREMITY OF THE TWO BONES OF THE FOREARM

The notable structures that can be detected by palpation are:

- The head (inferior extremity) of the ulna (*caput ulnae*) (Fig. 7.2); ulnar styloid process (*processus styloideus ulnae*) (Fig. 7.3).
- The inferior extremity of the radius (Fig. 7.4); medial (ulnar) border (Fig. 7.5); lateral surface and radial styloid process (*processus styloideus radii*) (Fig. 7.6).
- The dorsal tubercle of the radius (*tuberculum dorsale*): posterior view (Fig. 7.7).

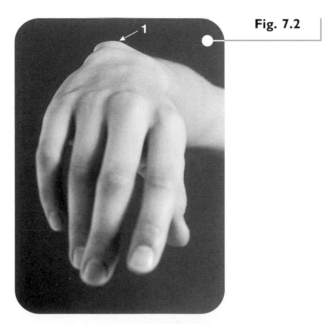

Fig. 7.2

The head (inferior extremity) of the ulna (*caput ulnae*)

This figure simply shows the position of the head of the ulna (1). It feels like a bulge beneath your fingers, overhanging the medial part of the proximal row of carpal bones. The inferior extremity of the ulna is cylindrical, formed of two raised features separated by a groove. These are the styloid process (Fig. 7.3) and a lateral prominence which articulates with the ulnar notch of the radius.

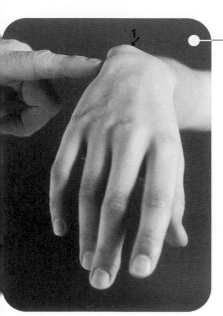

Fig. 7.3 | **The head (inferior extremity) of the ulna and ulnar styloid process (*processus styloideus ulnae*)**

On the inferior extremity of the ulna (1) is the styloid process, a protuberance that is easy to access using a pincer contact with thumb and finger. The styloid process is indicated here by the practitioner's index finger. It is separated from the lateral surface, which articulates with the ulnar notch of the radius, by a sagittal groove, through which the tendon of the extensor carpi ulnaris passes.

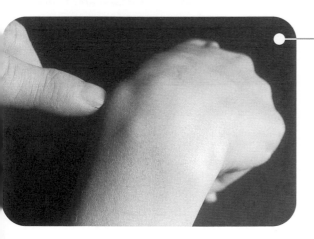

Fig. 7.4 | **The inferior extremity of the radius**

This figure shows the location of the inferior extremity of the radius; it overhangs the lateral part of the proximal row of carpal bones, as well as articulating with them. The inferior surface of the inferior extremity articulates laterally with the scaphoid and medially with the lunate.

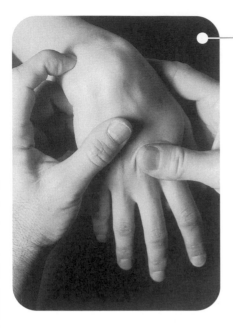

Fig. 7.5 | **The inferior extremity of the radius**
The medial (ulnar) border

The ulnar notch (*incisura ulnaris*) is situated at this border. It is a concave surface that articulates with the head of the ulna. The subject's wrist is in a neutral position. Place your index finger on the posterior surface of the head of the ulna, facing the distal end of the radius. Ask the subject to flex the wrist. The medial border will 'appear' beneath your finger.

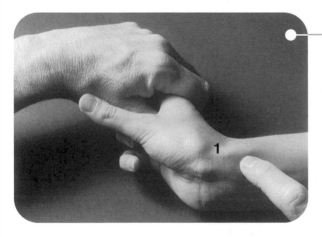

Fig. 7.6 | **The inferior extremity of the radius**
The lateral surface and radial styloid process (*processus styloideus radii*)

The practitioner's index finger indicates the lateral surface; across this run two vertical grooves. The tendons of the abductor pollicis longus and extensor pollicis brevis pass through the anterior groove, and the tendons of the extensor carpi radialis longus and brevis through the posterior one. Distally, the lateral surface terminates in the radial styloid process (1).

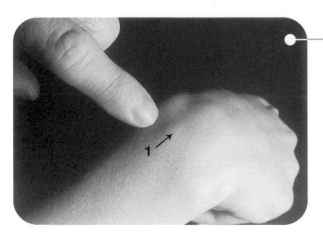

Fig. 7.7 | **The dorsal tubercle of the radius (*tuberculum dorsale*)**
Posterior view

This tubercle is an important landmark on the posterior part of the wrist. It separates two grooves; the tendon of the extensor pollicis longus passes through the lateral groove, and the tendons of the extensor digitorum and extensor indicis through the medial groove. The dorsal tubercle (1) is situated in the middle of the posterior surface of the inferior extremity of the radius. Its medial limit is marked by the ulnar border of the radius (see Fig. 7.5).

THE CARPAL BONES OF THE PROXIMAL ROW

The notable structures that can be detected by palpation are:

- The anatomical snuffbox (Fig. 7.9).
- The scaphoid (*os scaphoideum*) (Figs 7.10–7.17); the tubercle of the scaphoid (*tuberculum ossis scaphoidei*) (Fig. 7.14).
- The lunate (*os lunatum*) (Figs 7.18–7.20).
- The triquetrum (*os triquetrum*) (Figs 7.21–7.23).
- The pisiform (*os pisiforme*) (Figs 7.24 and 7.25).

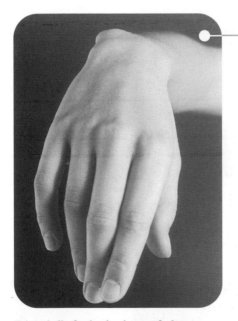

Fig. 7.8

Distal (inferior) view of the proximal row of the carpal bones

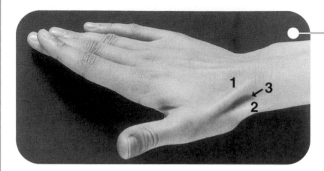
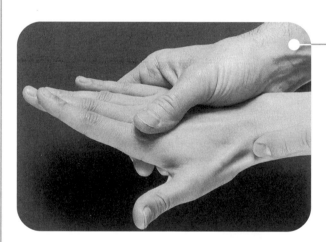

Fig. 7.9 | **The anatomical snuffbox**

The tendons of the extensor pollicis longus (1) and extensor pollicis brevis (2) gradually separate from each other in the region of the wrist, creating a triangular space with its base positioned proximally and its tip distally. This is called the anatomical snuffbox. The scaphoid (proximally) and the trapezium (distally) lie in the floor (3) of the snuffbox. The tendon of the abductor pollicis longus, which lies against that of the extensor pollicis brevis anteriorly, also forms part of the snuffbox. (See also Figs 7.72–7.74.)

Fig. 7.10 | **The scaphoid (os scaphoideum)**
Lateral approach
Step 1

The subject's hand is in a neutral position. Once you have located the anatomical snuffbox, the depression between the extensor tendons of the thumb (Fig. 7.9), slide your index finger down into the base of it. The figure alongside shows the practitioner's index finger in a contact that sits between the radial styloid process (Fig. 7.6) and the scaphoid.

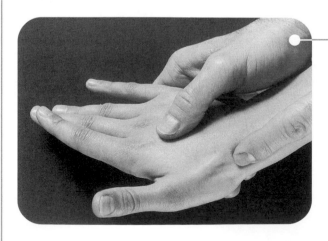

Fig. 7.11 | **The scaphoid**
Lateral approach
Step 2

Following the step shown in Figure 7.10, direct your index finger distally farther into the snuffbox (Fig. 7.9). With your other hand, incline the subject's hand in the ulnar direction. The lateral surface of the scaphoid will come into contact with your index finger.

Note: A groove runs across this surface of the scaphoid; the radial artery passes through it.

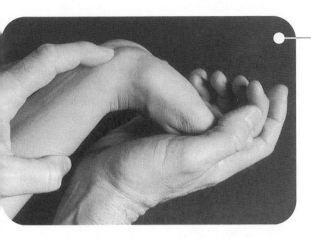

Fig. 7.12 | The scaphoid
Anterior approach

Place the subject's wrist in extension, as shown in the adjacent figure. This helps to 'disengage' the anterior (palmar) surface of the scaphoid. You should feel a convexity (a bulge) beneath your fingers. This indicates that you have contacted the scaphoid.

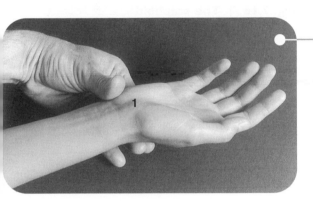

Fig. 7.13 | The scaphoid
Alternative anterior approach

Place the interphalangeal joint of your thumb on the radial part of the pisiform (Fig. 7.25), in line with the first cutaneous palmar fold. Flex your interphalangeal joint; your thumb will come into contact with the palmar surface of the scaphoid (1).

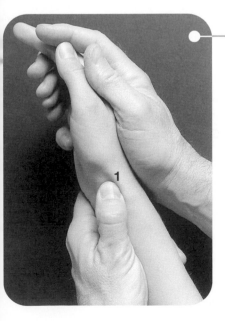

Fig. 7.14 | The tubercle of the scaphoid
(*tuberculum ossis scaphoidei*)

In the adjacent figure, the practitioner's left thumb is contacting the tubercle of the scaphoid, which is a lateral extension of the anterior (palmar) surface of the scaphoid.

In order to find and palpate this tubercle, position your contact on the anterior part of the tendon of the abductor pollicis longus (1). This is made easier if the subject's wrist is repeatedly inclined in the ulnar direction.

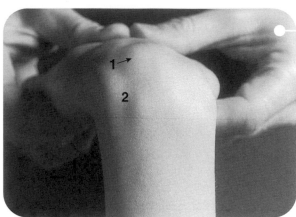

Fig. 7.15 | **The scaphoid**
Posterior approach
Step 1

Topographical location: To locate the dorsal surface of the scaphoid (1), begin from the lateral side of the inferior extremity of the radius (2) and extend this line distally.

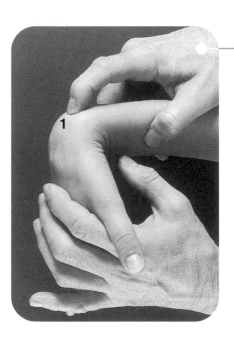

Fig. 7.16 | **The scaphoid**
Posterior approach
Step 2

Rest your index finger on the joint space of the subject's wrist. With your other hand, draw the subject's hand into palmar flexion. The dorsal surface of the scaphoid can be detected as a convex feature (1) below the joint space of the wrist.

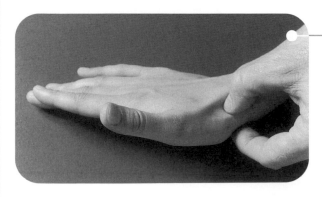

Fig. 7.17 | **The scaphoid**
Global approach

The adjacent figure shows an overall approach to the scaphoid. Use a pincer contact with your thumb and index finger to take hold of the palmar and lateral surfaces of the scaphoid. See Figures 7.12–7.14 for the location of the palmar surface. The practitioner's thumb is resting on the lateral surface in this photograph. It forms the floor of the anatomical snuffbox (see Figs 7.9–7.11).

Note: An alternative method for the global approach is to take hold of the palmar and dorsal surfaces between thumb and index finger.

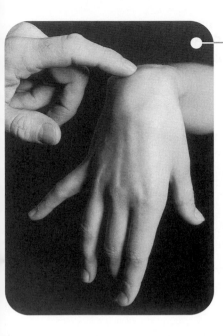

Fig. 7.18 | **The lunate (*os lunatum*)**
Topographical visualization

In the adjacent figure, the practitioner's index finger indicates the lunate. It can be made more prominent if you ask the subject to flex the hand. This 'disengages' the carpal articular surface (*facies articularis carpalis radii*) at the inferior extremity of the radius.

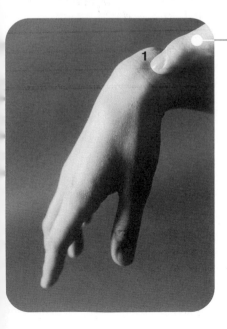

Fig. 7.19 | **The lunate**
Method 1
Proximal approach

The first step is to locate the dorsal tubercle of the radius (see Fig. 7.7). Then place your index finger on the medial (ulnar) side of the tubercle, on the wrist joint and pointing toward the fifth metacarpal. Ask the subject to flex the wrist in the palmar direction, and the lunate (1) will present itself to your contact.

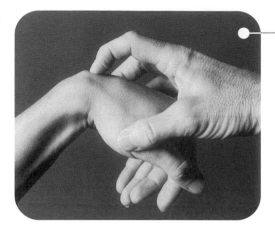

Fig. 7.20 **The lunate**
Method 2
Distal approach

Begin by locating the capitate (Figs 7.36–43). Place your index finger in the depression belonging to the body of the capitate and situated just above the base of the third metacarpal. Then slide your finger over the bulge of the head of the capitate, toward the distal extremity of the radius, between the tendon of the extensor digitorum medially (on the ulnar side) and, laterally (on the radial side), a hypothetical line extending distally from the dorsal tubercle of the radius (Fig. 7.7). When the subject's wrist is flexed, the lunate can be detected between the head of the capitate and the posterior border of the radius (toward the ulnar side).

Note:
— *If you slide the pad of your finger too far laterally (to the radial side), you will contact the dorsal surface of the scaphoid (see Figs 7.15 and 7.16).*
— *If you do not slide the pad of your finger far enough toward the radius, you will contact the head of the capitate (see Fig. 7.41).*

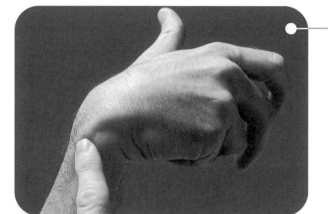

Fig. 7.21 **The triquetrum (*os triquetrum*)**
Step 1

Ask the subject to place the hand in palmar flexion and supinate the forearm. The practitioner's index finger indicates the ulnar styloid process (Fig. 7.3), the most distal bony prominence on the medial border of the wrist.

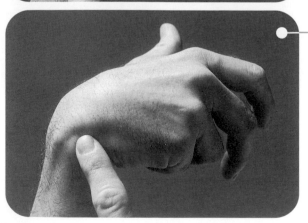

Fig. 7.22 **The triquetrum**
Step 2

The position of the subject's forearm and hand is the same as that described above. Here, the practitioner's index finger indicates the triquetrum, which is the first bony prominence you encounter on the medial border of the wrist, distal to the ulnar styloid process.

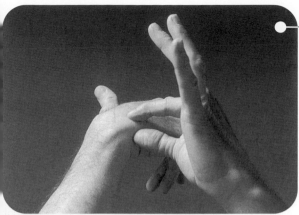

Fig. 7.23 | **The triquetrum**
Global approach

Once you have located the two bony structures described in Figures 7.21 and 7.22, take an overall hold of the triquetrum. The practitioner's thumb is on the medial (ulnar) surface of the triquetrum and his index finger on the dorsal surface.

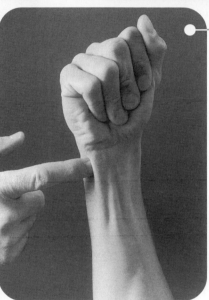

Fig. 7.24 | **The pisiform (*os pisiforme*)**

In the adjacent figure, the practitioner's index finger indicates the tendon of the flexor carpi ulnaris (Fig. 7.70), which is important for locating the pisiform because the tendon is inserted on the anterior surface of the bone. An additional guide to location is the fact that the pisiform is situated at the base of the hypothenar eminence (Fig. 7.83).

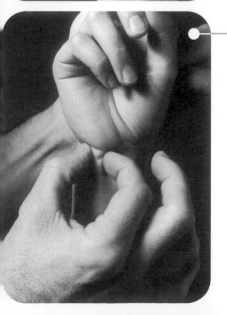

Fig. 7.25 | **The pisiform**

The posterior surface of the pisiform articulates with the triquetrum (Figs 7.21–7.23). Its anterior surface can be felt as a prominence under the skin. In the adjacent figure, the practitioner has taken hold of the pisiform between thumb and index finger.

Note: The subject's wrist should be allowed to fall naturally into a position of palmar flexion. This relaxes the tendon of the flexor carpi ulnaris, and makes the pisiform easier to mobilize and examine.

THE CARPAL BONES OF THE DISTAL ROW

The notable structures that can be detected by palpation are:

- The trapezium (*os trapezium*) (Figs 7.27–7.29).
- The tubercle of the trapezium (*tuberculum ossis trapezii*) (Figs 7.30–7.32).
- The trapezoid (*os trapezoideum*) (Figs 7.33–7.35).
- The capitate (*os capitatum*) (Figs 7.36–7.43).
- The hamate (*os hamatum*) (Figs 7.44–7.45).
- The hook of the hamate (*hamulus ossis hamati*) (Figs 7.46–7.48).

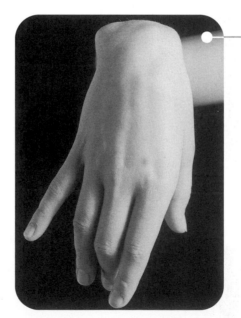

Fig. 7.26

Topographical localization of the distal row of the carpal bones

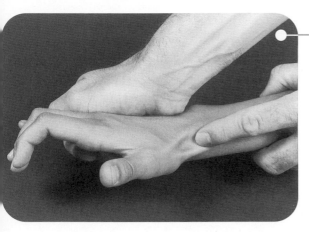

Fig. 7.27 | **The trapezium (*os trapezium*)**
Step 1: Localization of the
anatomical snuffbox

Begin by locating the anatomical snuffbox (Fig. 7.9). Place your finger into the snuffbox, the floor of which is formed by the scaphoid.

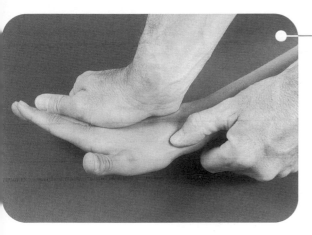

Fig. 7.28 | **The trapezium**
Step 2

Following the step shown in Figure 7.27, shift your thumb distally until you contact the base of the first metacarpal. You will detect the trapezium beneath your thumb.

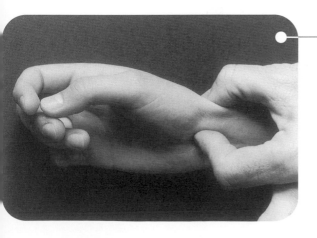

Fig. 7.29 | **The trapezium**
Global approach

In the adjacent figure, the practitioner has taken hold of the trapezium as a whole, between the thumb and index finger. Position your contact just above the base of the first metacarpal. Ask the subject to mobilize the first metacarpal; this will help confirm that you have made contact with the trapezium, as it remains immobile when the metacarpal is moved.

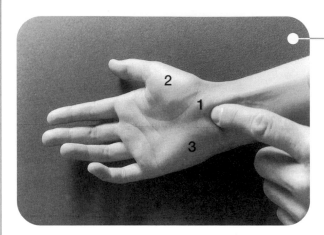

Fig. 7.30 | **The tubercle of the trapezium (*tuberculum ossis trapezii*) Step 1**

Begin by locating the scaphoid (1) (see also Figs 7.12 and 7.13), and the space between the thenar (2) and hypothenar (3) eminences at the fold created by the flexion of the wrist. The practitioner's index finger indicates the convexity on the anterior surface of the wrist created by the scaphoid.

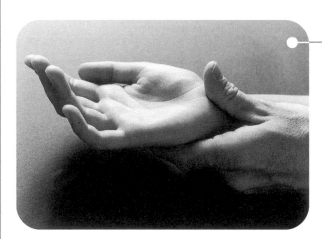

Fig. 7.31 | **The tubercle of the trapezium Step 2**

Place the interphalangeal joint of your thumb between the thenar and hypothenar eminences on the anterior part of the subject's wrist (Fig. 7.30), in contact with the scaphoid, and with your thumb in line with the column of the subject's thumb, as shown.

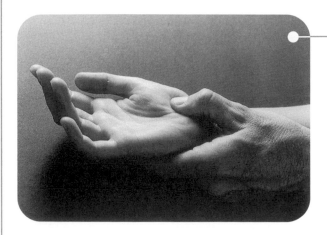

Fig. 7.32 | **The tubercle of the trapezium Step 3**

Once you have completed steps 1 and 2 (Figs 7.30 and 7.31), set down your thumb in line with the column of the subject's thumb, just above the base of the first metacarpal. The tubercle of the trapezium is directly beneath the pad of your thumb.

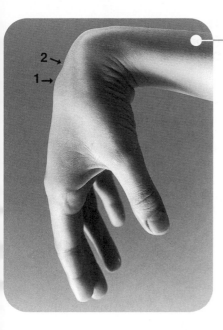

Fig. 7.33 | **The trapezoid (*os trapezoideum*)
Topographical location**

The adjacent figure shows the location of the base of the second metacarpal (1) and of the trapezoid (2) on the back of the hand.

Note: These two structures on the dorsal surface of the hand should not be confused. The bony prominence is the base of the second metacarpal; the dorsal surface of the trapezoid is recessed.

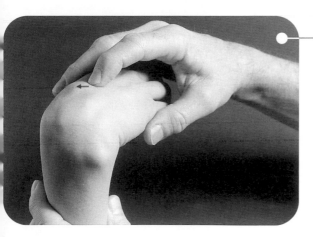

Fig. 7.34 | **The trapezoid
Step 1**

Place your index finger as shown in the adjacent figure (←) — flat against the base of the second metacarpal, the bony prominence indicated above.

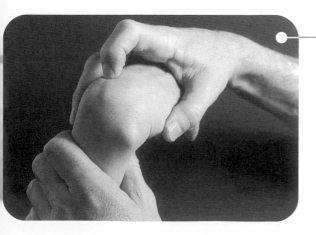

Fig. 7.35 | **The trapezoid
Step 2**

From the position shown in Figure 7.34, slide your index finger into the depression that lies proximal to it, slipping your contact in between the tendons of the extensor carpi radialis longus and extensor carpi radialis brevis (see Figs 7.76 and 7.77).

Note: Contact with the dorsal surface of the trapezoid is not always easy to achieve, because the bone is set back considerably relative to the base of the second metacarpal.

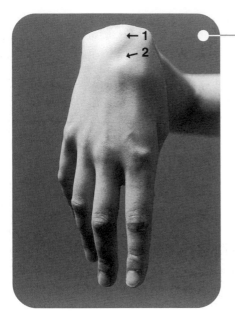

Fig. 7.36 | **The capitate (*os capitatum*)**
Form and location
Dorsal view

This is the largest of the bones of the wrist (also known as *os magnum*, the large bone), and its main axis lies in line with that of the hand. It consists of an enlarged, rounded superior part or head (1), an inferior part or body (2), and a transitional region between them, the neck.

Note: Proximally, the capitate fits in beneath the scaphoid and the lunate. Distally, it lies opposite the articular surfaces of the second, third, and fourth metacarpals. Its lateral (radial) surface articulates with the scaphoid superiorly and with the trapezoid inferiorly. Its medial (ulnar) surface articulates with the hamate.

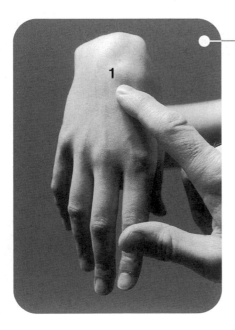

Fig. 7.37 | **The capitate**
Step 1
Dorsal view

The first step is to place a contact at the base of the third metacarpal (1). The capitate is situated proximally in line with this bone.

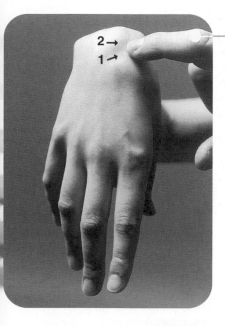

Fig. 7.38 | **The capitate**
Step 2
Dorsal view

Following the step shown in Figure 7.37, slide your index finger along from the base of the third metacarpal in the proximal direction. You will find a depression (1) just beyond it, belonging to the body of the capitate. The rounded feature (2) beyond that, rising above the depression, is the head of the capitate. (See also Figs 7.39–7.41.)

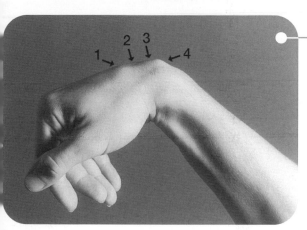

Fig. 7.39 | **Visualization of the notable**
features of the capitate
Lateral aspect

In this profile view, the base of the third metacarpal (1), the depression in the capitate (2), the head of the capitate (3), and the lunate (4) can all be clearly distinguished. The lunate becomes accessible if you flex the subject's wrist.

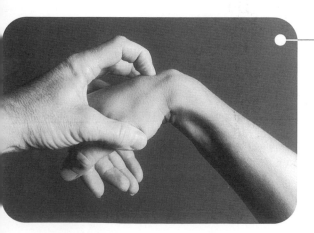

Fig. 7.40 | **The depression on the dorsal**
surface of the capitate
Lateral aspect

Place your index finger in the depression that lies in line with the base of the third metacarpal, on the radial side of the tendon of the extensor digitorum.

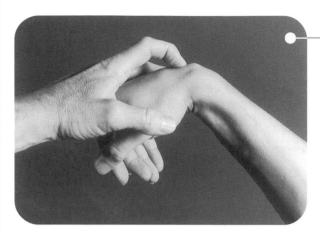

Fig. 7.41 | The head of the capitate
Lateral aspect

Once you have located the depression as described above (Fig. 7.40), shift your index finger proximally (but without sliding it over the skin) until you contact a convex structure. This is the head of the capitate.

Note: Do not confuse this structure with the lunate (Figs 7.18–7.20, 7.39, and 7.42).

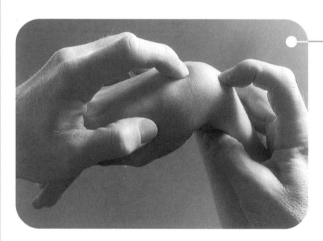

Fig. 7.42 | The capitate and lunate
(*os lunatum*)

The adjacent figure shows a global contact, between the practitioner's index fingers. The practitioner's two index fingers are in contact with the head of the capitate and the more proximally situated lunate. Do not confuse the capitate and the lunate (Figs 7.18–7.20, 7.39, and 7.41).

Note: One of the most commonly found fusions of the carpal bones is that involving the triquetrum and the lunate.

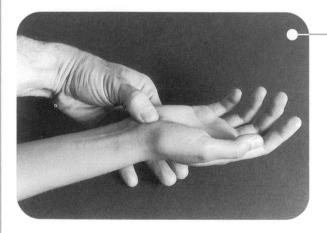

Fig. 7.43 | The capitate
Global approach

Begin by locating the pisiform (Figs 7.24 and 7.25). Then place the interphalangeal joint of your thumb on the pisiform, with your thumb pointing transversely, following the direction of the first palmar fold. Your index finger should rest on the back of the subject's hand, in the depression of the capitate (Figs 7.38–7.40), which is in line with the base of the third metacarpal (Fig. 7.37). Now flex the interphalangeal joint of your thumb. This contact provides an overall approach to the capitate.

Fig. 7.44 | **The hamate (*os hamatum*) Medial approach (i.e. from the ulnar side)**

Begin by locating the ulnar styloid process (1) (see also Fig. 7.3) and triquetrum (2) (see also Figs 7.21–7.23). Next, position your index finger on the medial surface of the hamate, between the base of the fifth metacarpal (3) and the triquetrum (2).

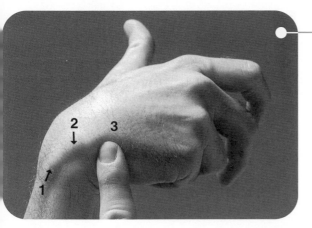

Fig. 7.45 | **The hamate Dorsal approach**

Begin with the contact described in Figure 7.44; then slide your index finger on to the dorsal surface of the hamate, between the bases of the fourth and fifth metacarpals (1) and the dorsal surface of the triquetrum (2).

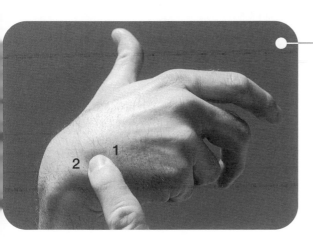

Fig. 7.46 | **The hook of the hamate (*hamulus ossis hamati*) Step 1**

Begin by locating the pisiform (indicated here by the practitioner's index finger), which lies at the base of the hypothenar eminence (1), at the ulnar extremity of the first anterior palmar fold (2). (See also Figs 7.24 and 7.25.)

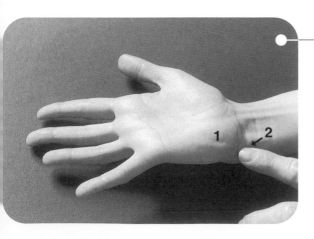

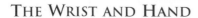

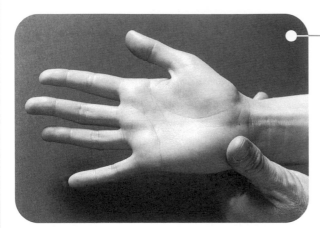

Fig. 7.47 | The hook of the hamate
Step 2

Once you have located the pisiform (Fig. 7.46), place the interphalangeal joint of your thumb on this bone.

Note: As shown here, your thumb should point toward the subject's index finger or the first commissure.

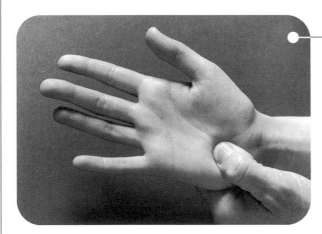

Fig. 7.48 | The hook of the hamate
Step 3

From the thumb position described above (Fig. 7.47), flex the distal phalanx on the proximal one, directing your thumb toward the subject's index finger or the first commissure. You will make contact with a fullness. This is the hook of the hamate.

THE METACARPUS AND PHALANGES

The notable structures that can be detected by palpation are:

- Metacarpals II–V (*ossa metacarpi; ossa metacarpalia II–V*): the heads of the metacarpals (Figs 7.50 and 7.51).
- The first metacarpal (*os metacarpi I*): base (*basis*) (Fig. 7.52), shaft or body (*corpus*) (Fig. 7.53), and head (*caput*) (Fig. 7.54).
- The sesamoid bones (*ossa sesamoidea*) (Fig. 7.55).
- The second metacarpal (*os metacarpi II*) (Fig. 7.56).
- The third metacarpal (*os metacarpi III*) (Fig. 7.57).
- The fourth metacarpal (*os metacarpi IV*) (Fig. 7.58).
- The fifth metacarpal (*os metacarpi V*) (Fig. 7.59).
- The proximal phalanx (*phalanx proximalis*) of the thumb (Fig. 7.60).
- The distal phalanx (*phalanx distalis*) of the thumb (Fig. 7.61).

Fig. 7.49

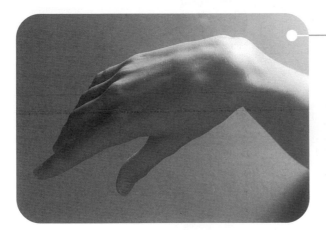

The metacarpals and phalanges: overall radial view

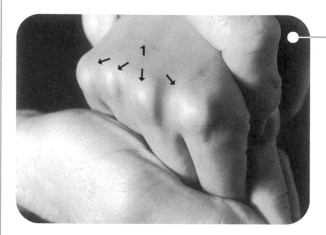

Fig. 7.50 | **Metacarpals II–V (*ossa metacarpi; ossa metacarpalia II–V*) The head (*caput*): dorsal view of heads**

The metacarpus is made up of five bones which articulate proximally with the carpal bones and distally with the proximal phalanges of the fingers. The adjacent figure shows how flexing the fingers at the metacarpophalangeal joints causes the heads of the metacarpals (1) to become prominent.

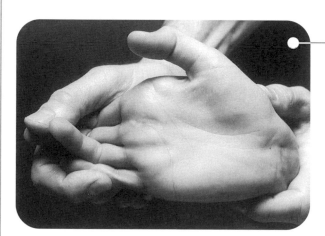

Fig. 7.51 | **The heads of metacarpals II – V Palmar view**

As shown in the adjacent figure, extension of the fingers at the metacarpophalangeal joints causes the palmar part of the heads of the metacarpals to become prominent.

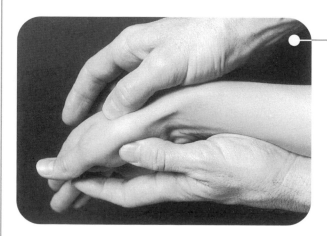

Fig. 7.52 | **The first metacarpal (*os metacarpi I*): base (*basis ossis metacarpi I*)**

The base of the first metacarpal is shaped like a saddle, and articulates only with the trapezium (not with the second metacarpal). Location of the first metacarpal is therefore not only important in its own right, but also when looking for the trapezium (see Figs 7.27–7.29).

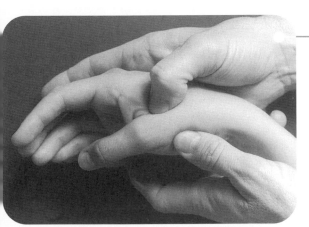

Fig. 7.53 | **The first metacarpal: shaft (body) (*corpus ossis metacarpi I*)**

This is the shortest and thickest of the metacarpals. Between the head (Fig. 7.54) and base (Fig. 7.52) of this bone lies the shaft or body.

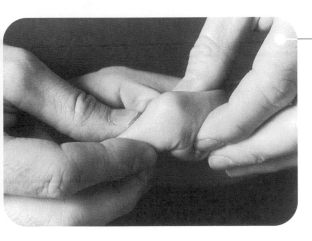

Fig. 7.54 | **The first metacarpal: head (*caput ossis metacarpi I*)**

This articulates with the base of the proximal phalanx. Ask the subject to flex the metacarpophalangeal joint to display the head.

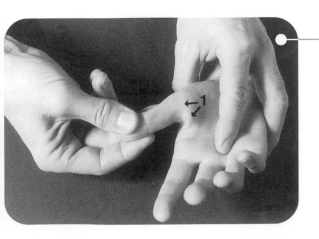

Fig. 7.55 | **The sesamoid bones (*ossa sesamoidea*) of the metacarpophalangeal joint**

Anteriorly, the head of the first metacarpal has two horns separated by a groove. The sesamoids are bony nodules that overlie these horns. There are always two sesamoid bones (1) (lateral and medial) at this joint.

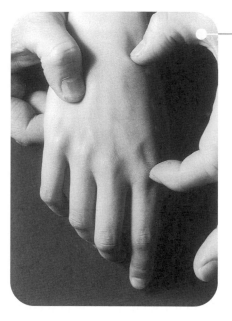

Fig. 7.56 | **The second metacarpal (os metacarpi II)**

This is the longest of the metacarpals. Location of the base of this metacarpal is important when palpating the trapezoid (see Figs 7.33–7.35). In the adjacent figure, the practitioner has taken hold of the second metacarpal; the practitioner's thumb is at the base and his index finger is at the head of the bone.

Note: The base of this bone articulates with the trapezoid, which is received by the center, with the trapezium on the radial side and with the capitate on the ulnar side.

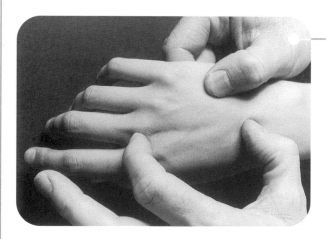

Fig. 7.57 | **The third metacarpal (os metacarpi III)**

The contact used for this bone is the same as that described above. The base of this metacarpal, which lies at the position of the practitioner's thumb in the pincer contact shown here, articulates with the capitate (see Figs 7.36–7.43).

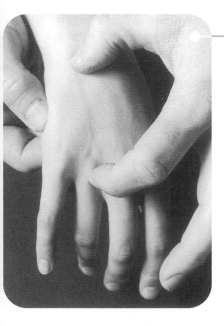

Fig. 7.58 | **The fourth metacarpal (*os metacarpi IV*)**

The contact used for this bone is the same as that described for Figure 7.56. The base of this metacarpal articulates with the capitate (see Figs 7.36–7.43) and with the hamate (see Figs 7.44–7.48).

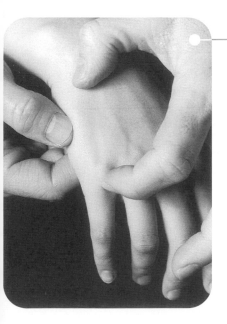

Fig. 7.59 | **The fifth metacarpal (*os metacarpi V*)**

This is the shortest of the metacarpals. The contact used for this bone is the same as that described for Figure 7.56. The base of this metacarpal therefore lies at the position of the practitioner's thumb in the pincer contact shown here. It articulates with the hamate (see Figs 7.44–7.48). The practitioner's index finger is at the head of the fifth metacarpal.

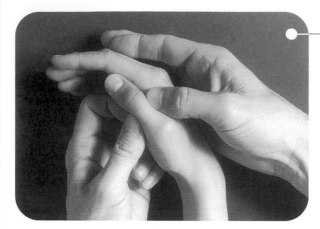

Fig. 7.60 | **The proximal phalanx (*phalanx proximalis*) of the thumb**

The base of this phalanx has a glenoid cavity articulating with the head of the first metacarpal. The head has a trochlea which occupies the palmar and inferior surfaces and articulates with the base of the distal phalanx.

Note: The head of the proximal phalanx of the other fingers articulates with the base of the middle phalanx (phalanx media).

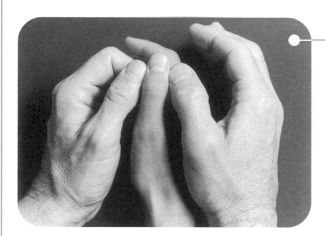

Fig. 7.61 | **The distal phalanx (*phalanx distalis*) of the thumb**

The thumb has only two phalanges, while the other fingers have three.

Note: The middle phalanx of the other fingers is shorter and thinner than the proximal one. The distal phalanx is the smallest of the three.

MYOLOGY

THE TENDONS OF THE ANTERIOR PART OF THE WRIST JOINT

The notable structures that can be detected by palpation are:

- The tendon of the flexor pollicis longus (*m. flexor pollicis longus*) (Fig. 7.63).
- The tendon of the flexor carpi radialis (*m. flexor carpi radialis*) (Fig. 7.64).
- The tendon of the palmaris longus (*m. palmaris longus*) (Fig. 7.65).
- The flexor digitorum superficialis (*m. flexor digitorum superficialis*):
    — The tendon to the fourth finger (Fig. 7.66)
    — The tendon to the third finger (Fig. 7.67)
    — The tendon to the fifth finger (Fig. 7.68)
    — The tendon to the index finger (Fig. 7.69).
- The tendon of the flexor carpi ulnaris (*m. flexor carpi ulnaris*) (Fig. 7.70).

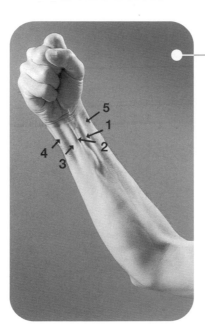

Fig. 7.62

Overall presentation of the tendons on the anterior surface of the wrist

1. The tendon of the flexor carpi radialis.
2. The tendon of the palmaris longus.
3. The flexor digitorum superficialis.
4. The tendon of the flexor carpi ulnaris.
5. Location of the tendon of the flexor pollicis longus.

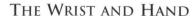
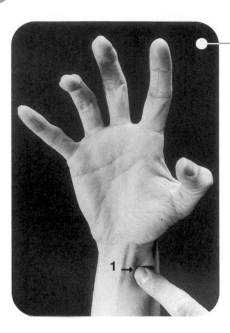

Fig. 7.63 | **The tendon of the flexor pollicis longus (*m. flexor pollicis longus, tendo*)**

Place the pads of one or two fingers just lateral to the tendon of the flexor carpi radialis (1) (Fig. 7.64). Ask the subject to flex the distal phalanx of the thumb briefly and repeatedly. You will sense the tendon of this muscle beneath your contact.

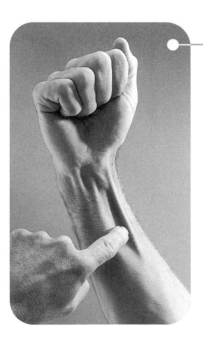

Fig. 7.64 | **The tendon of the flexor carpi radialis (*m. flexor carpi radialis, tendo*)**

Ask the subject to clench the fist. The tendon will appear on the radial side of the anterior surface of the wrist (indicated here by the practitioner's index finger), just outside the tendon of the palmaris longus (see Fig. 7.65). If it is difficult to display this tendon, ask the subject to flex and abduct the wrist (incline it to the radial side), at the same time slightly pronating the forearm.

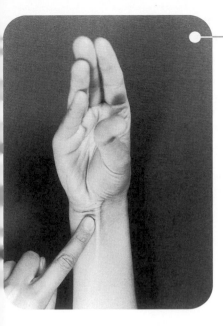

Fig. 7.65 | **The tendon of the palmaris longus (m. palmaris longus, tendo)**

This muscle is inconstant. Ask the subject to oppose the thumb and fifth finger. This will cause the tendon to appear in the middle of the anterior surface of the wrist, between the tendon of the flexor carpi radialis (Fig. 7.64), which lies laterally to it, and that of the flexor digitorum superficialis (Figs 7.66–7.69) medially.

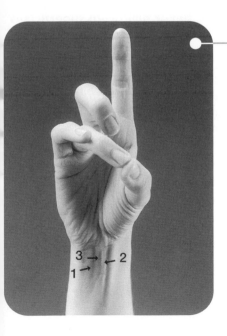

Fig. 7.66 | **The flexor digitorum superficialis (m. flexor digitorum superficialis) The tendon to the fourth finger (tendo)**

Clenching the fist causes this tendon (1) to become visible, medially to that of the palmaris longus (2) (Fig. 7.65). Should this not happen, ask the subject to oppose the thumb and fourth finger, perhaps together with palmar flexion of the wrist, to enable you to locate the tendon.

Note: In exceptional cases the tendon of the flexor digitorum superficialis going to the third finger (3) is also directly visible, as here.

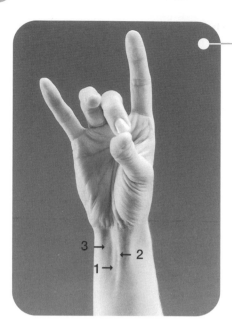

Fig. 7.67 | **The flexor digitorum superficialis
The tendon to the third finger**

This tendon (1) can be palpated behind the tendon of the palmaris longus (2) (see Fig. 7.65) and lateral to the tendon of the flexor digitorum superficialis going to the fourth finger (3) (Fig. 7.66). This can be done more easily if you ask the subject to oppose the thumb and middle finger, together with slight palmar flexion of the wrist.

Note: Take care not to damage the median nerve (see also Fig. 7.90), which is very close by.

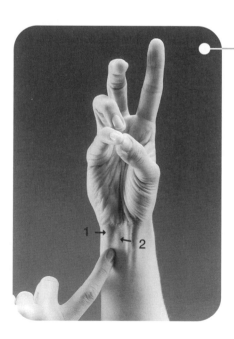

Fig. 7.68 | **The flexor digitorum superficialis
The tendon to the fifth finger**

This tendon is situated in the groove indicated here by the practitioner's index finger, between the tendon of the flexor carpi ulnaris medially (1) (see also Fig. 7.70) and the tendon of the flexor digitorum superficialis going to the fourth finger (2) laterally and anteriorly to it (see also Fig. 7.66). It becomes easier to detect if you ask the subject to oppose the thumb and fifth finger, together with slight palmar flexion of the wrist.

Fig. 7.69 | **The flexor digitorum superficialis**
The tendon to the index finger

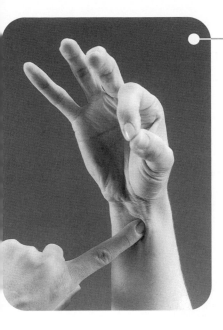

The tendon going to the index finger is the hardest to detect. It should be apparent if you push aside the palmaris longus laterally, as shown here, or if you seek it between the palmaris longus (see also Fig. 7.65) and the tendon of the flexor carpi radialis (Fig. 7.64). It becomes easier to detect if you ask the subject to oppose the thumb and index finger, together with slight flexion of the wrist.

Note: Take care not to damage the median nerve (see also Fig. 7.90), which is very close by.

Fig. 7.70 | **The tendon of the flexor carpi ulnaris (*m. flexor carpi ulnaris, tendo*)**

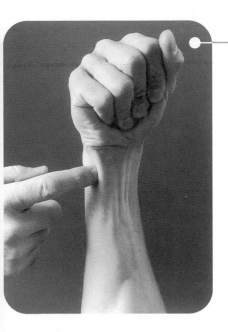

Ask the subject to flex the wrist slightly, inclining it to the ulnar side. The tendon of the flexor carpi ulnaris will appear on the part of the anterior surface of the subject's wrist farthest to the medial (ulnar) side.

THE TENDONS OF THE LATERAL PART OF THE WRIST

The notable structures that can be detected by palpation are:

- The tendon of the abductor pollicis longus (*m. abductor pollicis longus*) (Fig. 7.72).
- The tendon of the extensor pollicis brevis (*m. extensor pollicis brevis*) (Fig. 7.73).
- The tendon of the extensor pollicis longus (*m. extensor pollicis longus*) (Fig. 7.74).

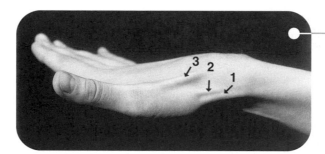

Fig. 7.71

Lateral view of the wrist

1. The tendon of the abductor pollicis longus.
2. The tendon of the extensor pollicis brevis.
3. The tendon of the extensor pollicis longus.

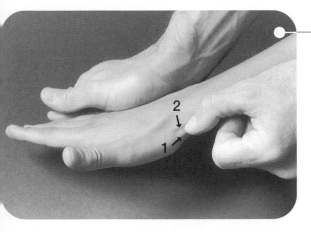

Fig. 7.72 | **The tendon of the abductor pollicis longus (*m. abductor pollicis longus, tendo*)**

This tendon can be displayed on some subjects as follows. The subject's wrist should be in a neutral position. As the thumb is drawn away from the plane of the rest of the hand, the tendon of the abductor pollicis longus (1) becomes apparent by the anterior (palmar) part of the tendon of the extensor pollicis brevis (2) (Figs 7.71 and 7.73). Ask the subject to incline the hand to the radial side while you resist this action. This will help you visualize the tendon.

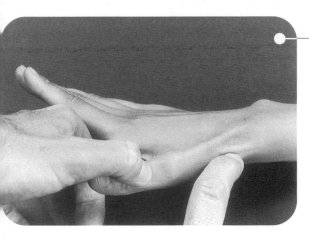

Fig. 7.73 | **The tendon of the extensor pollicis brevis (*m. extensor pollicis brevis, tendo*)**

The subject's wrist should be in a neutral position. Ask the subject to draw the thumb away from the plane of the rest of the hand. The tendon will appear on the radial part of the wrist, just behind the tendon of the abductor pollicis longus (see Figs 7.71 and 7.72).

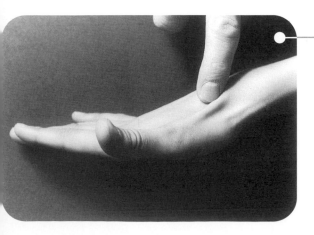

Fig. 7.74 | **The tendon of the extensor pollicis longus (*m. extensor pollicis longus, tendo*)**

The subject's wrist should be in a neutral position. Ask the subject to draw the thumb backward from the plane of the rest of the hand. The tendon will appear on the posterolateral part of the wrist.

THE TENDONS OF THE POSTERIOR PART OF THE WRIST JOINT

The notable structures that can be detected by palpation are:

- The tendon of the extensor carpi radialis longus (*m. extensor carpi radialis longus*) (Fig. 7.76).
- The tendon of the extensor carpi radialis brevis (*m. extensor carpi radialis brevis*) (Fig. 7.77).
- The tendon of the extensor digitorum (*m. extensor digitorum*) (Fig. 7.78).
- The tendon of the extensor digiti minimi (*m. extensor digiti minimi*) (Fig. 7.79).
- The tendon of the extensor carpi ulnaris (*m. extensor carpi ulnaris*) (Fig. 7.80).

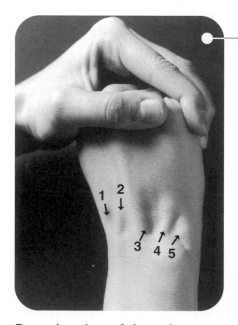

Fig. 7.75

Posterior view of the wrist

1. The tendon of the extensor carpi radialis longus.
2. The tendon of the extensor carpi radialis brevis.
3. The tendon of the extensor digitorum.
4. The tendon of the extensor digiti minimi.
5. The tendon of the extensor carpi ulnaris.

Note: The tendon of the extensor indicis (m. extensor indicis) is treated in Chapter 6.

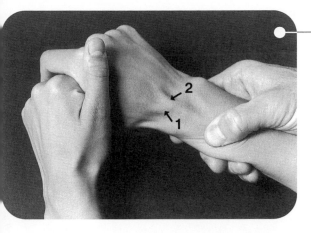

Fig. 7.76 | The tendon of the extensor carpi radialis longus (*m. extensor carpi radialis longus, tendo*)

This tendon (1) can sometimes be made to appear if the subject simply clenches the wrist tightly. The tendon of the extensor pollicis longus (see Fig. 7.74) overlies it. Place the subject's thumb on the palm of her hand; this will separate out the tendon you are looking for. Resist as shown here, as the subject tries to extend the wrist and incline it to the radial side.

Note: The tendon of the extensor carpi radialis brevis (2) lies medially to (on the ulnar side of) this tendon.

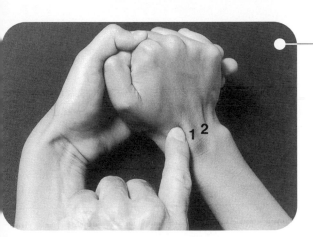

Fig. 7.77 | The tendon of the extensor carpi radialis brevis (*m. extensor carpi radialis brevis, tendo*)

This tendon (1) can sometimes be made to appear if the subject simply clenches the wrist tightly. It lies laterally to the tendons of the extensor digitorum (2) (Fig. 7.78) and medially to the tendon of the extensor carpi radialis longus (Fig. 7.76).

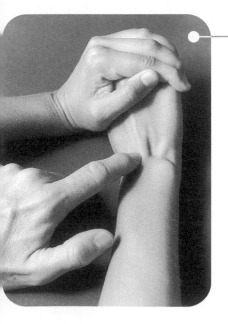

Fig. 7.78 | The tendon of the extensor digitorum (*m. extensor digitorum, tendo*)

Ask the subject to extend the wrist and metacarpophalangeal joints, while you resist this action; the subject's proximal and distal interphalangeal joints should remain flexed. This action is usually enough to make the tendon of the extensor digitorum prominent on the posterior, medial surface of the wrist.

Note: This tendon groups together the tendons going to the four individual fingers, and also that of the extensor indicis, which lies medially to (on the ulnar side of) the tendon of the extensor digitorum going to the index finger.

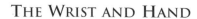
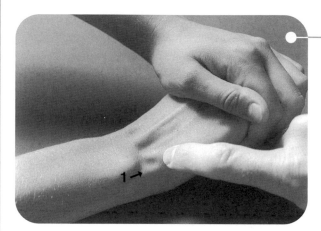

Fig. 7.79
The tendon of the extensor digiti minimi (*m. extensor digiti minimi, tendo*)

Ask the subject to extend the wrist and little finger while you resist these actions. The practitioner's index finger indicates this tendon, which appears on the posteromedial part of the wrist, laterally to (on the radial side of) the tendon of the extensor carpi ulnaris (1) (Fig. 7.80).

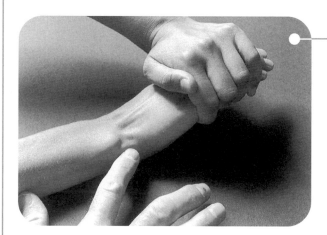

Fig. 7.80
The tendon of the extensor carpi ulnaris (*m. extensor carpi ulnaris, tendo*)

Ask the subject to incline the extended wrist to the ulnar side. Resist this action. The practitioner's index finger indicates the tendon, which will appear on the posteromedial part of the subject's wrist (on the ulnar side).

THE INTRINSIC MUSCLES OF THE HAND

The notable structures that can be detected by palpation are:

- The thenar eminence (*thenar; eminentia thenaris*) (Fig. 7.82).
- The hypothenar eminence (*hypothenar; eminentia hypothenaris*) (Fig. 7.83).
- The flexor tendons of the palm of the hand (Fig. 7.84).
- The lumbricals (*mm. lumbricales*) (Figs 7.85 and 7.86).
- The lumbricals (*mm. lumbricales*) and the dorsal and palmar interossei (*mm. interossei dorsales et palmares*) (Figs 7.86 and 87).

Actions

The muscles of the thenar eminence:

- The abductor pollicis brevis abducts the thumb.
- The opponens pollicis flexes the thumb and rotates it medially. This action enables the opposition of the thumb to the other fingers.
- The flexor pollicis brevis flexes the proximal phalanx of the thumb and draws it forward and medially, so assisting the opposition of the thumb.
- The adductor pollicis adducts the first metacarpal of the thumb.

The muscles of the hypothenar eminence:

- The palmaris brevis wrinkles the skin on the hypothenar eminence.
- The abductor digiti minimi abducts and flexes the little finger.
- The flexor digiti minimi brevis flexes the proximal phalanx of the little finger on the fifth metacarpal.
- The opponens digiti minimi draws the little finger anteriorly and laterally.

The muscles of the middle palmar region. The actions of the lumbricals and interossei complement each other:

- In the sagittal plane:
    — All flex the proximal phalanx and extend the middle and distal phalanges of the fingers.
- In the frontal plane:
    — The palmar interossei adduct the fingers (draw them together)
    — The dorsal interossei abduct the fingers (draw them apart).

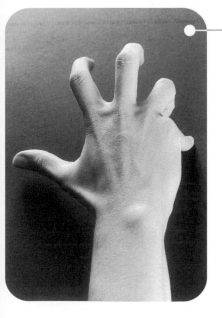

Fig. 7.81 | **Overall presentation of the intrinsic muscles of the hand**

The intrinsic muscles of the hand belong to three groups: the muscles of the thenar eminence, those of the hypothenar eminence, and the muscles of the middle palmar region.

- The muscles of the thenar eminence consist of the following, working from the superficial plane to the deepest:
    — The abductor pollicis brevis (*m. abductor pollicis brevis*)
    — The opponens pollicis (*m. opponens pollicis*)
    — The flexor pollicis brevis (*m. flexor pollicis brevis*)
    — The adductor pollicis (*m. adductor pollicis*).
- The muscles of the hypothenar eminence consist of the following, working from the superficial plane to the deepest:
    — The palmaris brevis (*m. palmaris brevis*)
    — The abductor digiti minimi (*m. abductor digiti minimi*)
    — The flexor digiti minimi brevis (*m. flexor digiti minimi brevis*)
    — The opponens digiti minimi (*m. opponens digiti minimi*).
- The muscles of the middle palmar region belong to three groups arranged one above the other. From palmar to dorsal, these are:
    — The lumbricals (*mm. lumbricales*)
    — The palmar interossei (*mm. interossei palmares*)
    — The dorsal interossei (*mm. interossei dorsales*).

THE WRIST AND HAND

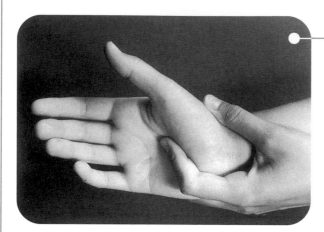

Fig. 7.82 | **The thenar eminence (***thenar; eminentia thenaris***)**

This eminence, which the practitioner is shown holding between the thumb and forefinger, centers on the bony framework provided by the first two metacarpals. It is made up of four muscles, arranged in three layers: the superficial layer, consisting of the abductor pollicis brevis; the middle layer, consisting of the opponens pollicis and the flexor pollicis brevis; and the deep layer, consisting of the adductor pollicis.

Attachments

The abductor pollicis brevis:

- This arises:
    — On the tubercle of the scaphoid
    — On the lateral part of the flexor retinaculum. (There is sometimes also a fibrous expansion from the abductor pollicis longus.)
- It is inserted on the radial border of the base of the proximal phalanx of the thumb and lateral sesamoid.

The opponens pollicis:

- This arises on the tubercle of the trapezium and on the flexor retinaculum.
- It is inserted on the lateral (radial) border of the first metacarpal

The flexor pollicis brevis muscle is composed of two heads: the superficial and deep portions:

- The superficial portion arises from the tubercle of the trapezium and the flexor retinaculum.
- The deep portion arises on the trapezoid and capitate.
- The two heads unite, creating a groove that is concave on the medial (ulnar) side and which gives passage to the tendon of the flexor pollicis longus. The muscle is inserted on the lateral (radial) part of the base of the first phalanx of the thumb and on the lateral sesamoid.

The adductor pollicis consists of an oblique head and a transverse head:

- The oblique head arises on the trapezoid and capitate.
- The transverse head arises:
    — On the third metacarpal
    — On the base of the second metacarpal
    — On the joint capsule of the second, third, and fourth metacarpophalangeal joints.
- The two heads have a common insertion by means of a tendon:
    — On the medial sesamoid
    — And on the medial (ulnar) part of the proximal phalanx of the thumb.

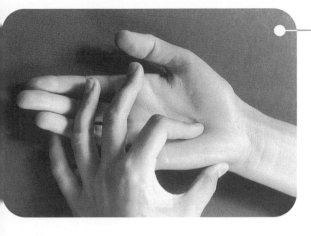

Fig. 7.83 | **The hypothenar eminence**
(*hypothenar; eminentia*
***hypothenaris*)**

This region, shown here held between the practitioner's thumb and forefinger, rests on the skeleton of the fifth metacarpal. It is made up of four muscles arranged as follows, working down from the superficial to the deep layer: palmaris brevis, abductor digiti minimi, flexor digiti minimi brevis, and opponens digiti minimi.

Attachments

The palmaris brevis:

- This small cutaneous muscle arises on the ulnar border of the palmar aponeurosis.
- It is inserted on the deep surface of the skin of the hypothenar eminence.

The abductor digiti minimi:

- The abductor muscle of the little finger arises on the inferior side of the pisiform and on the flexor retinaculum.
- It is inserted on the medial tubercle of the base of the first phalanx.

The flexor digiti minimi brevis:

- This arises on the hook of the hamate and on the flexor retinaculum.
- It is inserted on the medial tubercle of the base of the proximal phalanx of the little finger by a common tendon, together with the abductor digiti minimi.

Opponens digiti minimi:

- This arises on the hook of the hamate and flexor retinaculum.
- It is inserted on the border and ulnar surface of the fifth metacarpal along its entire length.

Note: The abductor digiti minimi can be palpated on the ulnar border of the fifth metacarpal if you ask the subject to abduct the little finger.

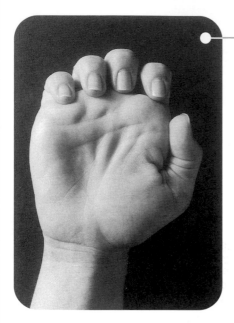

Fig. 7.84 | **The flexor tendons on the palm of the hand**

The tendons of the flexor muscles of the last four fingers are displayed on the palm of the hand as shown.

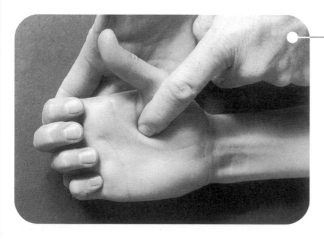

Fig. 7.85 | **The topographical location of the lumbricals (*mm. lumbricales*)**

In the adjacent figure, the practitioner's index finger is seen pushing aside the tendons of the flexor digitorum superficialis and profundus going to the index finger. The practitioner's index finger is positioned at the first lumbrical muscle, which arises on the radial side of the tendon of the flexor digitorum profundus going to the index finger.

Attachments of the intrinsic muscles of the hand (the muscles of the middle palmar region; see p. 235)

The lumbricals:

• Origin:
— The first and second lumbrical muscles arise on the radial border and anterior surface of the tendons of the flexor digitorum profundus to the second and third fingers.
— The third and fourth lumbrical muscles lie between the middle and ring fingers, and the ring and little fingers respectively. They arise on the radial and ulnar borders and on the anterior surface of the tendons of the flexor digitorum profundus going to the adjacent fingers between which that particular lumbrical muscle lies.
• They are inserted on the radial border of the extensor tendon of the corresponding finger, on the proximal, middle, and distal phalanges.

The palmar interossei:

• The origin of the palmar interosseous muscles is on the anterior part of the sides of the metacarpals. At the level of the fingers, these muscles form the so-called dorsal interosseous expansion.
— The first and second arise on the ulnar (medial) side of the first and second metacarpals[1]
— The third and fourth arise on the radial (lateral) side of the fourth and fifth metacarpals.
• Their insertion is by means of a deep part and a superficial part (note that there is no palmar interosseous muscle for the middle finger).
— The deep part is inserted:
— On the ulnar tubercle of the base of the proximal phalanx of the first and second metacarpals in the case of the first and second palmar interossei
— On the radial tubercle of the base of the proximal phalanx of the fourth and fifth metacarpals.
— The superficial part is inserted on the common extensor tendon of the corresponding fingers, on the proximal, middle, and distal phalanges.

The dorsal interossei:

• These arise on the posterior part of the adjacent sides of the metacarpals, and in each of the corresponding intermetacarpal spaces. At the level of the fingers, these muscles form the so-called dorsal interosseous expansion.
• Their insertion is by means of a deep part and a superficial part.
— The deep part is inserted:
— On the radial (lateral) tubercle of the base of the phalanges of the index and middle fingers, in the case of the first and second dorsal interossei
— On the ulnar (medial) tubercle of the base of the phalanges of the middle and ring fingers, in the case of the third and fourth dorsal interossei.
— The superficial part is inserted on the common extensor tendon of the corresponding fingers, on the proximal, middle, and distal phalanges.

[1] Other authors describe three palmar interossei, not four. The first palmar interosseus adducts the thumb, but it is often absent, and tends not to be included in most descriptions of this group of muscles. The muscles are numbered accordingly.

THE WRIST AND HAND

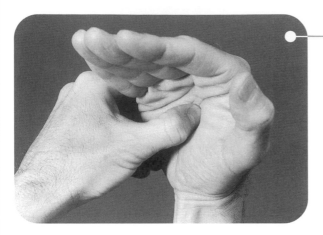

Fig. 7.86 | **The action of the lumbricals, the dorsal interossei (*mm. interossei dorsales*), and palmar interossei (*mm. interossei palmares*)**

In the sagittal plane, this set of muscles (see note below) is responsible for the flexion of the metacarpophalangeal joints of the last four fingers, and for the extension of the middle and distal phalanges of these fingers (see also Fig. 7.87).

Note: These twelve[1] muscles, the intrinsic muscles of the hand, comprise four lumbricals, four* palmar interossei, and four dorsal interossei.

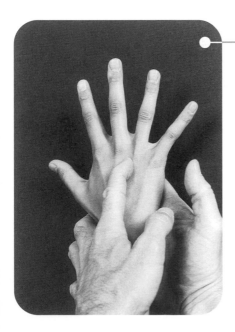

Fig. 7.87 | **The action of the dorsal and palmar interossei**

In addition to the action described above (Fig. 7.86), in the frontal plane, these muscles also abduct (draw apart) the fingers (dorsal interossei) and adduct them (draw them together) (palmar interossei). The contraction of the interossei can be palpated on the back of the hand, in the spaces between the metacarpals.

[1]See footnote on page 239.

NERVES AND BLOOD VESSELS

The notable structures that can be detected by palpation are:

- The radial pulse: taking the radial pulse at the wrist (Fig. 7.89).
- The median nerve (*n. medianus*) in the anterior part of the wrist (Fig. 7.90).
- The ulnar pulse: taking the ulnar pulse at the wrist (Fig. 7.91).
- The ulnar nerve (*n. ulnaris*) at the medial extremity of the anterior surface of the wrist (Fig. 7.92).

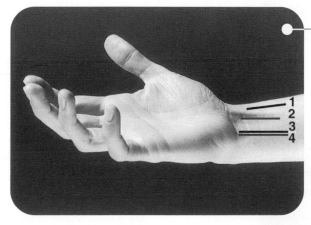

Fig. 7.88

The nerves and blood vessels in the anterior part of the wrist

1. The radial artery (*a. radialis*).
2. The median nerve.
3. The ulnar artery (*a. ulnaris*).
4. The ulnar nerve.

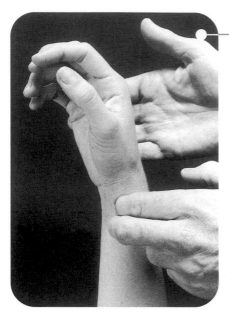

Fig. 7.89 | **The radial pulse: taking the radial pulse at the wrist**

Use a broad two- or three-finger contact on the inferior extremity of the anterior surface of the radius, lateral to (on the radial side of) the tendon of the flexor carpi radialis. You will feel the pulse of the radial artery beneath your fingers.

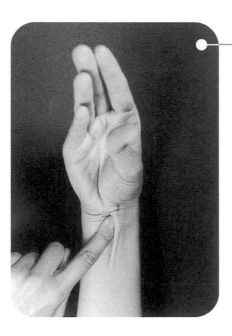

Fig. 7.90 | **The median nerve (*n. medianus*) in the anterior part of the wrist**

From the inferior third of the forearm, this nerve becomes very superficial. It runs behind the antebrachial aponeurosis between the tendon of the flexor carpi radialis (Fig. 7.64) laterally, the tendon of the flexor digitorum superficialis going to the third finger (Fig. 7.67) medially, and the tendon of the flexor digitorum superficialis going to the index finger behind. Push aside the tendon of the palmaris longus laterally (as shown here) in order to palpate the nerve.

Note: Take extreme care whenever you are palpating a nerve.

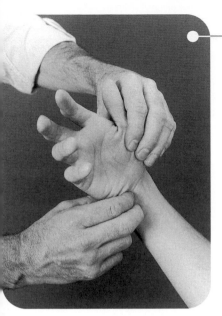

Fig. 7.91 | **The ulnar pulse: taking the ulnar pulse at the wrist**

Place the pads of two fingers on the medial extremity of the anterior surface of the wrist, at the cutaneous folds. Your fingers should be in contact with the lateral part of the pisiform (i.e. on the radial side of the bone) (see Figs 7.24 and 7.25). Slightly extend the subject's wrist in order to detect the pulse of the ulnar artery (*a. ulnaris*).

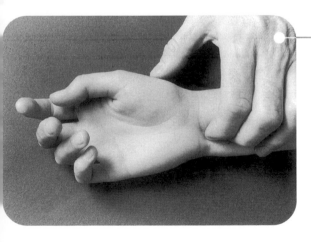

Fig. 7.92 | **The ulnar nerve (*n. ulnaris*) at the medial extremity of the anterior surface of the wrist**

Access to this nerve can be achieved at the lateral (radial) border of the tendon of the flexor carpi ulnaris (see Fig. 7.70). It is possible to roll the nerve on top of the tendon of the flexor digitorum superficialis going to the fifth finger (see Fig. 7.68).

Note: Great care should be taken in this investigation, as at any time when palpating a nerve.

CHAPTER 8

THE HIP

TOPOGRAPHICAL PRESENTATION OF THE HIP (*COXA*)

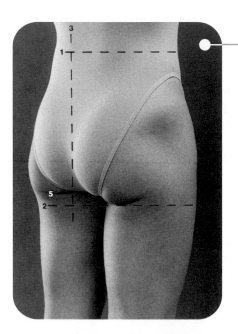

Fig. 8.1 | **Posteromedial view**

1. Superior boundary.
2. Inferior boundary.
3. Posteromedian boundary.
4. Anteromedian boundary.
5. Gluteal fold (sulius glutaeus).

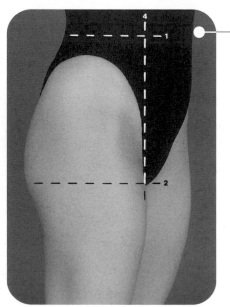

Fig. 8.2 | **Anterolateral view**

1. Superior boundary.
2. Inferior boundary.
3. Posteromedian boundary.
4. Anteromedian boundary.
5. Gluteal fold.

OSTEOLOGY

BONY ATTACHMENTS (ORIGINS AND INSERTIONS) OF THE HIP AND THIGH MUSCLES[1]

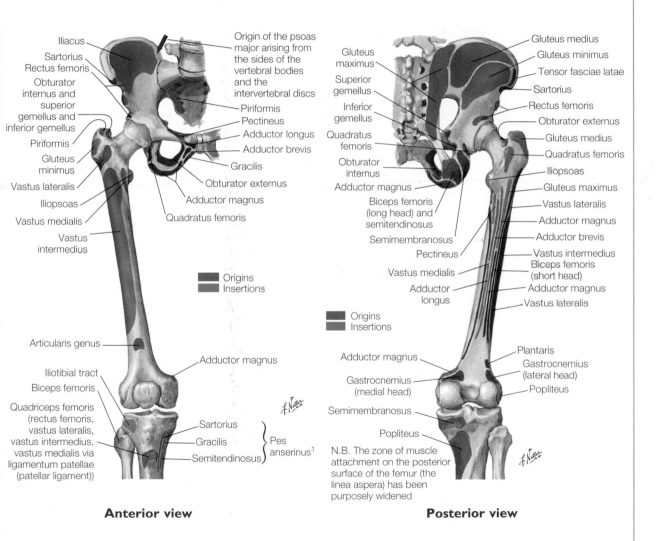

Iliacus
Sartorius
Rectus femoris
Obturator internus and superior gemellus and inferior gemellus
Piriformis
Gluteus minimus
Vastus lateralis
Iliopsoas
Vastus medialis
Vastus intermedius

Origin of the psoas major arising from the sides of the vertebral bodies and the intervertebral discs
Piriformis
Pectineus
Adductor longus
Adductor brevis
Gracilis
Obturator externus
Adductor magnus
Quadratus femoris

Articularis genus
Iliotibial tract
Biceps femoris
Quadriceps femoris (rectus femoris, vastus lateralis, vastus intermedius, vastus medialis via ligamentum patellae (patellar ligament))

Adductor magnus
Sartorius
Gracilis
Semitendinosus
} Pes anserinus[1]

■ Origins
■ Insertions

Anterior view

Gluteus maximus
Superior gemellus
Inferior gemellus
Quadratus femoris
Obturator internus
Adductor magnus
Biceps femoris (long head) and semitendinosus
Semimembranosus
Pectineus
Vastus medialis
Adductor longus

Gluteus medius
Gluteus minimus
Tensor fasciae latae
Sartorius
Rectus femoris
Obturator externus
Gluteus medius
Quadratus femoris
Iliopsoas
Gluteus maximus
Vastus lateralis
Adductor magnus
Adductor brevis
Vastus intermedius
Biceps femoris (short head)
Adductor magnus
Vastus lateralis

■ Origins
■ Insertions

Adductor magnus
Gastrocnemius (medial head)
Semimembranosus
Popliteus
N.B. The zone of muscle attachment on the posterior surface of the femur (the linea aspera) has been purposely widened

Plantaris
Gastrocnemius (lateral head)
Popliteus

Posterior view

[1] *Pes anserinus* means *goose's foot* in Latin. The term is used to highlight the resemblance between a goose's foot and the divergent nature of the tibial insertion of the distal tendons of the three thigh muscles (that is, sartorius, gracilis, and semitendinosus). These muscles are also called the anserine muscles.

PELVIC BONES AND LIGAMENTS

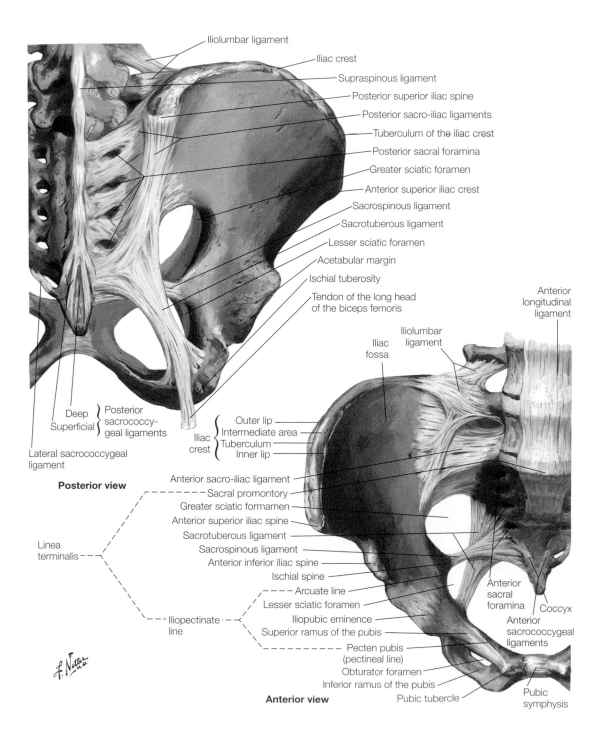

Iliolumbar ligament

Iliac crest

Supraspinous ligament

Posterior superior iliac spine

Posterior sacro-iliac ligaments

Tuberculum of the iliac crest

Posterior sacral foramina

Greater sciatic foramen

Anterior superior iliac crest

Sacrospinous ligament

Sacrotuberous ligament

Lesser sciatic foramen

Acetabular margin

Ischial tuberosity

Tendon of the long head
of the biceps femoris

Deep } Posterior
Superficial } sacrococcy-
geal ligaments

Lateral sacrococcygeal
ligament

Posterior view

Linea
terminalis

Iliac
fossa

Iliolumbar
ligament

Anterior
longitudinal
ligament

Outer lip
Intermediate area
Tuberculum
Inner lip

Iliac
crest

Anterior sacro-iliac ligament

Sacral promontory

Greater sciatic formamen

Anterior superior iliac spine

Sacrotuberous ligament

Sacrospinous ligament

Anterior inferior iliac spine

Ischial spine

Arcuate line

Lesser sciatic foramen

Iliopubic eminence

Superior ramus of the pubis

Pecten pubis
(pectineal line)

Obturator foramen

Inferior ramus of the pubis

Pubic tubercle

Anterior
sacral
foramina

Coccyx

Anterior
sacrococcygeal
ligaments

Pubic
symphysis

Iliopectinate
line

Anterior view

THE COXOFEMORAL REGION (*REGIO COXOFEMORALIS*)

The bony structures that can be detected by palpation are:

- The hip bone (*os coxae*):
    — The iliac crest (*crista iliaca*) (Fig. 8.4)
    — The tuberculum of the iliac crest (*tuberculum iliacum*) (Fig. 8.5)
    — The anterior superior iliac spine (*spina iliaca anterior superior*) (Fig. 8.6)
    — The pubic tubercle (*tuberculum pubicum*) (Fig. 8.13)
    — The posterior superior iliac spine (*spina iliaca posterior superior*) (Fig. 8.15)
    — The lesser innominate notch (Fig. 8.16)
    — The posterior inferior iliac spine (*spina iliaca posterior inferior*) (Figs 8.16 and 8.17)
    — The ischial spine (*spina ischiadica*) (Figs 8.18 and 8.19)
    — The lesser sciatic notch (*incisura ischiadica minor*) (Figs 8.18 and 8.19)
    — The greater sciatic notch (*incisura ischiadica major*) (Figs 8.20 and 8.21)
    — The ischial tuberosity (*tuber ischiadicum*) (Figs 8.22 and 8.23)
    — The inferior border of the hip bone (*os coxae, margo inferior*) (Figs 8.24 and 8.25).
- The femur (*femur*):
    — The femoral head (*caput ossis femoris*) (Figs 8.26–8.28)
    — The greater trochanter (*trochanter major*) (Figs 8.29 and 8.30)
    — The lesser trochanter (*trochanter minor*) (Figs 8.31 and 8.32).

Fig. 8.3

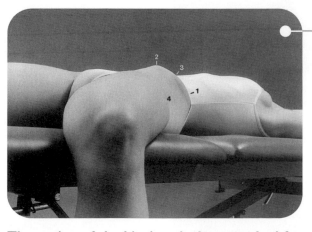

The region of the hip (*coxa*) photographed from below

(The subject is lying on her back with her knee facing the camera.)

The hip bone (*os coxae*):

1. Iliac crest.
2. Anterior superior iliac spine.
3. Iliac tuberosity.

Femur (*femur*):

4. Greater trochanter.

THE HIP

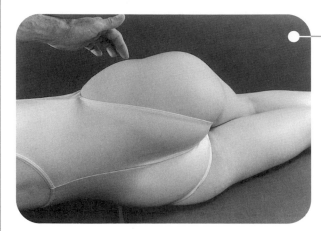

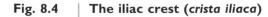

Fig. 8.4 | **The iliac crest (*crista iliaca*)**

This bone exhibits three easily visible curves:

- A medially concave anterior curve.
- A laterally concave posterior curve.
- A superiorly concave curve, whose apex lies almost midway between the two lower limbs.

Also visible are variations in thickness, which are more prominent at the two ends of the iliac crest, especially at the apex of the anterior curve (i.e. the tubercle of the crest; Fig. 8.5). To appreciate these two aspects of the iliac crest, just run over it anteroposteriorly and postero-anteriorly with the pads of two fingers or grip it between the thumb and the index. You must go over the crest as well as its lateral and medial lips.

Attachments
- The anterior part of the iliac crest gives attachment to the external oblique, the internal oblique, and the transverse muscles of the abdomen and the tensor fasciae latae.
- Its posterior part gives attachment to the latissimus dorsi, the quadratus lumborum, the sacrospinalis, and the iliocostalis.

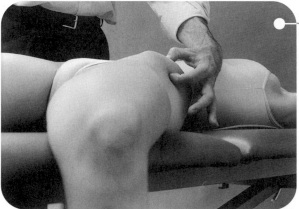

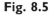

Fig. 8.5 | **The tubercle of the iliac crest (*tuberculum iliacum*)**

This lies at the apex of the anterior curve and projects toward the iliac fossa. Run over the iliac crest anteroposteriorly between your thumb and index finger and you will feel the thickening of the superior border of the base.

Note: In the figure the pad-to-pad grip holds the tuberculum with the index finger touching it.

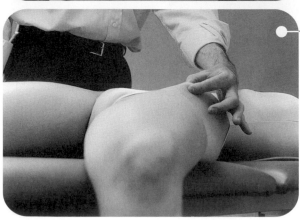

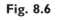

Fig. 8.6 | **The anterior superior iliac spine (*spina iliaca anterior superior*)**

This is easily accessible. You need only identify the most anterior part of the iliac crest and there it lies. Then grip it between thumb and index finger to bring it into focus.

Attachments
The tensor fasciae latae and the sartorius arise from its lateral surface.

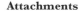

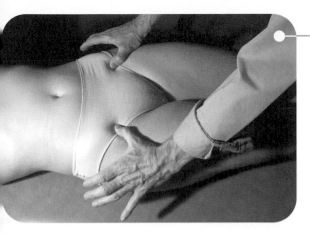

Fig. 8.7 | **The greater innominate notch**

This lies below the anterior superior iliac spine and is partly accessible.

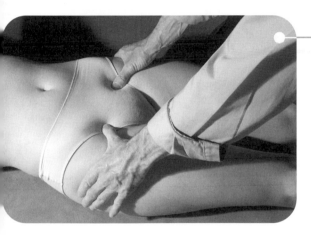

Fig. 8.8 | **The anterior inferior iliac spine**
(*spina iliaca anterior inferior*)

This is detected by the fingers as a fullness that lies about four finger-widths from the anterior superior iliac spine and at the inferior border of the notch. It is more or less accessible depending on the subject's body type. Ask the subject to tilt the pelvis anteriorly to facilitate its detection.

Attachment
This is the site of origin of the rectus femoris.

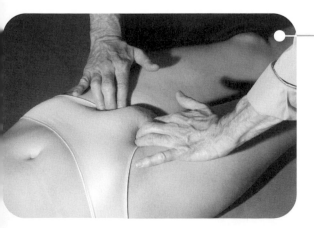

Fig. 8.9 | **The iliopectineal eminence and the pectineal surface**

The simplest approach is first to detect the pubic tubercle and then to move obliquely and laterally toward the anterior superior iliac spine.

Note: In men, take care with the spermatic cord during this procedure.

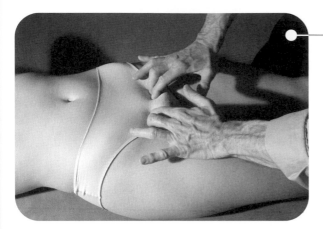

Fig. 8.10 | **The superior rami of the pubic bones**

Place your fingers in hook-like fashion over each of these rami as they lie on either side of the pubic symphysis.

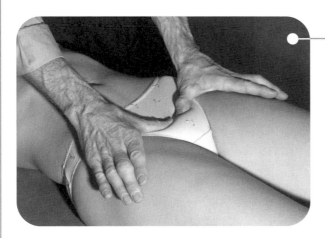

Fig. 8.11 | **The superior rami of the pubic bones: another approach**

Stand at the subject's head and place your thumb on the superior ramus of each pubic bone.

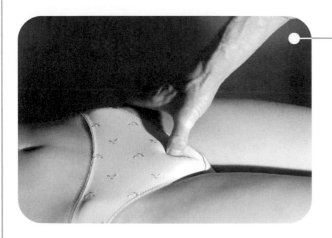

Fig. 8.12 | **The pubic symphysis (*symphysis pubica*)**

This is detected by the fingers as a depression between the two pubic bones filled by the fibrocartilaginous disc. The pubic symphysis is an amphi-arthrosis.

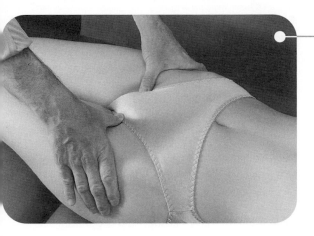

Fig. 8.13 | **The pubic tubercle (tuberculum pubicum)**

Place your hands flat on the greater trochanter, and move your thumbs horizontally and medially looking for a bony spine-like prominence in the pubic region (that is, the mons pubis in women). The pubic tubercle lies at the most medial part of the superior ramus of the pubic bone very close to the pubic symphysis or more precisely at the junction of the pectineal eminence and the obturator crest.

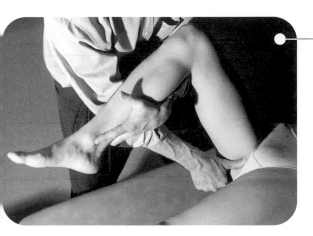

Fig. 8.14 | **The body of the pubic bone (quadrilateral surface)**

The obturator foramen is bounded superiorly by the superior ramus of the os pubis, medially and anteriorly by the quadrilateral body of the pubic bone, posteriorly by the ischial tuberosity, and inferiorly by the conjoined rami of the ischium and pubis. Place your thumb on the body of the pubis.

Note: The two bodies of the pubic bones are joined by the pubic symphysis (Fig. 8.12).

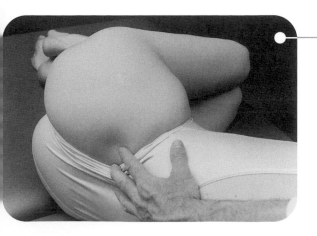

Fig. 8.15 | **The posterior superior iliac spine (*spina iliaca posterior superior*)**

This corresponds in general to the skin dimple more or less visible in everybody, and it faces the sacro-iliac joint.

You can also bring it out by finding the most posterior part of the iliac crest and following it down to its junction with the posterior margin of the hip bone, which is a shallow depression corresponding to the lesser innominate notch.

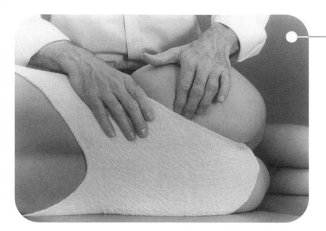

Fig. 8.16 | **The lesser innominate notch and the posterior inferior iliac spine (*spina iliaca posterior inferior*)**

The lesser innominate notch lies between the posterior superior and the posterior inferior iliac spines at two finger-widths from the latter and can be found between these two spines. Forward and backward tilting of the pelvis helps to localize it.

The posterior inferior iliac spine lies at the posterior margin of the iliac fossa. It can be detected by using the pads of two fingers placed about two finger-widths from the posterior superior iliac spine. You will feel it more easily if you ask the subject to tilt the pelvis forward and backward.

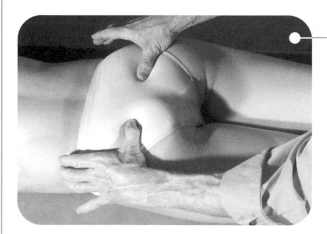

Fig. 8.17 | **The posterior inferior iliac spine in the prone position: another approach**

Just follow the lateral border of the sacrum until it joins the iliac bone. At this junction lies the posterior inferior iliac spine.

Note: Just above the spine is located the lesser innominate notch.

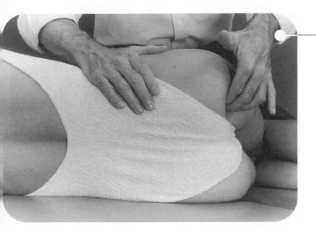

Fig. 8.18 | **The ischial spine (*spina ischiadica*) and the lesser sciatic notch (*incisura ischiadica minor*)**

To locate the ischial spine, the subject lies on the side with hip flexed. First, using the pads of two fingers, locate the ischial tuberosity and the lesser sciatic notch, which lies next to it superiorly. Then press on the ischial tuberosity and slide your fingers without losing contact with the skin (that is, by sliding the skin over the underlying tissues). The ischial spine lies at the proximal end of this notch.

Note: The gluteus maximus must be in a relaxed state.

Attachments
- The ischial spine gives origin to the superior gemellus on its lateral surface.
- It gives insertion to the sacrospinous ligament.

To locate the lesser sciatic notch, first use the pads of two fingers to find the ischial tuberosity (see Fig. 8.18). The depression that lies above it and runs toward the sacrum is the lesser sciatic notch. This is where the obturator internus is reflected.

Note: This notch lies between the ischial spine and the ischial tuberosity.

The gluteus maximus must be in a relaxed state. In some cases you may find it better to have the subject's hip in a less flexed position, since it lets you feel the muscle more easily through the body.

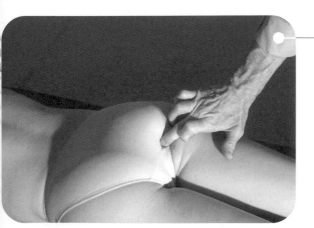

Fig. 8.19 | **The ischial spine and the lesser sciatic foramen in the prone position: alternative approach**

First locate the most distal part of the greater sciatic notch (as indicated in Fig. 8.20), maintaining the same grip and contact without sliding your fingers on the subject's skin. Then move your fingers up and down and you will feel a fullness under your fingers; this is the ischial spine.

The lesser sciatic notch is continuous with the greater sciatic notch and with the ischial spine. You can also approach the lesser notch by placing your fingers just above the superior pole of the ischial tuberosity.

Note: In the adjacent illustration the mode of approach uses only one hand.

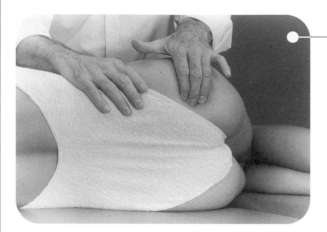

Fig. 8.20 | The greater sciatic notch (*incisura ischiadica major*)

First use the pads of two fingers to locate the posterior inferior iliac spine. Then press on the lateral surface of the iliac fossa and "bury" your fingers posteriorly toward the greater sciatic notch and the lateral border of the sacrum.

Note: The wide and deep greater sciatic notch lies between the posterior inferior iliac spine and the ischial spine. Feel for it through the body of the gluteus maximus. Remember that it is concave posteriorly and through it pass the piriformis and the sciatic nerve. This observation should influence your investigation of this notch.

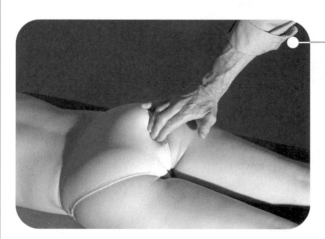

Fig. 8.21 | The greater sciatic notch in the prone position: alternative approach

Using the fingers of both hands placed very flat on the buttocks, try to identify a sharp border.

Note: In the adjacent illustration only one hand is used.

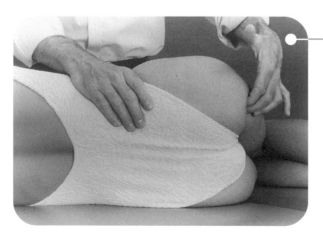

Fig. 8.22 | The ischial tuberosity (*tuber ischiadicum*)

It is oval with a bulky posterosuperior extremity and a narrow inferior extremity continuous with the inferior border of the hip bone. When the hip is flexed it is freed from the gluteus maximus.

You can also use the gluteal fold as a cutaneous landmark to palpate while the subject lies on the belly.

Note: We sit more often than not on our ischial tuberosities.

Attachments
- The inferior gemellus arises from the superior part of the ischial tuberosity just superior and lateral to the insertion of the sacrotuberous ligament.
- It is the origin of the hamstring muscles (the semimembranosus, the semitendinosus, and the biceps femoris).
- The sacrotuberous ligament is inserted into its medial border.

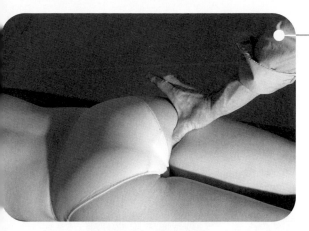

Fig. 8.23 | **The ischial tuberosity in the prone position: an alternative approach**

Place your thumb over the cutaneous landmark provided by the gluteal fold and you will touch the ischial tuberosity where the hamstring muscles take their origin.

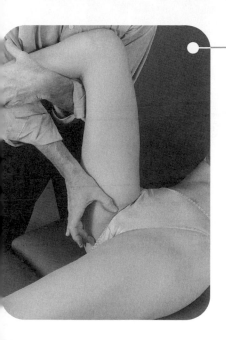

Fig. 8.24 | **The inferior border of the hip bone (*os coxae*)**

Locate the ischial tuberosity (Fig. 8.22) and the most anterior and medial part of the inferior ramus of the os pubis.

The inferior border of the hip bone has two parts:

- An anterior part, which articulates with that of the contra-lateral pubic bone to form the pubic symphysis.
- The rough-surfaced posterior part with two lips (inner and outer) and a groove.

Attachment

The gracilis arises from the external lip.

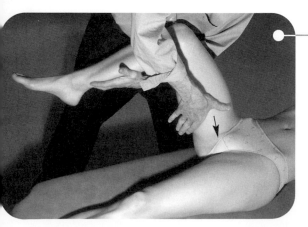

Fig. 8.25 | **The inferior border of the hip bone or the ischiopubic ramus**

Place your hand on the belly of the adductor longus and follow the muscle superiorly until it reaches the inferior border of the hip bone. You can make contact with the lateral border of your index finger or with your thumb (Fig. 8.19).

THE FEMUR (*FEMUR*)

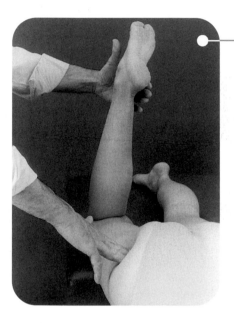

Fig. 8.26

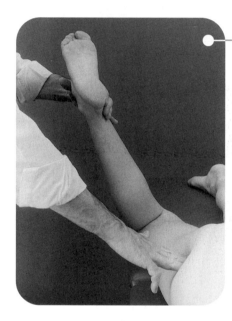

Fig. 8.27

Posterior approach to the femoral head (*caput ossis femoris*)

Medially rotate the hip so as to displace the femoral head posteriorly. It can be felt through the body of the gluteus maximus between the greater trochanter and the lateral surface of the hip bone.

In order to feel the femoral head more precisely under your fingers, ask the subject to rotate the hip several times.

Note: The femoral head bears a depression a little below and behind its center (that is, the fovea capitis). This pit is rugged and is pierced by a very large number of vascular foramina.

Attachment
The ligament of the femoral head is inserted in the fovea.

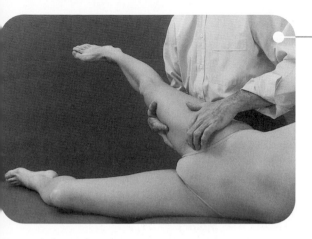

Fig. 8.28 | **Anterior approach to the femoral head**

With the subject lying on the side, stand behind and stabilize her pelvis in the anteroposterior plane with your hip.

Place your proximal hand on the anterolateral part of the subject's hip and use a thumb–index finger grip to hold the anterior part of the hip.

With your distal hand, cradle the anteromedial part of the thigh being examined and gently extend the subject's lower limb while keeping her pelvis steady with your hip.

Your proximal hand will gradually feel a fullness, which is the femoral head as it projects anteriorly.

Note: During this procedure you will be able to feel the femoral pulse, which has been displaced anteriorly by the protrusion of the femoral head.

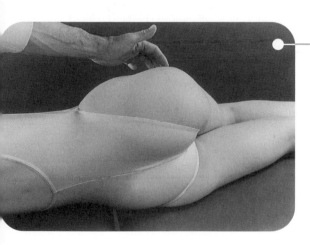

Fig. 8.29 | **Approach to the greater trochanter (*trochanter major*) with the subject lying on her side**

In this position the greater trochanter normally juts out on the lateral surface of the hip.

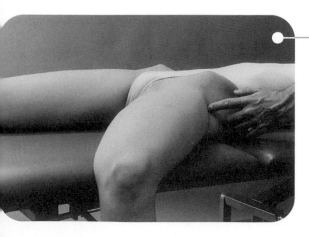

Fig. 8.30 | **Approach to the greater trochanter with the subject supine**

In this position, with the lower limb slightly abducted, the greater trochanter is directly accessible in the skin dimple caused by the hip abduction. This position provides optimal relaxation of the surrounding muscles and facilitates access to the different parts of the greater trochanter (that is, its superior, inferior, anterior, and posterior borders and its medial surface).

Attachments
- Superior border: insertion of the piriformis.
- Anterior border or surface: insertion of the gluteus maximus.
- External surface: insertion of the gluteus medius.

• Internal surface:
— Insertion of the obturator externus in the trochanteric fossa
— Above and in front of this fossa: insertion of the
obturator internus and of the gemellus muscles.
• The inferior border bounds its external surface inferiorly
and is also known as the crest of the vastus lateralis, which
is inserted there.

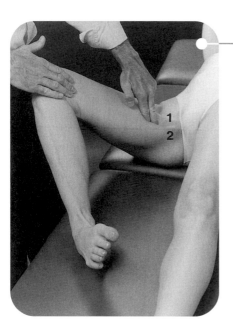

Fig. 8.31 | **The lesser trochanter (*trochanter minor*)**
Stage 1: demonstration of the adductor hiatus (1) and the gracilis (2)

The adjacent illustration shows the gracilis (2) and the long
adductor (1) lying posteromedial to the hip joint.

The subject lies on the back with hip and knee flexed. By
preventing the subject from adducting the thigh, you can
bring out the two muscles you are looking for. You can
contact the lesser trochanter in the gap between these two
muscles.

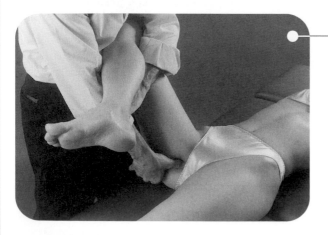

Fig. 8.32 | **The lesser trochanter**
Stage 2: direct contact

While the dorsal part of your hand cradles the medial aspect
of the subject's leg, you can displace the lesser trochanter
forward by laterally rotating the thigh. Slide the thumb of
your other hand into the depth of the soft tissues between the
adductor longus and the gracilis and look for a relatively
perceptible fullness.

Attachment

*The iliopsoas is inserted here either by a common tendon or by two tendons
separated by a synovial bursa.*

MYOLOGY

THE LATERAL INGUINOFEMORAL REGION (*REGIO FEMORALIS ANTERIOR — PARS LATERALIS ET SUPERIOR*)

With its apex located superiorly, this triangular region is bounded:

- Proximally by its apex consisting of the anterior superior iliac spine.
- Laterally by the tensor fasciae latae (*m. tensor fasciae latae*) (Fig. 8.34).
- Medially by the sartorius (*m. sartorius*) (Fig. 8.36).
- Deeply by its floor (that is, the rectus femoris (*m. rectus femoris*)), whose proximal extremity extends between the two above-mentioned muscles.

Note: The muscles demarcating this region belong topographically to the femoral region.

Actions of the muscles of the lateral inguinofemoral region
- Tensor fasciae latae: see Figure 9.14, page 297.
- Sartorius: see Figure 9.4, page 289.
- Rectus femoris: see Figure 9.8, page 292.

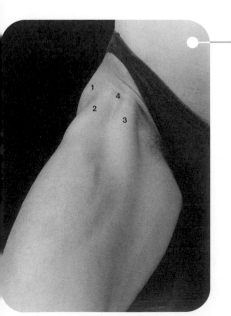

Fig. 8.33 | **Anteromedial view**

1. Gluteus medius.
2. Tensor fasciae latae.
3. Sartorius.
4. Rectus femoris.
5. Psoas major.
6. Iliacus.
7. Pectineus.
8. Adductor longus.

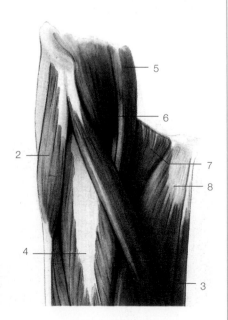

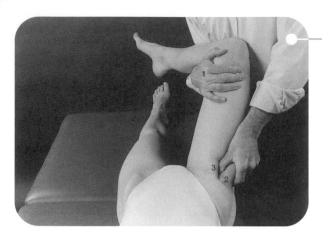

Fig. 8.34 | **The tensor fasciae latae (*m. tensor fasciae latae*)**

Press against the anteromedial surface of the flexed thigh (1), and two muscular bodies will appear in the proximal part of the thigh. The more lateral is the tensor fasciae latae (2).

Its body runs from the anterior superior iliac spine to the greater trochanter.

Attachment
See Figure 9.17, page 299.

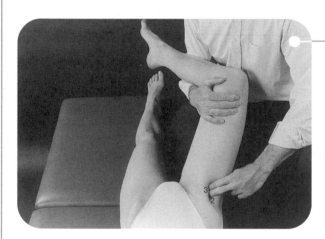

Fig. 8.35 | **The rectus femoris (*m. rectus femoris*)**

In the fossa between the tensor fasciae latae (2) laterally and the sartorius (3) medially you will be able to look for the most proximal part of the rectus femoris.

Even when it is relaxed you can easily feel its proximal extremity under your fingers. You can also ask the subject to contract and relax the muscle successively in order to feel its fibers better. The only additional movement required is extension of the knee.

Attachment
See Figure 9.13, page 296.

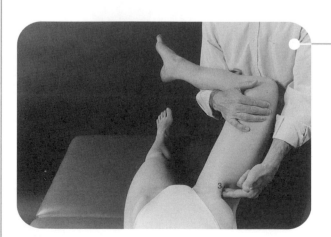

Fig. 8.36 | **The sartorius (*m. sartorius*)**

Use the same procedure as for the tensor fasciae latae.

This muscle is the more medial of the two muscle bodies that stand out in the proximal part of the thigh. The anterior superior iliac spine is the bony landmark, since the muscle arises from it.

Note: The sartorius is the medial border of the lateral inguinofemoral region. It is also the lateral border of the medial inguinofemoral region (or the femoral triangle).

THE MEDIAL INGUINOFEMORAL REGION OR THE FEMORAL TRIANGLE
(*REGIO FEMORALIS ANTERIOR/TRIGONUN FEMORALE*)

This region, called the femoral triangle, is triangular in shape with its apex located inferiorly and is bounded:

- Proximally by its base (that is, the inguinal ligament), which extends from the anterior superior iliac spine to the pubic tubercle.
- Laterally by the sartorius (*m. sartorius*) (Fig. 8.36).
- Medially by the adductor longus (*m. adductor longus*) (Fig. 8.38).
- At its apex distally (Fig. 8.37) by the junction of the sartorius and the adductor longus (Fig. 8.38).
- By its floor consisting of the pectineus (*m. pectineus*) (Fig. 8.39) medially and the iliopsoas (*m. iliopsoas*) laterally (Fig. 8.40).

This muscle complex forms a concave gutter that harbors the blood vessels and nerves for the lower limb.

Note: The sartorius, long adductor, and pectineus belong to the femoral region.

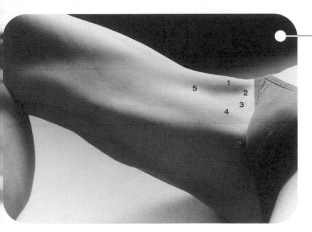

Fig. 8.37 | **Medial view**

1. Sartorius.
2. Iliopsoas.
3. Pectineus.
4. Adductor longus.
5. The apex of the femoral triangle (Scarpa's triangle), where the sartorius meets the adductor longus.

Actions of the muscles of the medial inguinofemoral region

Actions of the sartorius: see Figure 9.4, page 289.

Actions of the iliopsoas:

- When the fixed point is in the trunk:
    - It flexes the thigh over the pelvis and slightly rotates it laterally.
    - It also slightly adducts the thigh.
- When the fixed point is in the femur:
    - The iliacus produces flexion and anterior tilting of the pelvis.
    - The psoas major produces flexion, ipsilateral flexion, and contralateral rotation of the lumbar vertebral column.

Pectineus: see Figure 9.19, page 301.
Adductor longus: see Figure 9.19, page 301.
Gracilis: see Figure 9.26, page 306.

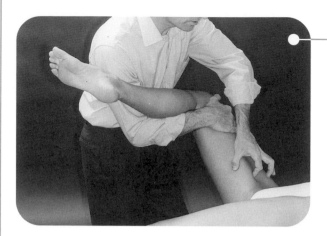

Fig. 8.38 | The adductor longus (*m. adductor longus*)

With the subject's hip and knee flexed, abduct the lower limb using a cradling hold. Ask the subject to adduct the thigh and resist his or her movement in order to make the adductor longus stand out in the superomedial part of the thigh.

Attachments
See Figure 9.21, page 303.

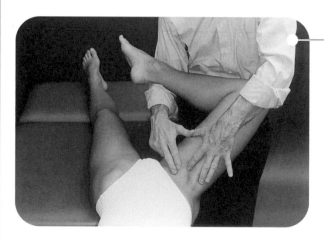

Fig. 8.39 | The pectineus (*m. pectineus*)

Look for this lateral to the adductor longus in the fossa that is continuous with it. It forms the medial portion of the floor of the femoral triangle. In the adjacent picture the sartorius lies between the index and the middle fingers of your left hand (that is, the hand that resists flexion and adduction of the hip). The other hand overlies the pectineus.

Attachments
See Figure 9.20, page 303.

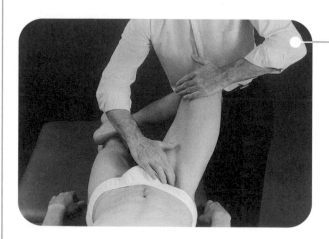

Fig. 8.40 | The iliopsoas (*m. iliopsoas*)

Place your contact medial to the medial portion of the sartorius near its origin from the anterior superior iliac spine. The iliopsoas is accessible at this point, since it is reflected on the iliopectineal surface and overlies the anterior aspect of the hip joint beyond that point of reflection. It is bordered medially by the pectineus. Make the muscle contract by opposing hip flexion with your distal hand, and your fingers can feel the contraction of the muscle fibers as they pass over the iliopubic eminence.

Note: This region is tender to the touch and must be approached with caution.

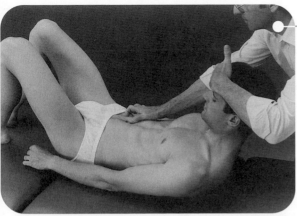

| Fig. 8.41 | **The iliopsoas in its proximal part Stage 1: looking for landmarks** |

When you resist the subject by placing a hand on his or her forehead, the strap-like abdominal muscles, including the lateral border of the rectus abdominis, stand out.

Place your hand on the subject's navel, your middle finger on the anterior superior iliac spine, and your index finger at the center of the line corresponding to the lateral border of the rectus abdominis.

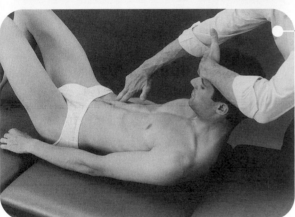

| Fig. 8.42 | **The iliopsoas in its proximal part Stage 2** |

The special point previously identified in the lateral border of the rectus abdominis (preceding figure) is the best point from which to approach the iliopsoas.

Once the landmark is identified, the subject should rest the head on a cushion to relax the abdominal muscles. You can change position and stand by the subject's hips in order to proceed. It is essential for you to feel through the abdominal muscles with care and by stages so as to overcome the defense mechanisms of the abdominal wall, which will certainly come into play.

Make the subject contract the muscles by actively flexing the hips and you will have a better appreciation of the body of the muscle you are looking for.

Note: The contact shown in the adjacent picture indicates the "point of entry" into the abdominal wall and not the method of palpation.

Attachments
- The psoas major arises from:
    — The intervertebral discs T12–L5
    — The lateral and adjacent parts of the vertebral bodies T12–L5
    — The fibrous arches running supero-inferiorly on the lateral aspects of these. These fibrous arches form a canal with the corresponding vertebrae, and through this canal the lumbar vessels and communicating rami of the sympathetic nerve pass
    — The anterior aspect of the transverse processes of the lumbar vertebrae
    — It is inserted into the apex of the lesser trochanter.
- The iliacus arises from:
    — The bulk of the internal surface of the iliac fossa
    — The inner lip of the iliac crest
    — The iliolumbar ligament and the base of the sacrum posteriorly.
- The iliacus and the psoas major are inserted into the lesser trochanter by a common tendon or by two tendons, which fuse at their insertion or remain separate.

THE GLUTEAL REGION (*REGIO GLUTEA*)

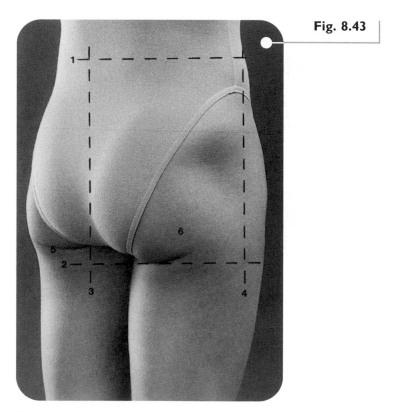

Fig. 8.43

Posterolateral view

1. Superior border: iliac crest.
2. Inferior border: gluteal fold.
3. Medial border: iliac crest and coccyx in continuity.
4. Lateral border: this is an imaginary vertical line running down from the anterior superior iliac crest to the greater trochanter and intersecting the most lateral part of the gluteal fold or its extension.

Note: This imaginary line has the remarkable property of corresponding more or less to the posterior border of the tensor fasciae latae.

5. The gluteal fold.
6. Gluteus maximus.

Gluteus maximus[1]

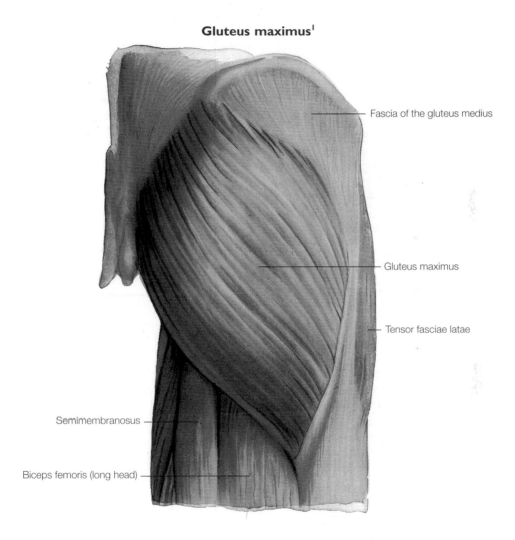

Fascia of the gluteus medius

Gluteus maximus

Tensor fasciae latae

Semimembranosus

Biceps femoris (long head)

1. The plates by H. Rouvière and A. Delmas are taken from Anatomie humaine descriptive, topographique et fonctionelle (see Bibliography).

THE HIP

Gluteal muscles, deep plane

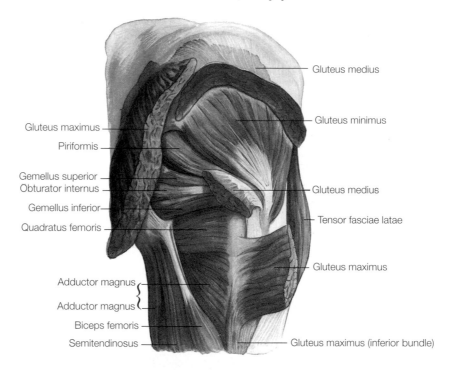

Gluteus medius

Gluteus minimus

Gluteus maximus

Piriformis

Gemellus superior
Obturator internus

Gluteus medius

Gemellus inferior

Tensor fasciae latae

Quadratus femoris

Gluteus maximus

Adductor magnus

Adductor magnus

Biceps femoris

Semitendinosus

Gluteus maximus (inferior bundle)

In this figure the gluteus medius masks the gluteus minimus

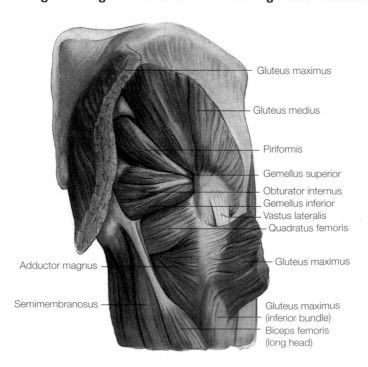

Gluteus maximus

Gluteus medius

Piriformis

Gemellus superior

Obturator internus
Gemellus inferior
Vastus lateralis
Quadratus femoris

Adductor magnus

Gluteus maximus

Semimembranosus

Gluteus maximus
(inferior bundle)
Biceps femoris
(long head)

THE SUPERFICIAL PLANE

The superficial plane of the gluteal region is occupied by one muscle: the gluteus maximus (Fig. 8.45).

Actions

- It extends the thigh over the pelvis.
- It laterally rotates the thigh over the pelvis.
- It stabilizes the pelvis in the sagittal plane.
- It tilts the pelvis posteriorly.

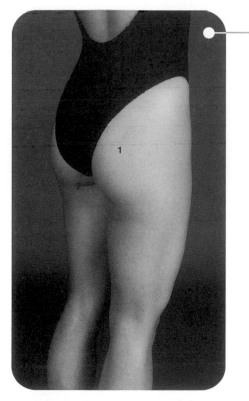

Fig. 8.44

Gluteus maximus (*m. gluteus maximus*)
Posterolateral view

1. Gluteus maximus.
2. Gluteal fold.

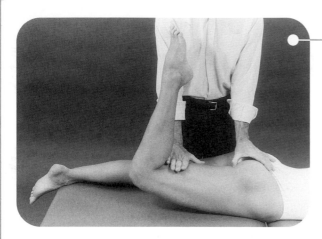

Fig. 8.45 | Gluteus maximus

The maneuver illustrated in this figure aims at displaying the gluteus maximus.

The iliac crest, the greater trochanter, and the ischial tuberosity are the essential bony landmarks that demarcate the gluteal region.

The gluteal fold is virtually horizontal and corresponds roughly to the inferior border of this muscle as it runs obliquely inferomedially.

Ask the subject to lift the anterior part of her thigh from the table with her knee flexed and without any compensation in the lumbar region.

Putting pressure on the postero-inferior part of the thigh prevents you from recruiting an intermediate joint (in this case, the knee), and allows you to bring out the muscle mass and to assess the quality of its contraction relative to that of the contralateral muscle.

Note: Knee flexion "shortens" the hamstring muscles and favors the specific activity of the gluteus maximus, which is to extend the hip.

THE MIDDLE PLANE

The middle plane of the gluteal region is filled by one muscle: the gluteus medius (Figs 8.47 and 8.48).

Actions of the gluteus medius
When the fixed point is in the pelvis:
- It abducts the thigh on the pelvis.
- Its anterior fibers flex and medially rotate the thigh on the pelvis.
- Its posterior fibers extend and laterally rotate the thigh on the pelvis.

When the fixed point is in the femur:

- It stabilizes the pelvis in the coronal plane.

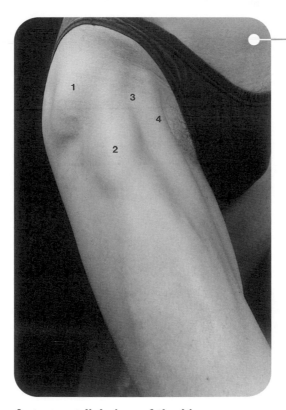

Fig. 8.46

Anteromedial view of the hip

1. Gluteus medius.
2. Tensor fasciae latae.
3. Rectus femoris.
4. Sartorius.

THE HIP

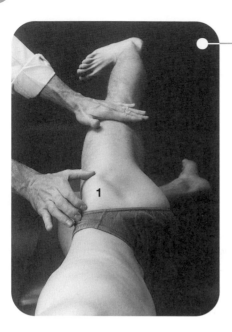

Fig. 8.47 | **Gluteus medius (*m. gluteus medius*)**

The essential bony landmarks are the anterior part of the iliac crest and the superior border of the greater trochanter.

Ask the subject to abduct the lower limb against resistance and to extend the hip slightly. The body of the muscle will tighten between your fingers.

Ask the subject to keep the hip abducted and flexed and then to rotate the hip medially in rapid successive bursts. Remember that the tensor fasciae latae lies below and in front of the gluteus medius.

Note: Your resisting hand is placed on the inferolateral part of the thigh above the knee in order to prevent recruitment of the intermediate joint (i.e. the knee in this case). The body of the muscle visible in the adjacent illustration is that of the tensor fasciae latae (1). The body of the gluteus medius lies behind and above the tensor fasciae latae.

Attachments

This muscle arises from the gluteal surface of the iliac fossa between the iliac crest and the anterior and posterior gluteal lines and from the lateral lip of the iliac crest.

It is inserted into the lateral surface of the greater trochanter.

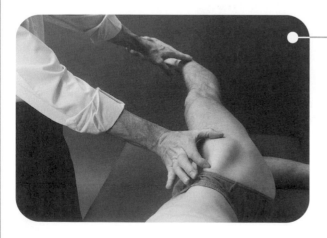

Fig. 8.48 | **Method for distinguishing the gluteus medius from the tensor fasciae latae**

Start from the same position and ask the subject to flex the hip slightly under your guidance while keeping it extended. The tensor fasciae latae will stand out between your fingers.

THE DEEP PLANE

The deep plane of the gluteal region contains the following:

- The gluteus minimus (*m. gluteus minimus*) (Fig. 8.50).
- The pelvitrochanteric muscles:
  — The piriformis (*m. piriformis*) (Figs 8.51 and 8.52)
  — The inferior and superior gemelli (*m. gemellus inferior* and *m. gemellus superior*) (Figs 8.54 and 8.55)
  — The obturator internus (*m. obturator internus*) (Figs 8.53–8.55)
  — The quadratus femoris (*m. quadratus femoris*) (Fig. 8.56)
  — The obturator externus (*m. obturator externus*) (Fig. 8.57).

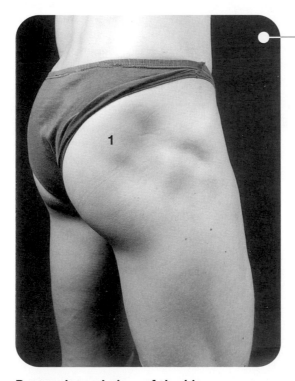

Fig. 8.49

Posterolateral view of the hip

Note: The gluteus minimus is covered by the body of the gluteus medius (Fig. 8.47). To approach the other muscles of the deep plane you must go through the gluteus maximus (1) (Fig. 8.45).

Actions

Actions of the gluteus minimus: see Figure 8.50.

Actions of the pelvitrochanteric muscles:

- They all laterally rotate the thigh on the pelvis.
- The piriformis abducts and stabilizes the hip when the fixed point of its action is at femoral level.
- The quadratus femoris is an adductor.

Note: The pelvitrochanteric muscles are lateral rotators when the hip is extended. They are horizontal abductors when the hip is flexed.

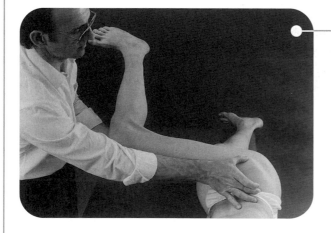

Fig. 8.50 | **The gluteus minimus (*m. gluteus minimus*)**

Place your proximal hand (the palpating hand) between the superior border of the greater trochanter and the most anterior part of the iliac crest. In this position you will encompass the tensor fasciae latae between your thumb and your other fingers. In the palm of your distal hand cradle the medial part of the knee and support the entire leg.

From this starting position (hip and knee flexed at 90°) ask the subject to rotate her hip medially. In effect this movement will raise the leg. Under your fingers you will feel a muscle mass that corresponds to the tensor fasciae latae. The gluteus minimus and the gluteus medius lie behind and above it.

Note: You cannot gain direct access to this muscle because it is masked by the anterior fibers of the gluteus medius, whose action is similar to that of the gluteus minimus.

Attachments

The gluteus minimus arises from the gluteal surface of the iliac fossa in front of and below the curved semicircular anterior gluteal line and is inserted into the anterior surface of the greater trochanter.

Actions

- It medially rotates the thigh on the pelvis.
- It abducts the thigh on the pelvis.
- It stabilizes the pelvis in the coronal plane.
- It helps in flexing the thigh on the pelvis.

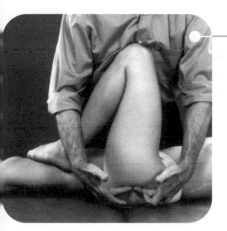

Fig. 8.51 | **The piriformis (*m. piriformis*)**

Place both your hands flat on the superior border of the greater trochanter to come into contact with the insertion of the piriformis.

Attachments

The muscle arises from the anterior surface of the second and third sacral vertebrae and adheres distally to the gemellus superior before being inserted into the superior border of the greater trochanter.

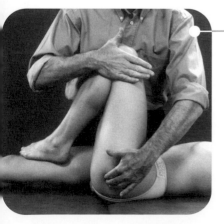

Fig. 8.52 | **The piriformis**

You can palpate the piriformis in the gluteal region. For precise location of the direction of this muscle, which is concealed by the gluteal muscles, you must keep in mind the following two bony landmarks: the superior border of the greater trochanter and the lateral border of the sacrum. The piriformis bridges these two landmarks.

THE HIP

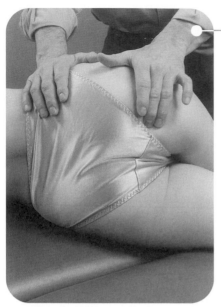

Fig. 8.53 | The obturator internus (*m. obturator internus*)

When you touch the lesser sciatic notch with the pads of your fingers, you will be in contact with the obturator internus, since the muscle is reflected at the level of this bony landmark.

Attachments

The obturator internus arises from the internal surface of the obturator membrane, the internal surface of the ischiopubic ramus above the insertion of the obturator membrane and the internal surface of the iliac bone between the obturator foramen and the arcuate line. It is inserted with the two gemelli in front and above the trochanteric fossa where the obturator externus is also inserted.

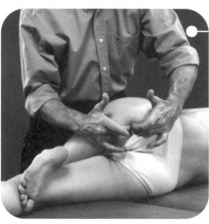

Fig. 8.54 | The inferior and superior gemelli (*m. gemellus inferior* and *m. gemellus superior*) and the obturator internus

Using both hands press hard on the lesser sciatic notch. From this point of reference you can then move your hands toward the greater trochanter in order to contact the muscles under investigation (that is, the gemelli accompany the obturator internus right down to its femoral insertion).

Attachments

- The gemellus superior arises from the lateral surface of the ischial spine.
- The gemellus inferior arises from the superior pole of the ischial tuberosity.
- These two muscles join the tendon of the obturator internus before being inserted together into the medial surface of the greater trochanter.

Fig. 8.55 | The inferior and superior gemelli and the obturator internus

In the adjacent illustration the practitioner has moved his hand into the gluteal region looking for the contraction of the muscles under investigation. These muscles are thrown into contraction by putting pressure on the lateral surface of the subject's knee while she abducts her flexed hip horizontally.

Note: These three muscles lie caudal to the piriformis.

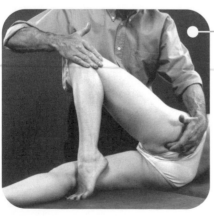

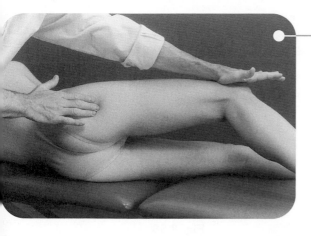

Fig. 8.56 | **The quadratus femoris**
(*m. quadratus femoris*)

You cannot directly study this muscle, for it lies deep to the gluteus maximus. The essential bony landmarks are the ischial tuberosity medially and the greater trochanter laterally.

The essential muscular landmark is the inferior border of the gluteus maximus.

Place the subject on her side with the hip slightly flexed, and prevent her from laterally rotating and abducting the hip by pressing on the lateral surface of her knee. The body of the muscle you are looking for contracts under your fingers and is felt through the body of the totally relaxed gluteus maximus, near its inferior border and between the two notable landmarks previously described.

Palpation of this muscle is difficult in normal subjects.

Attachments

The quadratus arises from the lateral surface of the ischial tuberosity and is inserted into the posterior surface of the greater trochanter lateral to the intertrochanteric line.

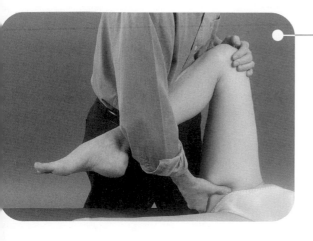

Fig. 8.57 | **The obturator externus**
(*m. obturator externus*)

With the subject's hip and knee flexed at 90°, place the thumb of your palpating hand between the adductor longus and the gracilis (see Fig. 9.29). With your right forearm resist the subject's lateral hip rotation, which you have asked him or her to perform repeatedly. As a result of the subject's muscular action, you can feel the muscle you are looking for contract under your fingers. Your other hand helps support the lower limb.

Attachments

The obturator externus arises from the external surfaces of the margins of the obturator foramen and of the obturator membrane and from the superior border of the ischiopubic ramus. It is inserted by tendon into the trochanteric fossa on the medial surface of the greater trochanter.

NERVES AND BLOOD VESSELS

THE MEDIAL INGUINOFEMORAL REGION OR THE FEMORAL TRIANGLE
(*REGIO INGUINOFEMORALIS ANTERIOR/TRIGONUM FEMORALE*)

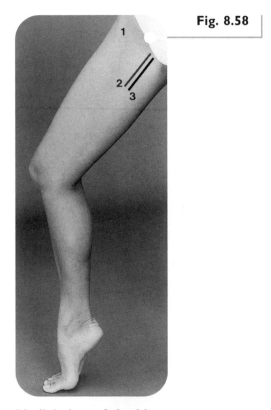

Fig. 8.58

Medial view of the hip

1. Sartorius.
2. Femoral nerve.
3. Femoral artery.

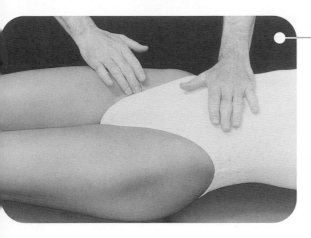

Fig. 8.59 | **The femoral artery (*a. femoralis*)**

With two of your fingers press lightly on the artery at a point in the middle of an imaginary line running from the anterior superior iliac spine to the pubic tubercle. You can feel the arterial pulse better when the hip is in the neutral position or is slightly extended.

Caution: Adjacent to the artery and medial to it, your fingers can feel two more or less round structures on the surface; they are the superficial inguinal lymph nodes.

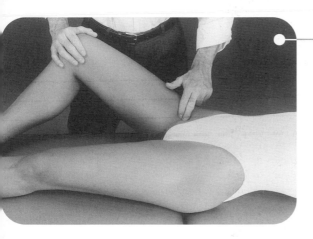

Fig. 8.60 | **The femoral nerve (*n. femoralis*) Stage 1**

As you did for the femoral pulse (figure above), place the pads of two of your fingers in the middle of an imaginary line running from the anterior superior iliac spine to the pubic tubercle.

Note: The subject can keep her lower limb in the neutral position for hip flexion–extension, (that is, lying flat on the table, not as in the figure, where she has her hip and knee flexed).

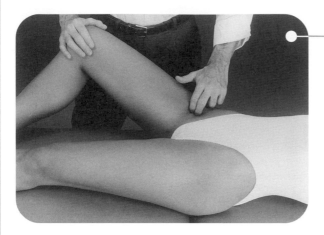

Fig. 8.61 | **The femoral nerve Stage 2**

Next move your hand laterally by one finger-width toward the sartorius and you will reach the structure you are after. You must approach it with the pads of your fingers, using a hook-like grip with all the care needed for such a structure. Your fingers will feel the nerve as a solid cylindrical cord.

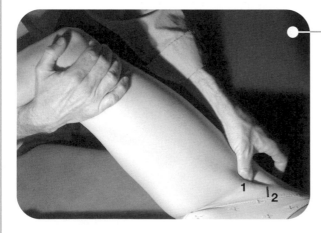

Fig. 8.62 | **The lateral cutaneous nerve of the thigh**

Most commonly, this nerve arises from L2 (the second lumbar nerve root) and then leaves the abdominal cavity by passing under the inguinal ligament and medial to the sartorius. It then crosses this muscle mediolaterally at the level of the greater innominate notch (the space between the two anterior iliac spines). In order to palpate the nerve, make the sartorius (1) contract by resisting the subject as she flexes the hip. Under your fingers roll the nerve (2), which crosses the anterior surface of that muscle before supplying the gluteal region (that is, the posterior aspect of the thigh and the anterolateral aspect of the thigh down to the knee).

THE GLUTEAL REGION (*REGIO GLUTEA*)

THE SCIATIC NERVE (*N. ISCHIADICUS*)

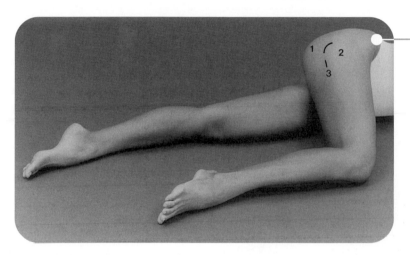

Fig. 8.63

Lateral view of the gluteal region

1. Ischial tuberosity.
2. Greater trochanter.
3. Sciatic nerve.

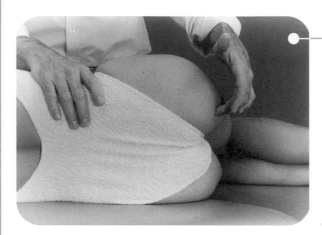

Fig. 8.64 | **Locating the sciatic nerve**
Stage 1: looking for the ischial
tuberosity (*tuber ischiadicum*)

In the position shown the subject's hip is flexed, and the ischial tuberosity is normally free of the gluteus maximus. Place the pads of your middle and ring fingers over it.

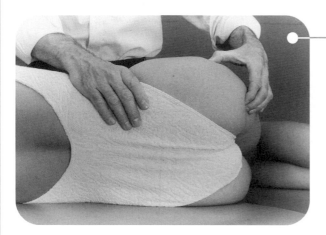

Fig. 8.65 | **Locating the sciatic nerve**
Stage 2: looking for the greater
trochanter

Keeping your two fingers in the same place, place your thumb on the greater trochanter.

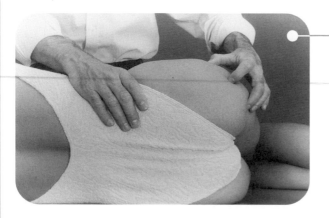

Fig. 8.66 | **Locating the sciatic nerve**
Stage 3

Imagine a line running between the two bony structures you have located and position your index finger roughly at the midpoint, where the sciatic nerve lies.

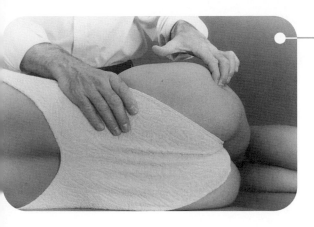

Fig. 8.67 | **The sciatic nerve (*n. ischiadicus*) Stage 4**

At this point the nerve measures about one finger-width.

You must approach it cautiously from the side, with the pads of two fingers.

Note: You can only gain access to this nerve through the gluteus maximus (if the shape of the subject's body allows it) when it is in a state of perfect relaxation. Then you will feel it as a solid cylindrical cord.

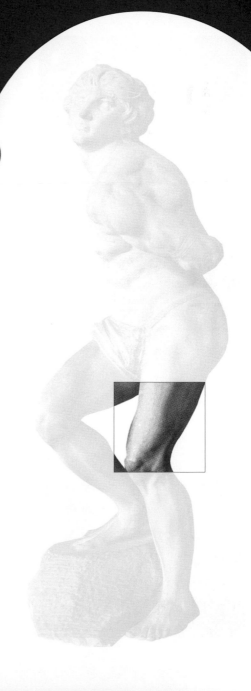

CHAPTER 9

THE THIGH

TOPOGRAPHICAL PRESENTATION OF THE THIGH (*FEMUR*)

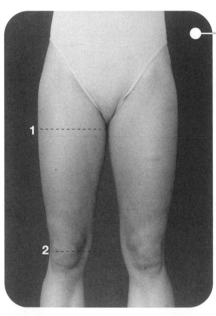

Fig. 9.1   **Anterior view**

1. Superior boundary.
2. Inferior boundary.

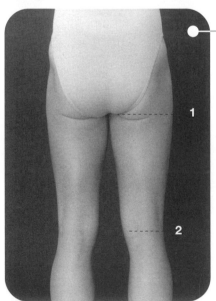

Fig. 9.2   **Posterior view**

1. Superior boundary.
2. Inferior boundary.

MYOLOGY

THE ANTERIOR FEMORAL REGION (*REGIO FEMORALIS ANTERIOR*): THE MUSCLES OF THE ANTERIOR COMPARTMENT

This region contains the muscles of the anterior compartment:

- The sartorius (*m. sartorius*) (Figs 9.5–9.7).
- The quadriceps femoris, which comprises:
  — The vastus medialis (*m. vastus medialis*) (Fig. 9.10)
  — The vastus lateralis (*m. vastus lateralis*) (Fig. 9.11)
  — The rectus femoris (*m. rectus femoris*) (Figs 9.12 and 9.13)
  — The vastus intermedius (*m. vastus intermedius*) and the articularis genus (*m. articularis genus*) (these muscles are not dealt with in this book).
- The tensor fasciae latae (*m. tensor fasciae latae*) and the iliotibial tract (*tractus iliotibialis*) (Figs 9.14–9.17).

Note: The tensor fasciae latae can logically be classified as belonging to the superficial plane of muscles of the gluteal region along with the gluteus maximus.

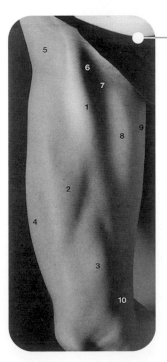

| **Fig. 9.3** | **Anteromedial view of the thigh** |

1. Sartorius.
2. Rectus femoris.
3. Vastus medialis.
4. Vastus lateralis.
5. Tensor fasciae latae.
6. Iliopsoas.
7. Pectineus.
8. Adductor longus.
9. Gracilis.
10. The distal tendon of the adductor magnus inserting into the medial tibial condyle on the adductor tubercle.

Anterior muscles of the thigh

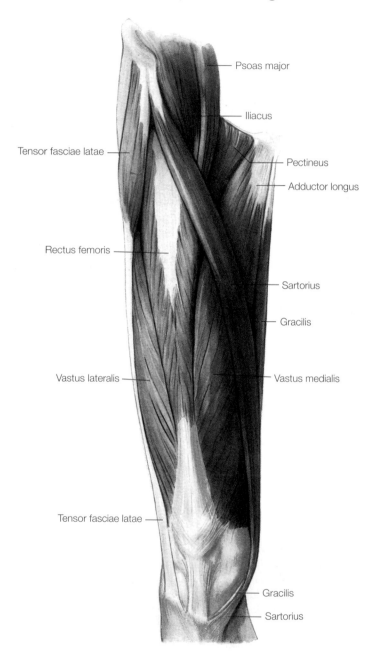

Psoas major

Iliacus

Tensor fasciae latae

Pectineus

Adductor longus

Rectus femoris

Sartorius

Gracilis

Vastus lateralis

Vastus medialis

Tensor fasciae latae

Gracilis

Sartorius

The sartorius (m. sartorius)

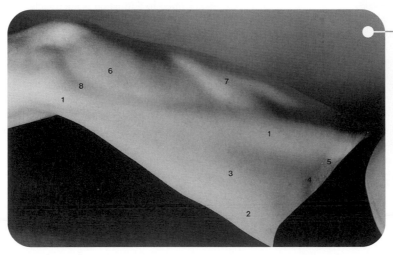

Fig. 9.4

Medial view of the sartorius and display of its relations with the other thigh muscles

1. Sartorius.
2. Gracilis.
3. Adductor longus.
4. Pectineus.
5. Iliopsoas.
6. Vastus medialis.
7. Rectus femoris.
8. Distal tendon of the adductor magnus inserted into the medial condyle on the adductor tubercle.

Actions of the sartorius
- It flexes, abducts, and laterally rotates the thigh on the pelvis.
- It flexes and medially rotates the leg on the thigh.
- It stabilizes the pelvis in the sagittal plane.
- It tilts the pelvis anteriorly.
- It stabilizes the knee laterally with the other muscles of the pes anserinus (the semitendinosus and the gracilis).

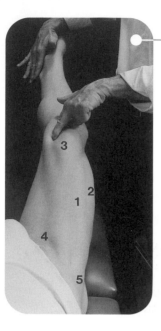

Fig. 9.5 | The sartorius in its medial part

Ask the subject to extend the knee almost fully and to flex the hip slightly, and then to maintain these positions isometrically.

Proceed by slightly rotating the subject's hip, and apply a resistance on the inferomedial end of the leg so as to counter the hip adduction isometrically.

Note: The practitioner's proximal hand is seen detaching the sartorius from the vastus medialis (3).

Attachment

This muscle is inserted into the anteromedial surface of the tibia along the tibial crest below the insertion of the patellar ligament. Its tendon of insertion also lies in front of the tendons of the gracilis and semitendinosus, the other two muscles of the pes anserinus.

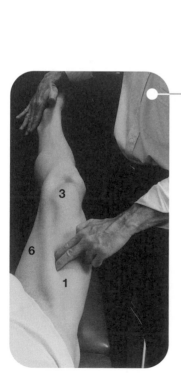

Fig. 9.6 | The sartorius in the thigh

Use the method described above to make the muscle contract. When the muscle is not made to stand out, it appears as a flat muscle forming a "depression" at the meeting point of the anterior and medial compartments of the thigh. It is bordered by the obturator muscles medially, by the vastus medialis distally (3) and by the rectus femoris (1) proximally and laterally.

Legend for Figures 9.5–9.7

1. Rectus femoris.
2. Vastus lateralis.
3. Vastus medialis.
4. Pectineus.
5. Tensor fasciae latae.
6. Adductor muscles.

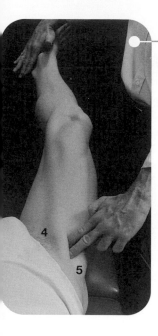

Fig. 9.7 | **The sartorius in its proximal part**

Use the method described in Figure 9.5 to make the muscle contract. The proximal part then stands out near the anterior superior iliac spine. (See also the hip region.)

In order to displace the sartorius medially, place your two fingers in the depression between the sartorius and the tensor fasciae latae (5). It is bordered medially by the iliopsoas (not shown in the figure) and the pectineus (4).

Attachment

This muscle arises from the lateral surface of the anterior superior iliac spine in front of the origin of the tensor fasciae latae.

*The quadriceps femoris (*m. quadriceps femoris*)*

Fig. 9.8

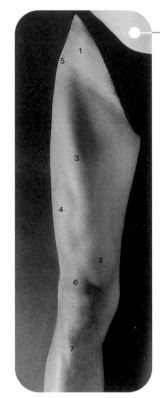

Anterior view of the thigh

1. Sartorius.
2. Vastus medialis.
3. Rectus femoris.
4. Vastus lateralis.
5. Tensor fasciae latae.
6. Quadriceps tendon.
7. Patellar ligament.

Note: The vastus intermedius, which is the deepest muscle of the quadriceps femoris, is no visible in Figure 9.8.

Actions of the quadriceps femoris
- It extends the leg on the thigh.
- The direct and crossed fibers of the vastus muscles contribute to knee stability in the coronal plane.
- The rectus femoris extends the leg on the thigh and flexes the thigh on the pelvis.

Quadriceps femoris and adductor muscles

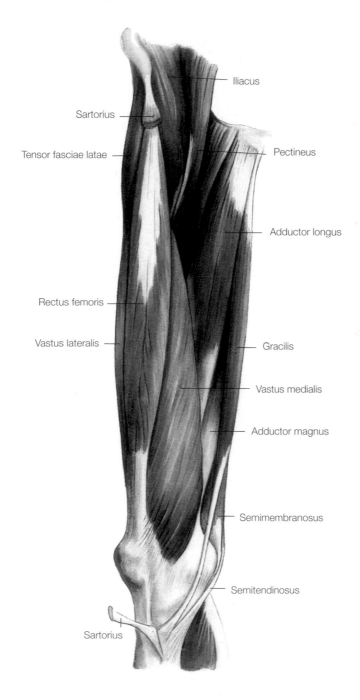

Iliacus

Sartorius

Pectineus

Tensor fasciae latae

Adductor longus

Rectus femoris

Vastus lateralis

Gracilis

Vastus medialis

Adductor magnus

Semimembranosus

Semitendinosus

Sartorius

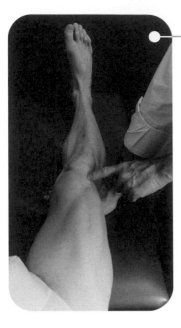

Fig 9.9 | The tendon of the quadriceps femoris (*m. quadriceps femoris, tendo*)

Place your distal hand under the subject's knee to make sure that the muscle contracts properly.

Ask the subject to contract and relax his quadriceps a few times in succession, checking that he flattens your hand against the table. Then look for the muscle above the patella and between the vastus muscles (see Fig. 9.10).

Note: For the patellar ligament, see Figure 10.51, page 343.

Attachments

The tendon is formed by the meeting of the four heads of the quadriceps: the vasti lateralis, medialis and intermedius, and the rectus femoris. This common tendon is inserted into the base of the patella.

The rectus femoris, which lies in the superficial plane of this common tendon, and the vastus lateralis and vastus medialis, which lie in its intermediate plane, contribute to the formation of the patellar ligament, which is inserted into the tibial tuberosity. The tendon of the vastus intermedius forms the deep plane of this common tendon and is inserted into the posterior part of the base of the patella.

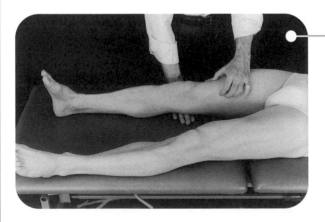

Fig. 9.10 | The vastus medialis (*m. vastus medialis*)

To bring out this muscle ask the subject to extend the knee

Place one hand under the knee with the back of your hand touching the subject's popliteal fossa and ask him to flatten your hand against the table.

Use the other hand to locate the vastus medialis on the inferomedial part of his thigh.

Note: The main feature of the vastus medialis is that it extends farther down than the lateralis. (There is a distance of about four finger-width between their distal ends.)

Attachments

It arises from the entire medial lip of the linea aspera and from its proximal medial trifurcation, which extends into the pectineal line up to the inferior border of the intertrochanteric line.[1]

[1] According to the author, the linea aspera of the femur trifurcates or divides proximally into three branches or lips (that is, medial, intermediate, and lateral). Currently, the linea aspera is considered to bifurcate or divide proximally into a medial and a lateral lip.

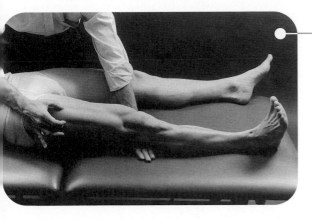

Fig. 9.11 | The vastus lateralis (*m. vastus lateralis*)

This lies in the lateral compartment of the thigh lateral to the vastus intermedius, and its lateral part is covered by the iliotibial tract (Figs 9.15 and 9.16).

To make it contract, use the same procedure as for the vastus medialis (Fig. 9.10).

Note: Remember that this muscle extends slightly posteriorly beyond the iliotibial tract.

Attachment

This muscle arises from a crest that bounds the anterior surface of the greater trochanter medially and inferiorly and from the entire lateral lip and lateral border of the linea aspera.

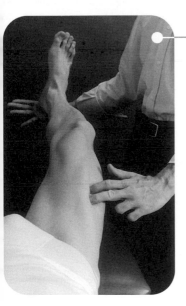

Fig. 9.12 | The rectus femoris (*m. rectus femoris*) in the thigh

Ask the subject to flex the hip slightly and to extend the knee partially. Place your hand under the subject's heel in order to modulate these two movements.

Ask the subject to contract his quadriceps femoris isometrically and to maintain this contraction.

In most subjects the muscle stands out in the midline of the thigh between the vastus medialis on the inside and the vastus lateralis on the outside. In other subjects you must look for the contracted muscle through rather a thick layer of adipose tissue.

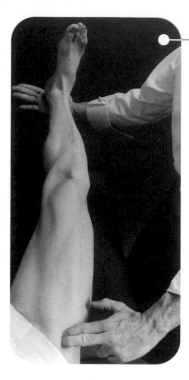

Fig. 9.13 | The rectus femoris in its proximal part

Ask the subject to flex the hip and partially extend the knee to make the muscle stand out better.

Place your distal hand under the heel to control these movements.

Ask the subject to raise the heel slightly from your supporting hand, and the muscle will contract between the sartorius on the inside and the tensor fasciae latae on the outside. (See also the gluteal region.)

Note: At this level the body of the muscle slides between the two above-mentioned muscles and forms the floor of the lateral iliofemoral region.

Attachments

It arises from the anterior inferior iliac spine and from the floor of the groove above the acetabulum, and is inserted into the base of the patella and the tibial tuberosity (Fig. 9.9).

*The tensor fasciae latae (*m. tensor fasciae latae)

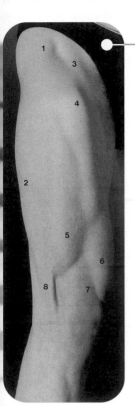

Fig. 9.14 | **Anterolateral view of the thigh**

1. Tensor fasciae latae.
2. Iliotibial tract.
3. Sartorius.
4. Rectus femoris.
5. Vastus lateralis.
6. Vastus medialis.
7. Tendon of the quadriceps femoris.
8. Tendon of the iliotibial tract.
9. Gluteus maximus.
10. Biceps femoris.

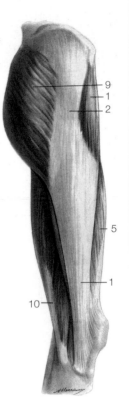

Actions of the tensor fasciae latae
- It flexes, abducts, and medially rotates the thigh on the pelvis.
- It extends the leg on the thigh and laterally rotates the leg on the thigh when the knee is flexed.
- It stabilizes the knee in the transverse plane by balancing the action of the anserine muscles.

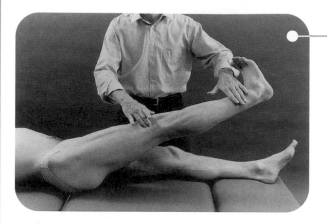

Fig. 9.15 | **The iliotibial tract (*tractus iliotibialis*) in its distal part**

With the subject's knee extended and the hip slightly flexed, prevent him from abducting the hip medially by placing your hand above the lateral malleolus on the distal extremity of the lower limb you are examining; this will widen the lateral part of the knee joint. As a result the tract is stretched, since it is inserted distal to the knee joint. As it nears the knee, this tract forms a veritable tendon, which stands out prominently, especially in male subjects.

Note: You can also ask the subject to rotate the hip, and this will make it even easier for you to feel this tract in some subjects.

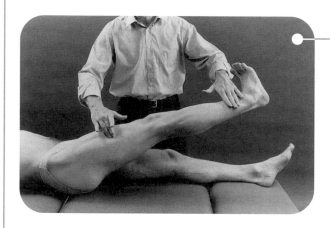

Fig. 9.16 | **The iliotibial tract in the thigh**

Use the same technique as the one described in Figure 9.15.

It is important to remember that the tract lies in the lateral part of the thigh with the vastus lateralis projecting beyond it anteriorly and posteriorly.

Note: The resisting action of your distal hand on the subject's leg makes the tract stand out more prominently.

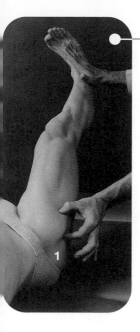

Fig. 9.17 | The tensor fasciae latae (*m. tensor fasciae latae*)

With the subject's hip slightly flexed and medially rotated, you need only isometrically resist the hip abduction by placing a resisting hand (as shown above) above the lateral malleolus at the distal extremity of the subject's lower limb. In this position, the muscle is preferentially recruited as an abductor and flexor of the hip. As you recruit its third action (that is, as a medial rotator) by asking the subject to perform repeated medial rotations of the hip, the body of the muscle becomes easier to localize.

It is felt between the anterior superior iliac spine and the anterior border of the greater trochanter in front of the gluteus medius.

Note: Take care not to mistake the tensor fasciae latae for the gluteus medius. In the figure the practitioner's grip demarcates the most distal part of the tendon, which lies below the gluteus medius (1).

Attachments

It arises from the external surface of the anterior superior iliac spine and from the anterior extremity of the lateral lip of the iliac crest.

Its body joins the superior quarter of the anterior border of the iliotibial tract, which acts as its tendon of insertion into the infracondylar tubercle (Gerdy's tubercle) on the lateral tibial condyle.

THE POSTERIOR FEMORAL REGION (*REGIO FEMORALIS POSTERIOR*)

This region includes the medial and posterior muscle groups.

The medial muscle group consists of:

- The four adductor muscles:
    - The pectineus (*m. pectineus*) (Fig. 9.20)
    - The adductor longus (*m. adductor longus*) (Fig. 9.21)
    - The adductor brevis (*m. adductor brevis*) (Fig. 9.22)
    - The adductor magnus (*m. adductor magnus*) (Figs 9.23–9.25).
- The gracilis (*m. gracilis*) (Figs 9.27–9.29).
  The posterior group consists of:
- The two medial ischiocrural muscles:
    - The semitendinosus (*m. semitendinosus*) (Figs 9.33, 9.34, 9.40)
    - The semimembranosus (*m. semimembranosus*) (Figs 9.35, 9.36, 9.40).
- The lateral ischiocrural muscle:
    - The biceps femoris (*m. biceps femoris*) with its long and short heads (Figs 9.38–9.40).

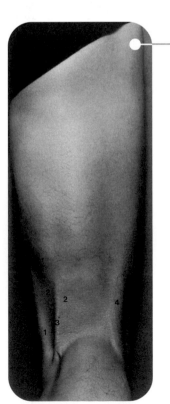

Fig. 9.18 | **Posterior view of the thigh**

1. Gracilis.
2. Semimembranosus.
3. Semitendinosus.
4. Tendon of the biceps femoris.

THE MEDIAL MUSCLE GROUP

This lies in the posterior femoral region and consists of:

- The four adductor muscles arranged in three planes:
    — The superficial plane, made up of the pectineus (*m. pectineus*) (Fig. 9.20) and the adductor longus (*m. adductor longus*) (Fig. 9.21)
    — The intermediate plane, made up of the adductor brevis (*m. adductor brevis*) (Fig. 9.22)
    — The deep plane, made up of the adductor magnus (*m. adductor magnus*) (Figs 9.23–9.25).
- The gracilis (*m. gracilis*) (Figs 9.27–9.29).

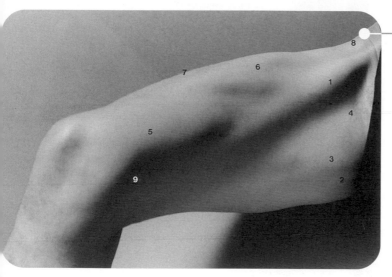

Fig. 9.19

Medial view of the hip

1. Sartorius.
2. Gracilis.
3. Adductor longus.
4. Pectineus.
5. Vastus medialis.
6. Rectus femoris.
7. Vastus lateralis.
8. Tensor fasciae latae.
9. Tendon of insertion of the adductor magnus into the adductor tubercle on the medial tibial condyle.

Actions of the adductor muscles

- They adduct the thigh on the pelvis.
- They laterally rotate the thigh on the pelvis, except for the medial or vertical bundle of the adductor magnus, which takes part in medial rotation.
- Apart from this vertical bundle, all these muscles contribute to thigh flexion on the pelvis and can become extensors beyond a certain degree of flexion (45°).
- They stabilize the pelvis by balancing the abductors.

Quadriceps femoris and thigh adductors

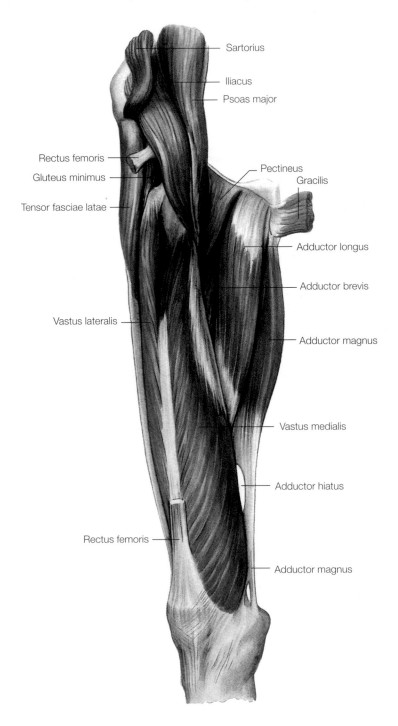

Sartorius

Iliacus

Psoas major

Rectus femoris

Gluteus minimus

Tensor fasciae latae

Pectineus

Gracilis

Adductor longus

Adductor brevis

Vastus lateralis

Adductor magnus

Vastus medialis

Adductor hiatus

Rectus femoris

Adductor magnus

The adductor muscles

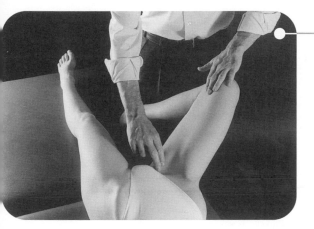

Fig. 9.20 | **The pectineus (*m. pectineus*)**

This lies in front of the adductor brevis between the iliopsoas on the outside and the adductor longus on the inside.

With the subject's knee and hip flexed, gently and isometrically resist any hip adduction.

A triangular depression with its base lying superiorly will appear at the proximal end of the thigh; it corresponds overall to the pectineus.

Attachments

- Proximally it arises in two planes: superficial and deep.
  — Its superficial fibers arise from the iliopectineal line between the iliopubic eminence and the pubic tubercle.
  — The deep fibers arise from the anterior lip of the groove in the superior pubic ramus.
- Distally it is inserted into the superior intermediate trifurcation of the linea aspera.

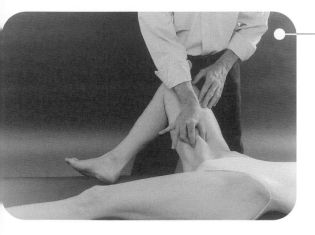

Fig. 9.21 | **The adductor longus (*m. adductor longus*)**

The subject flexes the knee and hip and abducts the hip horizontally. The practitioner places the right hand on the medial surface of the subject's thigh and uses the forearm to resist the subject as she adducts the hip horizontally at the practitioner's request.

This double maneuver brings out on the medial surface of her thigh a sizable muscular mass, which is the adductor longus.

Attachments

- It arises from the angle of junction of the body of the pubis with the symphysis and from the inferior surface of the pubic tubercle by a narrow, thick, flat tendon (that is, medial and inferior to the pectineus and above the adductor brevis).
- It is inserted into the middle third of the linea aspera.

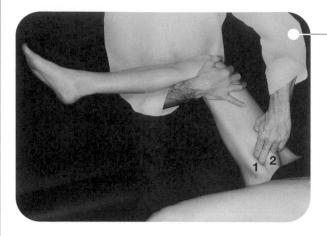

Fig. 9.22 | The adductor brevis (*m. adductor brevis*)

Using a cradling hold, progressively abduct the subject's thigh against a slight resistance on his or her part. The gracilis shows up as a rope along the medial surface of the thigh. You must then slide your fingers between this muscle (1) and the adductor longus (2) as far as possible proximally in order to come close to the adductor brevis, particularly its inferior bundle.

Note: In female subjects adipose tissue generally masks the gracilis muscular landmark, but the approach remains the same. You need only abduct the subject's lower limb maximally, and in this extreme position you must then resist hip abduction. This modification allows you to localize the gracilis better and to slide your fingers between the gracilis and the adductor longus.

Attachments
- Proximally the adductor brevis arises in front of and above the adductor magnus from the femoral surface of the pubic bone and on the adjacent ischiopubic ramus between the origins of the obturator externus and the gracilis.
- Distally it is inserted via two bundles:
  — A proximal bundle inserted into the superior intermediate trifurcation of the linea aspera.
  — A distal bundle inserted into the proximal part of the linea aspera.

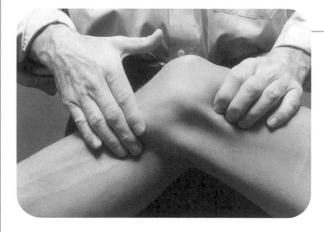

Fig. 9.23 | The adductor magnus (*m. adductor magnus*): the distal end of its medial portion (its inferior or vertical bundle)

The bony landmark is the adductor tubercle (see Chapter 10), and the important muscle landmark is the vastus medialis (Fig. 9.10).

After localizing the posterior part of the vastus medialis, look for the tendon of the adductor magnus, which your fingers will feel as a full cylindrical cord.

Note: You can increase the tension in this muscle by isometrically resisting the subject as he adducts his hip while keeping his knee and hip flexed.

Attachments
- It arises from the postero-inferior part of the ischial tuberosity.
- It is inserted into the adductor tubercle.

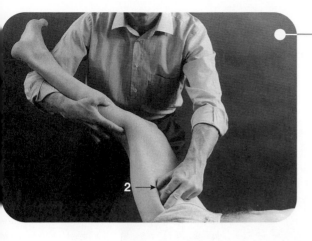

Fig. 9.24 | **The adductor magnus: the upper bundle of its lateral part**

The technique of tightening the landmark muscles is the same as that described previously. As your proximal hand slides between the adductor longus (see Fig. 9.21) and the gracilis (2), you need only go posteriorly round the medial border of the thigh to encounter the adductor magnus.

Note: Remember the origin of the muscle on the ischial tuberosity, which is a very posterior structure.

Attachments
The lateral part of the muscle splits into two bundles, superior and intermediate (see next figure).

The superior bundle arises from the middle third of the ischiopubic ramus and is inserted into the medial lip of the superior lateral trifurcation of the linea aspera.

Legend for Figures 9.24 and 9.25

1. Adductor longus.
2. Gracilis.

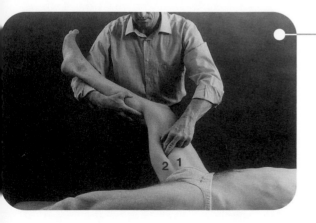

Fig. 9.25 | **The adductor magnus: the intermediate bundle of its lateral part**

Using a cradling hold, abduct the subject's hip so as to stretch the relevant adductor muscles, especially the adductor longus (1) and the gracilis (2).

Slide your palpating hand between these two muscles and, as shown in the adjacent figure, it will encounter the lateral part (the intermediate bundle) of the adductor magnus, which overshoots the adductor longus distally and is plastered against the intermediate part of the medial portion (the inferior or vertical bundle) of the adductor magnus.

Attachments
The intermediate bundle of the lateral portion of the muscle (see the previous figure) arises from the ischiopubic ramus and the external surface of the ischium and is inserted into the full length of the groove of the linea aspera.

The gracilis (m. gracilis)

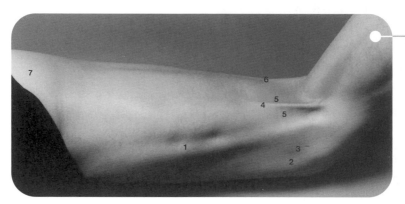

Fig. 9.26

Posteromedial view of the thigh

1. Gracilis.
2. Vastus medialis.
3. Tendon of insertion of the adductor magnus into the adductor tubercle on the medial condyle.
4. Semitendinosus.
5. Semimembranosus.
6. Biceps femoris.
7. Gluteus maximus.

Actions of the gracilis
- It flexes and medially rotates the leg on the thigh.
- It adducts and medially rotates the thigh on the pelvis.

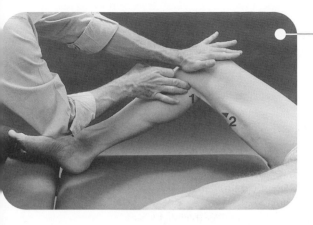

Fig. 9.27 | The gracilis: its distal part on the medial border of the tibia

The subject lies on her back with knees flexed. Ask her to rotate the right knee medially while producing an isometric flexion of the same joint by dragging the heel on the table toward the buttocks. Make contact with the posteromedial border of the medial tibial condyle and place your middle finger on the tendon you are looking for. Your ring finger encounters the semitendinosus (1); the semimembranosus (2) lies on either side of the semitendinosus tendon and in front of it.

Attachment

The semimembranosus is inserted into the superior part of the medial aspect of the tibia behind the sartorius, which hides it, and above the semitendinosus.

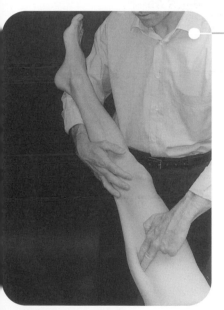

Fig. 9.28 | The gracilis in the thigh

Using a cradling hold, grasp the lower limb with your distal hand and move it passively into hip abduction. Ask the subject to adduct the hip, and then resist the movement in order to bring out the body of the muscle, which is more or less visible, depending on the subject. As shown in the adjacent figure, you simply have to detach the muscle from the underlying muscles by using the pads of two of your fingers.

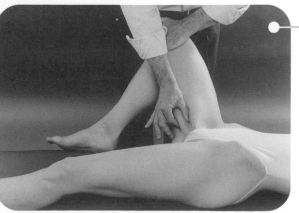

Fig. 9.29 | The gracilis: its proximal part

The subject's knee is flexed, and the hip is flexed and laterally rotated. Place your distal hand flat on the medial surface of the knee to resist the subject's horizontal hip adduction. With your proximal hand take hold of the gracilis on the medial aspect of the thigh.

Note: The adipose tissue, quite abundant in women, can somewhat hamper this approach.

Attachment

The gracilis arises by a large, flat tendon from the body of the pubis along the margin of the pubic arch.

THE POSTERIOR MUSCLE GROUP

It lies in the posterior compartment of the thigh and comprises:

- The two medial ischiocrural muscles:
  - The semitendinosus (*m. semitendinosus*) (Figs 9.33, 9.34, 9.40)
  - The semimembranosus (*m. semimembranosus*) (Figs 9.35, 9.36, 9.40).
- The lateral ischiocrural muscle:
  - The biceps femoris (*m. biceps femoris*) with its:
    Long head (caput longum)
    Short head (caput breve) (Figs 9.38–9.40).

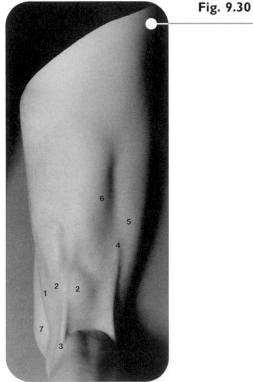

Fig. 9.30

Posterior view of the thigh

1. Gracilis.
2. Semimembranosus.
3. Semitendinosus.
4. Tendon of the biceps femoris.
5. The short head of the biceps femoris.
6. The long head of the biceps femoris.
7. Vastus medialis.

Posterior muscles of the thigh

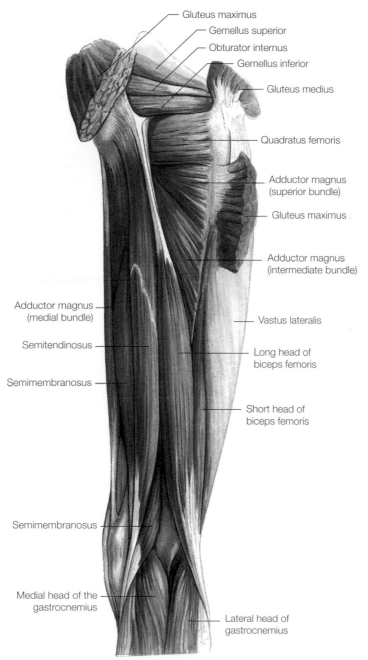

Gluteus maximus

Gemellus superior

Obturator internus

Gemellus inferior

Gluteus medius

Quadratus femoris

Adductor magnus
(superior bundle)

Gluteus maximus

Adductor magnus
(intermediate bundle)

Adductor magnus
(medial bundle)

Semitendinosus

Semimembranosus

Vastus lateralis

Long head of
biceps femoris

Short head of
biceps femoris

Semimembranosus

Medial head of the
gastrocnemius

Lateral head of
gastrocnemius

The medial ischiocrural muscles
(semitendinosus and semimembranosus)

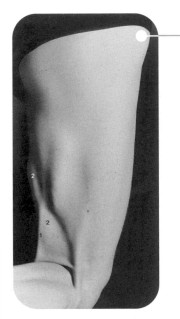

Fig. 9.31

Fig. 9.32

Posterolateral view of the thigh

1. Semitendinosus.
2. Semimembranosus.

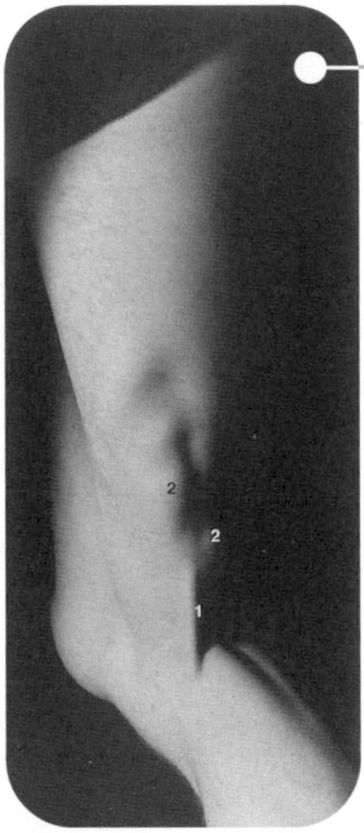

Posteromedial view of the thigh

1. Semitendinosus.
2. Semimembranosus.

Actions of the semitendinosus and the semimembranosus

- On the knee:
  — They flex the leg on the thigh.
  — The semitendinosus medially rotates the knee along with the weaker semimembranosus.
  — The ischiocrural muscles globally stabilize the knee during rotational movements.
- On the hip:
  — They extend the thigh on the pelvis, especially when the knee is extended.
- On the pelvis:
  — They stabilize the pelvis in the sagittal plane.
  — They tilt the pelvis posteriorly.

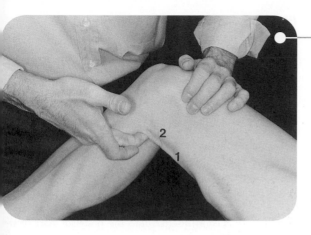

Fig. 9.33 | **The tendon of the semitendinosus (*m. semitendinosus, tendo*) on the medial border of the tibia**

As shown in the adjacent figure, apply your finger pads along the medial border of the tibia, and with your middle finger hook the semitendinosus (1). In this position, with the knee flexed, the tendon of the gracilis (2) lies in front of the semitendinosus tendon.

Attachments

- It arises from the posterior surface of the ischial tuberosity (see Fig. 9.40) by a common tendon with the long head of the biceps femoris medial to the origin of the semimembranosus.
- It is inserted into the superior part of the medial surface of the tibia behind the sartorius and below the gracilis.

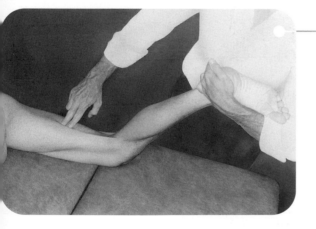

Fig. 9.34 | **The semitendinosus on the posterior surface of the thigh**

Your distal hand cups the subject's heel and lies flat on the medial border of his or her foot so as to resist knee flexion and medial rotation at the same time. You will find the body of the muscle as an extension of the tendon you localized in the figure above.

The muscle lies in the posterior part of the thigh medial to the biceps femoris and behind the semimembranosus.

Note: The peculiar feature of this muscle is the fact that its tendon extends very high proximally on the posterior surface of the thigh. This is clearly seen in the adjacent figure. Another peculiar feature is the fact that it is fleshy above and tendinous below, unlike the semimembranosus.

For its site of origin from the ischial tuberosity, see Figure 9.40.

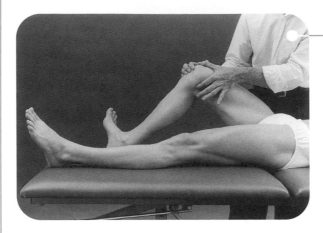

Fig. 9.35 | **The semimembranosus (*m. semimembranosus*): its distal part (medial view)**

With your distal hand passively rotate the subject's leg laterally so as to free the distal end of the tendon adequately. You will feel the tendon under your fingers as a large cylindrical cord near its insertion into the posteromedial part of the upper border of the medial tibial condyle.

Attachments

It is inserted via three tendons:

- A straight tendon inserted into the posterior part of the medial tibial condyle.
- A reflected tendon, which under cover of the collateral tibial ligament slides into the horizontal groove on the medial tibial condyle before being inserted into the anterior edge of this groove.
- A recurrent tendon (also known as the oblique popliteal ligament), which is inserted into the thickened portion of the capsule of the knee.

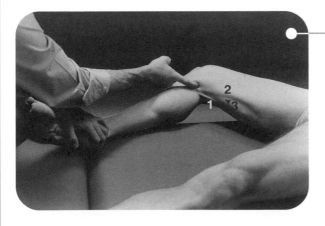

Fig. 9.36 | **The semimembranosus: its distal part (posteromedial view)**

In addition to the approach described above, you may find it useful to ask the subject to flex and medially rotate the knee while you resist these movements, the better to feel the tendon under your fingers.

With your index placed on the semimembranosus at its tibial insertion you will notice, as shown in the adjacent figure, that the gracilis (2) crosses it posteriorly in order to come to lie above the semitendinosus (1) on the medial border of the tibia.

Attachment

It arises from the lateral part of the ischial tuberosity medial to the quadratus femoris and lateral to the common tendon of the long head of the biceps femoris and of the semitendinosus (see Fig. 9.40).

The lateral ischiocrural muscle or the biceps femoris

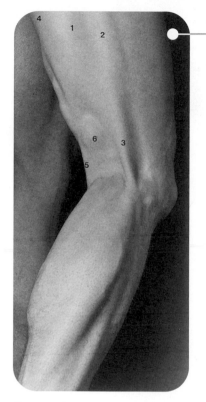

Fig. 9.37

Posterolateral view of the thigh

1. Biceps femoris — long head.
2. Biceps femoris — short head.
3. Tendon of the biceps femoris.
4. Semitendinosus.
5. Tendon of the semitendinosus.
6. Semimembranosus.

Actions of the biceps femoris
- On the knee:
    — It flexes the leg on the thigh and laterally rotates the knee when flexed.
    — It stabilizes the knee during rotational movements.
- On the hip:
    — It extends the thigh over the pelvis, especially when the knee is extended.
- On the pelvis:
    — It helps to stabilize the pelvis in the sagittal plane.
    — It tilts the pelvis posteriorly.

THE THIGH

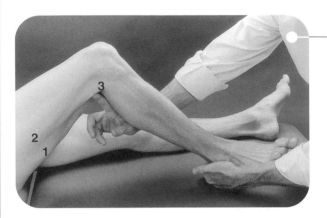

Fig. 9.38 | **The biceps femoris: its distal part**

With your hand cupping the subject's heel resist his knee flexion, and with the anterior surface of your forearm resting on the lateral border of the subject's foot resist his lateral knee rotation.

The tendon, shown by the practitioner's index finger, stands out in the lateral part of the knee just before its insertion into the head of the fibula.

Attachment

It is inserted into the head of the fibula outside the insertion of the collateral fibular ligament, from which it is separated by a bursa. It also is inserted into the lateral tibial condyle.

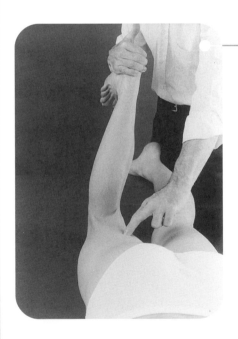

Fig. 9.39 | The biceps femoris: on the posterior surface of the tibia

While the subject lies on the belly, your resisting hand cups his heel and lies flat on the lateral border of the foot in order to resist knee flexion and lateral rotation. On the posterior surface of the thigh the long head of the biceps femoris joins the medial ischiocrural muscles (semimembranosus and semitendinosus).

Legend for Figures 9.38–9.40

1. Biceps femoris: long head.
2. Biceps femoris: short head.
3. Tendon of the biceps femoris.
4. Gluteal fold.

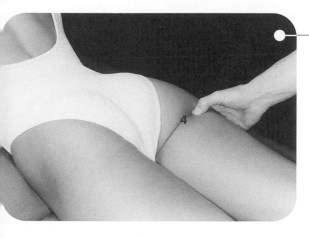

Fig. 9.40 | **The tendons of origin of the ischiocrural muscles from the ischial tuberosity (*tuber ischiadicum*)**

With the subject lying on the belly, use a cutaneous landmark: the gluteal fold (4). Through it you can feel the origins of these muscles from the ischial tuberosity. In the adjacent figure the thumb is slightly displaced laterally with respect to the origin of these muscles from the ischial tuberosity.

Attachments

- The long head of the biceps femoris arises from the ischial tuberosity by a tendon shared with the semitendinosus. This common site of origin lies medial to that of the semimembranosus.
- The short head of the biceps femoris arises from the groove of the linea aspera and from its lateral distal bifurcation (the lateral supracondylar line).

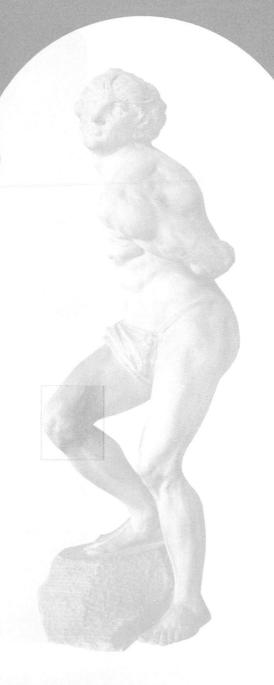

CHAPTER 10

THE KNEE

TOPOGRAPHICAL PRESENTATION OF THE KNEE

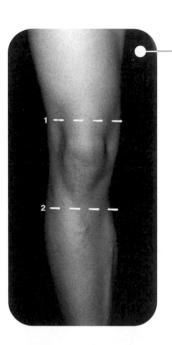

Fig. 10.1 | **Anterior view**

1. Superior boundary.
2. Inferior boundary.

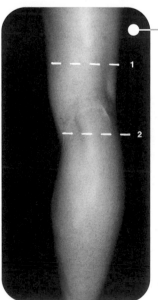

Fig. 10.2 | **Posterior view**

1. Superior boundary.
2. Inferior boundary.

OSTEOLOGY

THE ANTERIOR COMPARTMENT

The bony structures that can be detected by palpation are:

- The suprapatellar fossa (*fossa suprapatellaris*) (Fig. 10.4).
- The patella (*patella*):
  — The base (*basis patellae*) (Fig. 10.5)
  — The anterior surface (*facies anterior*) (Fig. 10.6)
  — The apex (*apex patellae*) (Fig. 10.7)
  — The lateral border (*margo lateralis*) (Fig. 10.8)
  — The lateral approach to the posterior articular surface (*facies articularis*) (Fig. 10.9)
  — The medial approach to the posterior articular surface (*facies articularis*) (Fig. 10.10).
- The femur (*femur*):
  — The articular surfaces of the condyles (*femur, condyli medialis et lateralis, facies articulares*) (Fig. 10.13)
  — The oblique grooves in the condyles (*femur — condyli medialis et lateralis, facies articularis, sulci medialis et lateralis*) (Figs 10.14 and 10.15).
- The tibia (*tibia*):
  — The superior articular surface (*tibia — facies articularis superior*) and the tibiofemoral joint (Fig. 10.12)
  — The tibial tuberosity (*tuberositas tibiae*) (Fig. 10.11).

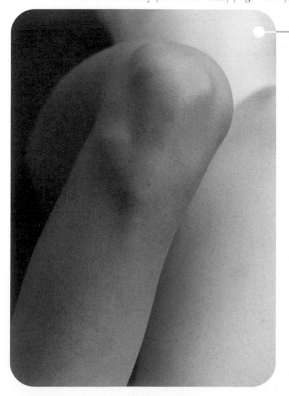

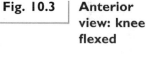

Fig. 10.3 | **Anterior view: knee flexed**

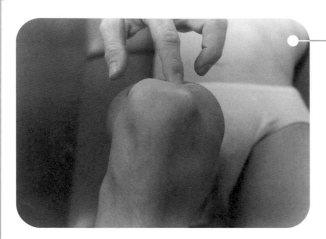

Fig. 10.4 | **The suprapatellar fossa (*fossa suprapatellaris*)**

This triangular fossa lies above the condyles on the anterior surface of the distal end of the femur and receives the superior portion of the patella during knee extension.

Maximally flex the subject's knee to be able to feel it optimally, starting from the easily located base of the patella (Fig. 10.5).

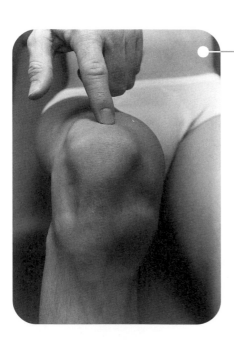

Fig. 10.5 | **The patellar base (*basis patellae*)**

This is triangular with its base located inferiorly and its apex superiorly, and it can be felt under the fingers as a sloping surface.

Attachments

The quadriceps tendon is inserted into its anterior half, and the articular capsule is attached posteriorly near its articular surface.

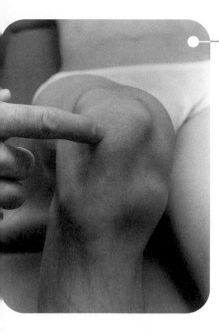

Fig. 10.6 | **The anterior surface of the patella (*patella, facies anterior*)**

Curved and pitted by many vascular openings, this has an uneven surface with vertical bumps and depressions formed by contact with the quadriceps tendon.

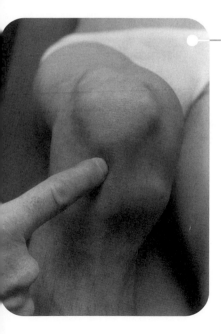

Fig. 10.7 | **The patellar apex (*apex patellae*)**

This points toward the distal extremity of the lower limb and receives the insertion of the patellar ligament. You can approach it with the knee flexed or extended.

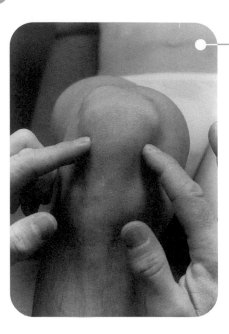

Fig. 10.8 | **The medial and lateral borders of the patella (*patella, margo lateralis*)**

These two borders run supero-inferiorly and lateromedially, with reference to the median axis of the patella. They are directly accessible to palpation.

Attachments
The borders of the patella, or more accurately their junctions with the base, provide attachment to the medial and lateral patellar retinacula.

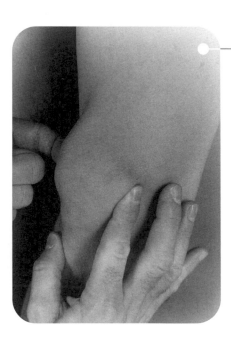

Fig. 10.9 | **The lateral approach to the lateral articular surface of the patella (*patella, facies articularis*)**

Only the most medial part of this facet is accessible. Hyper-extend the subject's knee, keeping the quadriceps femoris in a perfectly relaxed state, and you can feel it by displacing the patella laterally.

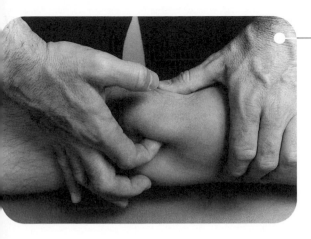

Fig. 10.10 | **The medial approach to the medial articular surface of the patella**

Hyperextend the knee, keeping the quadriceps femoris in a perfectly relaxed state, and you gain access to it by displacing the patella medially.

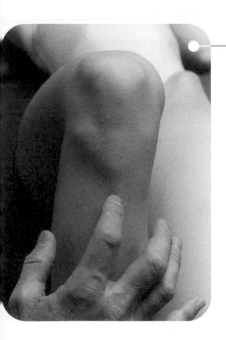

Fig. 10.11 | **The tibial tuberosity (*tuberositas tibiae*)**

This is triangular, with its apex located distally; it separates anteriorly the medial and lateral condyles of the tibia.

It is easy to access and gives insertion to the patellar ligament.

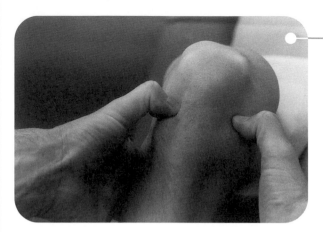

Fig. 10.12 | **The superior articular surface of the tibia (*tibia, facies articularis superior*)**

With the subject's knee flexed at 90°, place your thumbs on either side of the patellar ligament in the tibiofemoral joint space. Move your thumbs down to touch the non-articular border of the superior tibial surface. Palpate this border up to the point where it meets the femur.

Note: This approach also allows you to come into contact with the tibiofemoral joint space.

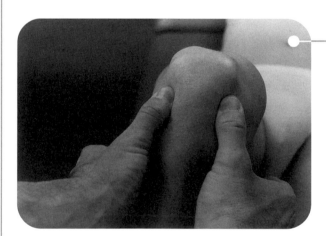

Fig. 10.13 | **The articular surfaces of the femoral condyles (*femur, condyli medialis et lateralis, facies articulares*)**

With the subject's knee flexed at 90°, place your thumbs on either side of the patellar ligament in the tibiofemoral joint space, and then move them upward to reach these surfaces. If you have any difficulty, flex the knee even more, and this will make access much easier.

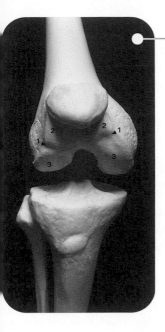

Fig. 10.14 | **Display of the oblique grooves (*sulci medialis et lateralis*)**

These two grooves in the distal cartilage-lined articular surface of the femur divide it into two parts: the articular surfaces in front of and above these grooves form part of the patellar surface or the trochlea; the articular surfaces behind and below these grooves are called the tibial articular surfaces.

1. Condylopatellar (trochleocondylar) grooves.
2. Patellar surface (trochlea).
3. Tibial articular surfaces of the femur.

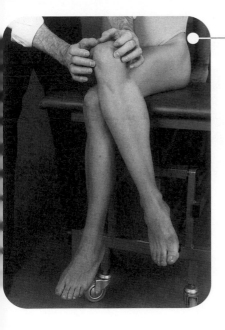

Fig. 10.15 | **Approach to the oblique grooves (*sulci medialis et lateralis*)**

For this the ideal position is with the knee flexed a little beyond 90°.

Run your fingers along the articular surface between the patella and the condylar articular surfaces themselves, and you will feel these two grooves (see (1) on Fig. 10.14).

Note: The lateral oblique groove is often the much easier one to feel with the fingers, since it is more pronounced.

THE MEDIAL COMPARTMENT

The bony structures that can be detected by palpation are:

- The femur (*femur*):
  - The medial epicondyle (*femur, epicondylus medialis*) (Figs 10.17 and 10.18)
  - The medial border of the patellar articular surface (*condylus medialis, facies patellaris, margo medialis*) (Fig. 10.19)
  - The medial oblique groove (*condylus medialis, sulcus*) (Fig. 10.19)
  - The patellar articular surface (*condylus medialis, facies patellaris*) (Fig. 10.20)
  - The adductor tubercle (*tuberculum adductorium*) (Fig. 10.21).
- The tibia (*tibia*):
  - The medial part of the superior articular surface (*tibia, facies articularis superior, pars medialis*) (Fig. 10.22)
  - The inferior border of the medial condyle (*tibia, condylus medialis*) (Fig. 10.23)
  - The superior part of the medial border (*tibia, margo medialis*), which is the crucial structure for the localization of the anserine muscles (Fig. 10.24).

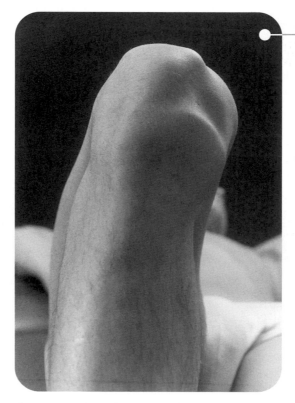

Fig. 10.16

Anteromedial view: knee flexed

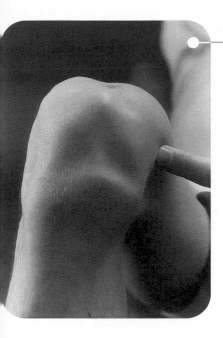

Fig. 10.17 | The medial epicondyle of the femur (*femur, epicondylus medialis*): anterior view

This is a subcutaneous structure directly accessible to palpation and represents the most prominent bony projection on the rough medial surface of the medial condyle.

Note: Its posterior aspect has a depression for the insertion of the tibial collateral ligament of the knee.

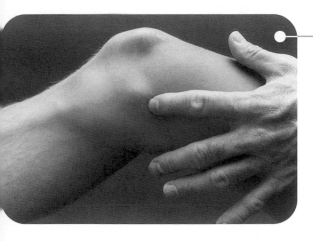

Fig. 10.18 | The medial epicondyle of the femur: medial view

A medial view allows a more precise display and localization of this structure.

Attachments

Behind the medial epicondyle there are the following:

- A depression for the insertion of the tibial collateral ligament.
- The adductor tubercle, which lies at the distal end of the medial branch of the distal bifurcation of the linea aspera and receives the insertion of the adductor magnus.

Below and behind this tubercle there is a depression from which arises the medial head of the gastrocnemius.

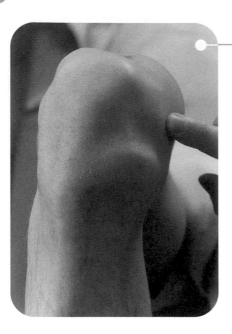

Fig. 10.19 | **The medial border of the patellar articular surface of the femur (*condylus medialis, facies patellaris*)**

This border is the lateral boundary of the patellar surface (trochlea) and of the medial tibial articular surface of the femur.

When the knee is maximally flexed there is easy access to this structure.

The medial oblique groove (*condylus medialis—sulcus*) is the lower border of the medial aspect of the condylar articular surface of the femur, which feels rough to the touch, and it is deeper posteriorly than anteriorly. Flex the subject's knee to free it from the adjacent musculotendinous structures.

Note: Remember that, when the knee is flexed, a large part of the distal articular surface of the femur is in front of you.

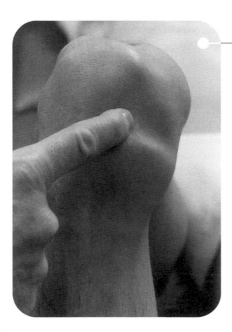

Fig. 10.20 | **The medial patellar articular surface of the femur (*condylus medialis, facies patellaris*)**

With your thumb and index finger locate the medial part of the tibiofemoral joint space. Starting from this point, run over the joint space, which you will feel as a smooth surface under your fingers, and which is bounded by the medial border of the medial patellar articular surface.

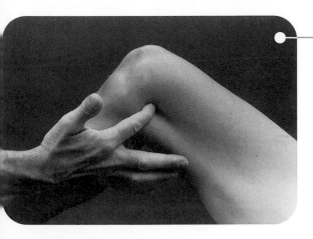

Fig. 10.21 | **The adductor tubercle (*tuberculum adductorium*)**

This structure is difficult to locate, but you can find it by first localizing the tendon of the vertical bundle of the adductor magnus (see Fig. 10.69).

You need only follow this tendon to its insertion and you will feel a projection, which is the adductor tubercle.

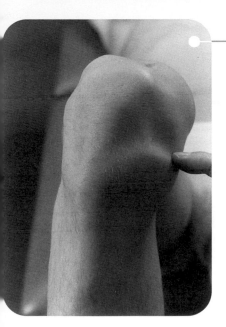

Fig. 10.22 | **The medial part of the superior articular surface of the tibia (*tibia, facies articularis superior, pars medialis*)**

With the knee flexed at 90° it is easy to locate this structure. Viewed from the front, the most medial part of this articular surface is important, since it is the site of approach to the tibial collateral ligament.

Note: Only the margin, and not the articular surface itself, is accessible to palpation.

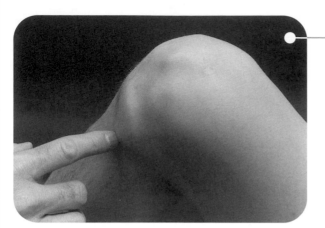

Fig. 10.23 | **The inferior border of the medial condyle of the tibia (*tibia, condylus medialis, margo inferior*)**

With the subject's knee flexed, you need only locate the medial border of the tibia and follow it up to its superior extremity. You will then easily get hold of the inferior border of the medial condyle using the pads of one or two fingers.

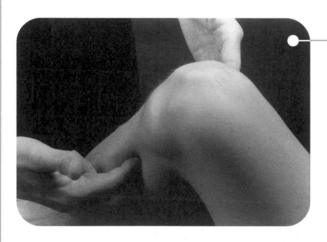

Fig. 10.24 | **The superior part of the medial border of the tibia (*tibia, margo medialis*)**

This is a notable bony structure where you can locate the three anserine muscles (that is, the semitendinosus, the gracilis, and the sartorius), which are inserted more distally into the anteromedial surface of the tibia close to its anterior border.

THE LATERAL COMPARTMENT

The bony structures that can be detected by palpation are:

- The femur (*femur*):
    — The lateral border of the suprapatellar fossa (*fossa suprapatellaris, margo lateralis*) (Fig. 10.26)
    — The lateral border of the patellar articular surface (*condylus lateralis, facies patellaris, margo lateralis*) (Fig. 10.27)
    — The lateral epicondyle (*femur, epicondylus lateralis*) (Fig. 10.28)
    — The lateral oblique groove (*condylus lateralis, sulcus*) (Fig. 10.29)
    — The lateral part of the patellar articular surface (*condylus lateralis, facies patellaris*) (Figs 10.29 and 10.30).
- The tibia (*tibia*):
    — The lateral part of the superior articular surface (*tibia: facies articularis superior, pars medialis*) (Fig. 10.31)
    — The infracondylar tubercle (Gerdy's tubercle) (*tuberculum infracondylare*) (Figs 10.32 and 10.33)
    — The oblique line (*tibia, linea obliqua*) (Fig. 10.34).
- The fibula (*fibula*):
    — The head (*caput fibulae*) (Fig. 10.35)
    — The neck (*collum fibulae*) (Fig. 10.36).

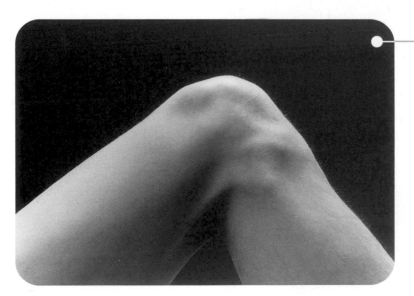

Fig. 10.25

Lateral view: knee flexed

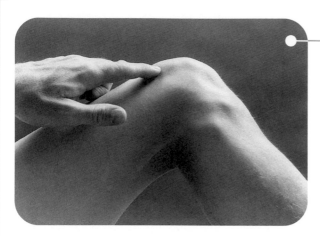

Fig. 10.26 | **The lateral border of the suprapatellar fossa of the femur (*fossa suprapatellaris, margo lateralis*)**

This is more marked than the medial border, the more so as the knee is brought into full flexion.

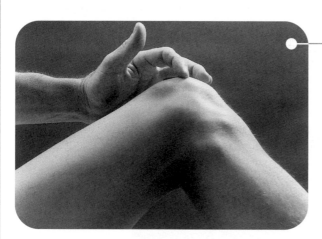

Fig. 10.27 | **The lateral border of the lateral patellar articular surface**

This lies very far laterally because the patella is markedly thrown off centre when the knee is flexed.

Note: As a result, the patellar articular surface is more exposed medially than laterally when the knee is flexed.

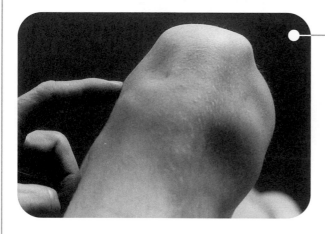

Fig. 10.28 | **The lateral epicondyle of the femur (*femur, epicondylus lateralis*)**

This is less prominent than the medial epicondyle and occupies the middle part of the lateral surface of the condyle.

If you have any difficulty finding it, stretch the fibular collateral ligament by opening the lateral part of the tibiofemoral joint space with the knee kept in flexion (see Fig. 10.39).

The lateral epicondyle is the femoral site of attachment of the above-mentioned ligament.

Attachments
- Below and behind the lateral epicondyle there is a depression from which the popliteus arises.
- Above and behind there is another depression giving origin to the lateral head of the gastrocnemius.
- Between the two depressions there is a crest to which the fibular collateral ligament is attached.

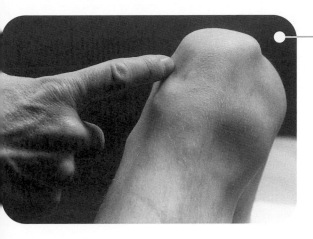

Fig. 10.29 | The lateral border of the lateral surface of the patellar articular surface of the femur (*condylus lateralis, facies articularis*)

This border laterally bounds the femoral trochlea (patellar articular surface) and the tibial articular surface of the lateral condyle.

When the knee is fully flexed it is easily accessible.

The lateral oblique groove *(condylus lateralis, sulcus)* is the lower boundary of the rough lateral surface of the lateral condyle. It is much deeper posteriorly than anteriorly.

Flex the knee to free it from the adjacent musculotendinous structures.

Note: Remember that, when the knee is flexed, the distal articular surface of the femur faces you.

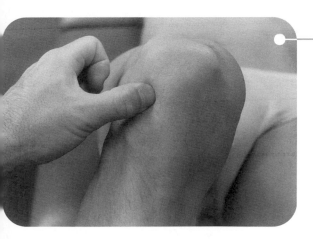

Fig. 10.30 | The lateral surface of the patellar articular surface of the femur

With your thumb find the lateral part of the tibiofemoral joint space. Starting from this point, run over the articular surface, which feels smooth under your fingers. This articular surface is bounded medially by the patellar ligament and the lateral border of the patella, and laterally by the lateral border of the patellar articular surface.

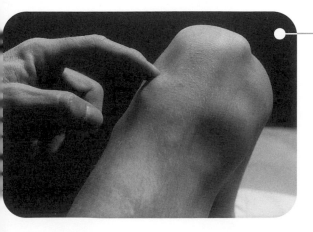

Fig. 10.31 | The lateral part of the superior articular surface of the tibia (*tibia, facies articularis superior, pars lateralis*)

When the knee is flexed this structure can easily be found. Viewed from the front the most lateral part of this articular surface is important, since it is the site of approach for the fibular collateral ligament at the knee joint.

Note: Its margin is accessible to palpation, but not the articular surface itself.

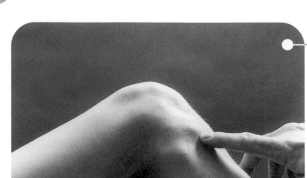

Fig. 10.32 | **The infracondylar tubercle (Gerdy's tubercle) (*tuberculum infracondylare*): lateral view**

This is the most prominent projection on the lateral tibial condyle. With the subject's knee flexed at 90°, look for it just below the lateral part of the superior articular surface of the tibia and lateral to the tibial tuberosity.

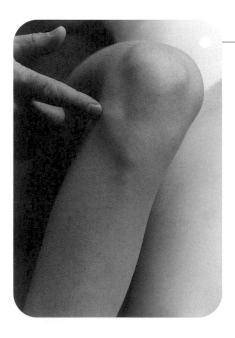

Fig. 10.33 | **The infracondylar tubercle: anterior view**

This additional anterior view provides a more precise display and localization of the tubercle. A further bony landmark is the fibular head, which is a bony structure lying behind and below the tubercle.

Attachment

It is the site of insertion of the tensor fasciae latae.

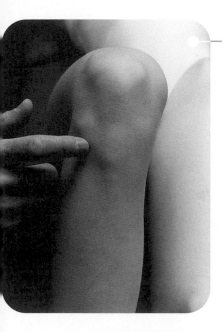

Fig. 10.34 | The oblique line of the tibia (*tibia, linea obliqua*): anterior view

This is a bony ridge running between the infracondylar tubercle (see Figs 10.32 and 10.33) and the lateral border of the tibial tuberosity (see Fig. 10.11). It is oblique supero-inferiorly and postero-anteriorly, and is directly accessible under the skin.

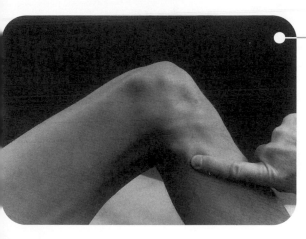

Fig. 10.35 | The fibular head (*caput fibulae*): lateral view

There is easy access to the fibular head. To bring it out further, you can first place the leg in medial rotation.

Note: The styloid process is a bony projection that arises posteriorly and laterally from the articular surface of the fibular head.

Attachment
The biceps femoris and the fibular collateral ligament are inserted into the apex of the fibular head near the styloid process.

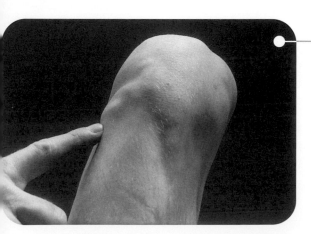

Fig. 10.36 | The fibular neck (*collum fibulae*): anterior view

This lies between the proximal end of the fibula and its shaft, and is notable in so far as the common peroneal nerve curves round it before entering the leg.

Knee joint, medial aspect

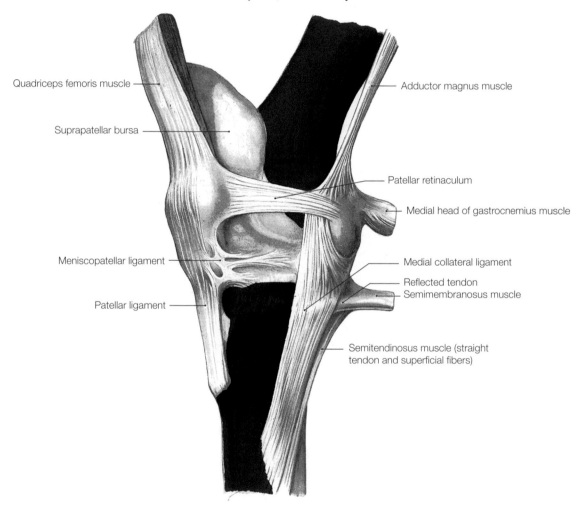

Quadriceps femoris muscle

Suprapatellar bursa

Meniscopatellar ligament

Patellar ligament

Adductor magnus muscle

Patellar retinaculum

Medial head of gastrocnemius muscle

Medial collateral ligament

Reflected tendon
Semimembranosus muscle

Semitendinosus muscle (straight tendon and superficial fibers)

Knee joint, lateral aspect

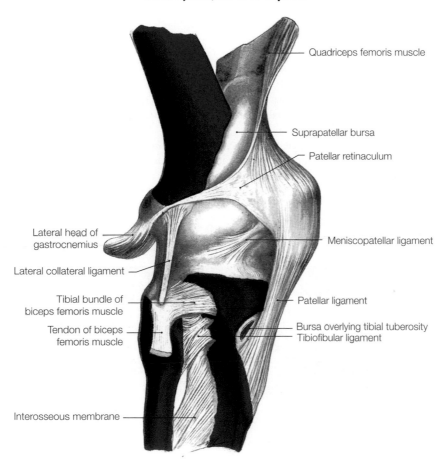

Quadriceps femoris muscle

Suprapatellar bursa

Patellar retinaculum

Lateral head of gastrocnemius

Lateral collateral ligament

Tibial bundle of biceps femoris muscle

Tendon of biceps femoris muscle

Meniscopatellar ligament

Patellar ligament

Bursa overlying tibial tuberosity
Tibiofibular ligament

Interosseous membrane

THE LIGAMENTS

The ligamentous structures that can be detected by palpation are:

- The fibular collateral ligament (*lig. collaterale fibulare*): method for displaying and stretching it (Figs 10.38 and 10.39).
- The lateral patellar retinaculum (*retinaculum patellae laterale*) (Figs 10.40–10.42).
- The tibial collateral ligament (*lig. collaterale tibiale*): method for displaying and stretching it (Figs 10.43–10.46).
- The medial patellar retinaculum (*retinaculum patellae mediale*) (Figs 10.47–10.49).
- The infrapatellar fat pad (*corpus adiposum infrapatellare*): how to display and approach it (Fig. 10.50).
- The patellar ligament (*lig. patellae*) (Fig. 10.51).

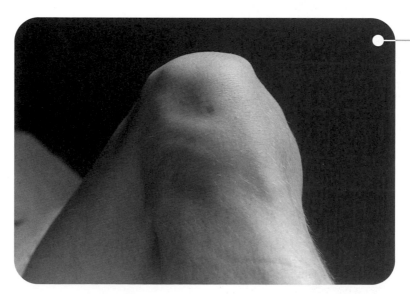

Fig. 10.37

Anterior view of the knee

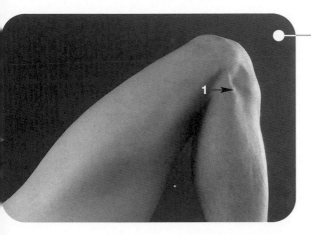

Fig. 10.38 | **Display of the fibular collateral ligament (*lig. collaterale fibulare*)**

This ligament (1) runs from the lateral femoral epicondyle to the anterolateral part of the fibular head in front of the styloid process.

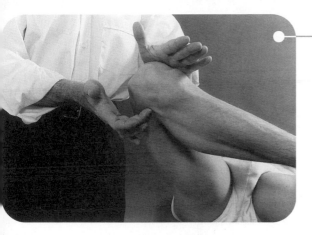

Fig. 10.39 | **Method for stretching the fibular collateral ligament**

In order to locate it under the best conditions it is preferable to stretch this ligament. Once located, it is easy to investigate in all positions of the knee joint.

Have the subject adopt a posture as indicated in the adjacent illustration. With one of your hands resting on the medial surface of the knee under investigation, apply some pressure mediolaterally in order to open up the lateral part of the joint space and stretch the ligament. Place your other hand to face the joint space between the fibular head and the lateral femoral epicondyle.

Note: Your fingers will feel the ligament as a solid cylindrical cord of variable thickness depending on the individual. Those with genu varum (knock knees) will obviously have a stronger and thicker ligament, because it is constantly stretched.

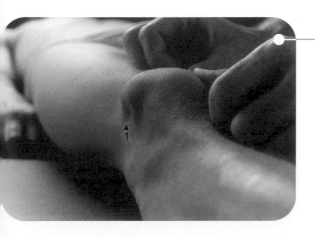

Fig. 10.40 | **Display of the lateral patellar retinaculum (*retinaculum patellae laterale*)**

When the knee is fully extended the quadriceps femoris is relaxed.

You can push the patella laterally and stretch the ligament (1), or you can push it medially with the same effect. Approach the retinaculum in a plane perpendicular to its course.

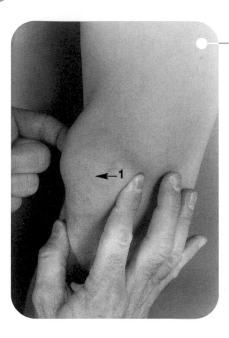

Fig. 10.41 | **Palpation of the lateral patellar retinaculum: transverse bundle**

In this maneuver, pushing the patella mediolaterally (1) brings the retinaculum as displayed in Figure 10.40 into a plane closer to the strict sagittal plane. It is a reinforcement of the capsule and is felt under your fingers as a fibrous band.

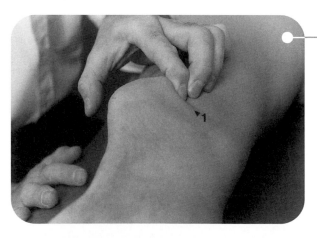

Fig. 10.42 | **Method for stretching the medial and lateral patellar retinacula simultaneously**

As you pull the patella laterally the medial retinaculum stands out (1), while the lateral retinaculum is stretched (not shown in the adjacent figure; see Fig. 10.40).

Note: During this procedure the medial retinaculum is stretched in a plane that gets progressively closer to the strict sagittal plane, whereas the lateral retinaculum is stretched in a progressively more horizontal plane. The adjacent figure provides an inferomedial view.

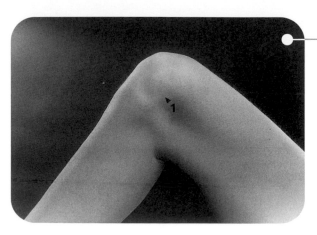

Fig. 10.43 | **Display of the tibial collateral ligament (*lig. collaterale tibiale*)**

This ligament (1) runs from the top of the medial femoral epicondyle and the depression just behind it to the superior part of the medial border of the tibia and its adjacent antero-medial surface.

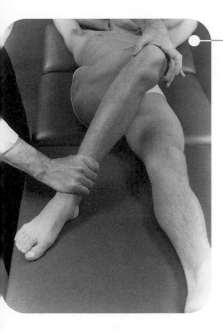

Fig. 10.44 | **Method for stretching the tibial collateral ligament**

Two steps are needed to stretch this ligament optimally.

First flex the subject's knee to 90° and laterally rotate the leg to stretch the ligament.

Next place your hand on the knee and push it medially while the foot stays still on the table. The joint space will gape medially and the ligament will be stretched more tightly.

Note: The same hand, whose fingers face the joint space, will feel the ligament as a fairly flat fibrous band.

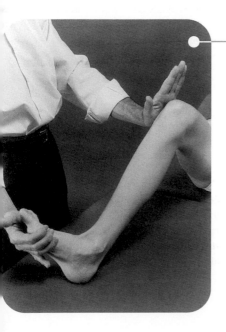

Fig. 10.45 | **Alternative method for stretching the tibial collateral ligament**

With the subject's heel lying on the table, take hold of the medial border of the foot in the palm of your hand so as to rotate the leg laterally.

Then use your other hand positioned flat on the lateral part of the knee to push the knee medially so as to open up the joint space and as a result stretch the ligament.

Note: The ligament stands out very clearly at the level of the joint space (see next figure).

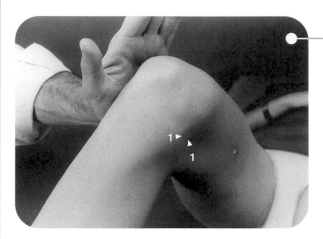

Fig. 10.46 | **Alternative method for stretching the tibial collateral ligament, similar to the previous one but shown in close-up**

This figure shows an anteromedial close-up view of the knee that demonstrates very clearly the stretching of the ligament.

Note: The ligament stands out very clearly at the level of the joint.

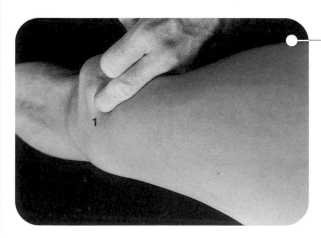

Fig. 10.47 | **Display of the transverse fibers of the medial patellar retinaculum: knee extended, medial view**

The knee is fully extended and the quadriceps femoris is relaxed.

Push the patella laterally so as to stretch the ligament (adjacent figure), or push it medially (Fig. 10.48) and you will again stretch the ligament.

Palpate the medial patellar retinaculum (1) in the same way, in both cases using a transverse approach.

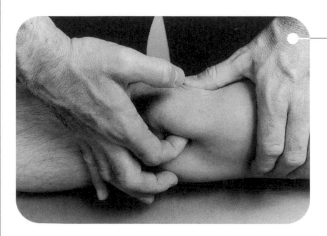

Fig. 10.48 | **Palpation of the medial patellar retinaculum (*retinaculum patellae mediale*)**

This maneuver stretches the retinaculum in a plane that gets progressively closer to the strict sagittal plane. The capsule is reinforced by the retinaculum, which is felt by the fingers as a fibrous band.

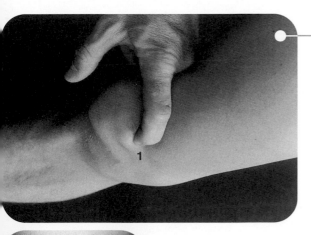

Fig. 10.49 | Method for stretching the transverse fibers of the medial patellar retinaculum by pulling the patella laterally

This procedure, similar to the one described in Figure 10.42, stretches the medial patellar retinaculum (1) in a plane that progressively approaches the horizontal plane. It is a reinforcement of the capsule, which is felt by the fingers as a fibrous band.

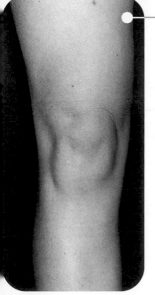

Fig. 10.50 | Display of the infrapatellar fat pad (*corpus adiposum infrapatellare*)

This is a large fat pad lying between the patellar ligament and the posterior non-articular portion of the patella, and above the anterior intercondylar area of the superior articular surface of the tibia. Laterally it extends halfway between the medial and lateral borders of the patella as folds of fat. It is easily visible and becomes more obvious when the subject is asked to extend the knee, as in the adjacent figure.

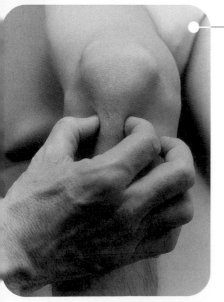

Fig. 10.51 | The patellar ligament (*ligamentum patellae*)

You can approach this ligament with the subject's knee flexed or extended. Take hold of its medial and lateral borders using a thumb–index pincer. You will feel it better thus as it runs obliquely supero-inferiorly and postero-anteriorly.

MYOLOGY

THE ANTEROLATERAL REGION

The muscular and tendinous structures that can be detected by palpation are:

In the thigh:

- The vastus lateralis (*m. vastus lateralis*) (Fig. 10.53).
- The iliotibial tract (*tractus iliotibialis*) (Fig. 10.54).
- The tendon of the biceps femoris (*m. biceps femoris*) (Fig. 10.55).

In the leg:

- The tibialis anterior (*m. tibialis anterior*) (Figs 10.56–10.58).
- The extensor digitorum longus (*m. extensor digitorum longus*) (Figs 10.56, 10.57, and 10.59).
- The peroneus longus (*m. peroneus longus*) (Figs 10.56, 10.57, 10.60).

(The approach to the proximal part of the peroneus longus is described in the section on the lateral compartment.)

Note: Since the patellar ligament is not an "active structure" it is dealt with in Figure 10.51, page 343.

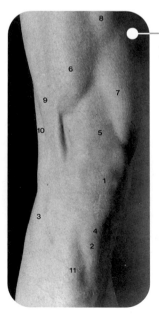

Fig. 10.52 | **Anterolateral view of the knee**

1. Patella.
2. Tibial tuberosity.
3. Head of the fibula.
4. Patellar ligament.
5. Quadriceps femoris tendon.
6. Vastus lateralis.
7. Vastus medialis.
8. Rectus femoris.
9. Iliotibial tract (Maissiat's band).
10. Biceps femoris tendon.
11. Tibialis anterior.

THE THIGH

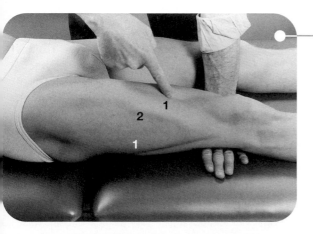

Fig. 10.53 | **The vastus lateralis (*m. vastus lateralis*)**

Ask the subject to press hard on your hand placed between his popliteal fossa and the table. The vastus lateralis (1) stands out in the anterolateral part of the thigh in front of and behind the iliotibial tract (2).

See also the figure below.

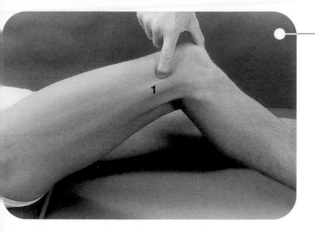

Fig. 10.54 | **The iliotibial tract (*tractus iliotibialis*)**

With the subject's knee flexed and foot resting on the table, ask him to start extending the knee, and the iliotibial tract (1) will appear or will be felt under your fingers on the lateral aspect of the knee. Active medial rotation of the leg will bring it out further, since it is stretched by this movement. You can equally well ask the subject to extend the knee fully so that you can feel the tract even better (see Figs 9.15 and 9.16.).

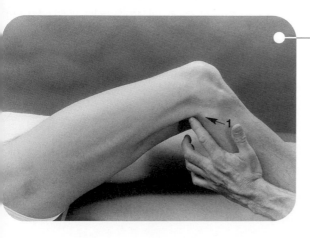

Fig. 10.55 | **The distal tendon of the biceps femoris (*m. biceps femoris, tendo distalis*)**

The main bony landmark is the fibular head (1).

Take hold of the subject's heel with the palm of one hand and resist his knee flexion; with the other hand positioned in the vicinity of the fibular head, you can approach the biceps, which in effect forms the superolateral border of the popliteal fossa (see also Figs 10.75 and 10.76.)

THE LEG

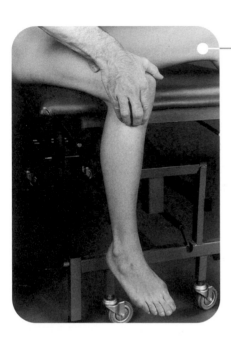

Fig. 10.56 | **Global localization of the tibialis anterior (*tibialis anterior*), the extensor digitorum longus (*m. extensor digitorum longus*) and the peroneus longus (*m. peroneus longus*)**

The subject sits on the edge of the table, and can also have the legs crossed. The foot hangs down in a relaxed state. (Subjects can also lie on their back with the trunk partly raised so that they can visually control the movements of the foot.)

With your thumb and fingers palpate the superolateral portion of the leg between the fibular head and the tibial tuberosity.

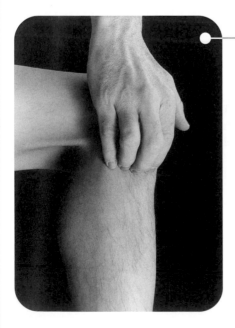

Fig. 10.57 | **Close-up of the global localization described above**

To be more precise, place your fourth and fifth fingers flat against the anterior part of the fibular head and your second and third fingers on the lateral border of the tibial tuberosity, just below the oblique line of the tibia and the infracondylar tubercle (Gerdy's tubercle).

While this global contact is in place, your little finger faces the peroneus longus, your ring finger the extensor digitorum longus, and your middle and index fingers the tibialis anterior.

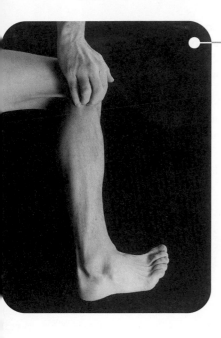

Fig. 10.58 | **Localization of the proximal part of the tibialis anterior**

From the starting position described in Figures 10.56 and 10.57, ask the subject to adduct, supinate, and dorsiflex the foot; these movements correspond to the actions of the tibialis anterior. You will feel the muscle contracting under your fingers: more precisely, under your second and third fingers.

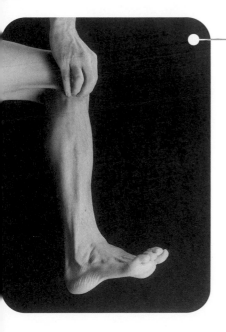

Fig. 10.59 | **Localization of the proximal part of the extensor digitorum longus**

From the starting point described in Figures 10.56 and 10.57, ask the subject to abduct, pronate, and dorsiflex the foot; these movements correspond to the actions of this muscle. You will feel the muscle contracting under your fingers: more precisely, under your ring finger.

Note: This muscle is not necessarily easily detected at this level. It can be masked by a well-developed tibialis anterior or peroneus longus, or both.

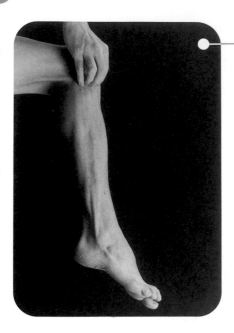

Fig. 10.60 | **Localization of the proximal part of the peroneus longus**

From the starting point described above, ask the subject to abduct, pronate, and plantarflex the foot; these movements correspond to the actions of this muscle. You will feel the muscle contracting under your fingers: more precisely, under your ring and little fingers.

THE ANTEROMEDIAL REGION

With the knee flexed at 90°, the muscular and tendinous structures that can be detected by palpation are, distoproximally:

- The tendon of the semitendinosus (*m. semitendinosus*) (Figs 10.62–10.65).
- The tendon of the gracilis (*m. gracilis*) (Figs 10.62–10.64, 10.66).
- The semimembranosus (*m. semimembranosus*) (Fig. 10.68).
- The sartorius (*m. sartorius*) (Figs 10.62–10.64, 10.67).
- The distal tendon of the vertical bundle of the adductor magnus (*m. adductor magnus*) (Fig. 10.69).
- The body of the vastus medialis (*m. vastus medialis*) (Fig. 10.70).

Note: The global approach to the anserine muscles is dealt with on the next page.

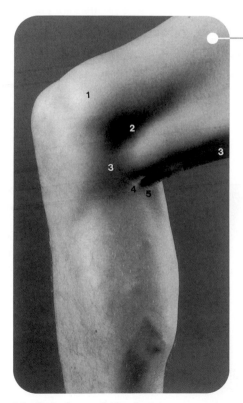

Fig. 10.61

Medial view of the knee

1. Vastus medialis.
2. Tendon of the adductor magnus.
3. Semimembranosus, lying on both sides of the semitendinosus.
4. Tendon of the gracilis.
5. Tendon of the semitendinosus.

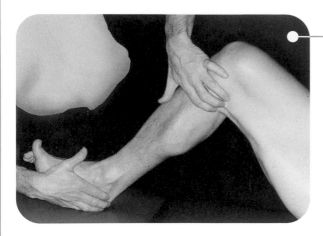

Fig. 10.62 | **Global localization of the anserine muscles (*pes anserinus*) on the medial tibial border**

First locate the distal end of the medial border of the tibia and position your fingers as shown in the figure. With your other hand, resist the subject's isometric flexion and medial rotation of the knee. Ask the subject to contract and relax these muscles in succession in order to bring out the muscles and their topographic distribution.

• The tendon of the semitendinosus is the lowest and is easily felt under the index finger.
• The tendon of the gracilis lies above the former and is felt under the middle finger.
• The distal part of the sartorius overlies the gracilis. Contraction of this muscle is felt under the ring finger (see also Fig. 10.67), and even better if the subject is asked to flex the knee slightly.

Note: If the tendons on the medial tibial border are difficult to feel, palpate them more proximally by moving your fingers slightly posteriorly. This is the case with women, whose subcutaneous fat hampers palpation of these muscles at this level.

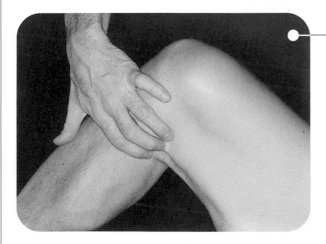

Fig. 10.63 | **Close-up of the global localization described above**

This figure is of interest as it clearly shows the relative positions of the different tendons and muscle bodies. The practitioner's index finger faces the tendon of the semitendinosus, the middle finger faces the tendon of the gracilis, and the ring finger faces the tendon of the sartorius, which is not shown in this figure and is better felt if the subject is asked to extend the knee slightly.

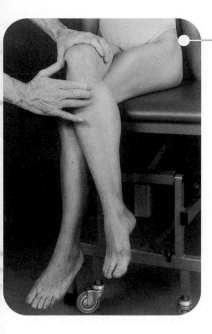

Fig. 10.64 | **Simultaneous detection of the contraction of the anserine muscles on the anterior and medial part of the tibia**

Use a large surface of contact and place all your fingers together under the medial tibial condyle while holding in your palm the tibial tuberosity, which is continuous with these tendons (Figs 10.62 and 10.63). Subjects activate the same muscles as in Figure 10.62. As they flex the knee isometrically against the contralateral lower limb, they also medially rotate the leg by moving the tips of the toes medially, since the anserine muscles are also medial rotators of the leg. You can then feel the contraction of these muscles directly under your fingers.

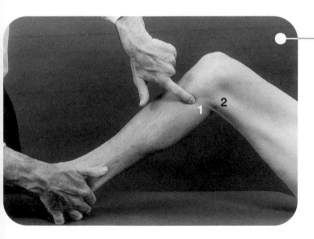

Fig. 10.65 | **The distal tendon of the semitendinosus (*m. semitendinosus, tendo distalis*)**

The main bony landmark is the proximal end of the medial border of the tibia.

With the subject's knee flexed at about 90°, place one of your hands flat on the posterior surface of the calcaneus and the medial border of the foot; resist the subject's flexion and medial rotation of the knee, while your other hand goes up the medial border of the tibia until it reaches the semitendinosus tendon (1).

You can also ask the subject to press the heel against the table, thus causing an isometric flexion of the knee. Then ask the subject to perform a succession of rapid medial rotations of the leg. Your two hands are then free to investigate.

Warning: Locating this tendon is relatively easy in men, but much more difficult in women because of their subcutaneous fat. In case of difficulty, look for it more posteriorly in the fleshy mass of the upper calf, and even in the popliteal region (see Fig. 10.72).

Legends for Figures 10.65 and 10.66

1. Semitendinosus
2. Gracilis

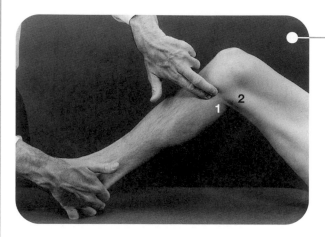

Fig. 10.66 | **The distal tendon of the gracilis (*m. gracilis, tendo distalis*)**

The bony landmark is the same: the medial tibial border, where you place the fingers of one hand.

With the other hand, resist the subject's knee flexion and medial rotation by holding the heel in your palm and placing your forearm against the medial border of the subject's foot.

You will feel the tendon you are looking for (2) (see also Fig. 10.73) above that of the semitendinosus and below the sartorius (see also Fig. 10.67), which can partially overlap it.

Warning: The same difficulty arises as with the tendon of the semitendinosus (Fig. 10.65).

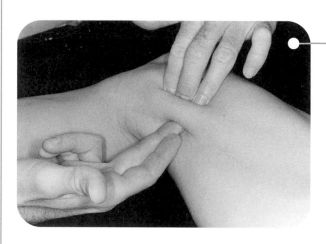

Fig. 10.67 | **The distal part of the sartorius (*m. sartorius*): medial view, knee semiflexed**

Extend the subject's knee almost completely and rotate his hip slightly laterally to bring out the body of the muscle on the medial surface of the knee.

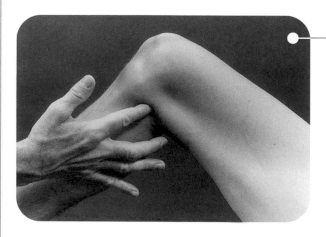

Fig. 10.68 | **The tendon of the semimembranosus (*m. semimembranosus, tendo*)**

The main bony landmark is the angle at the junction of the medial and posterior surfaces of the medial tibial condyle. Rotate the leg laterally in order to bring out this bony landmark. With one of your hands, resist the subject's knee flexion and medial rotation; with the other look for a tendon that your fingers can feel as a full, fairly thick, cylindrical cord. More anteriorly the reflected tendon of this muscle slides under the tibial collateral ligament in the horizontal groove on the medial tibial condyle.

Warning: Avoid difficulty by placing the leg correctly in lateral rotation and thus freeing the tendon.

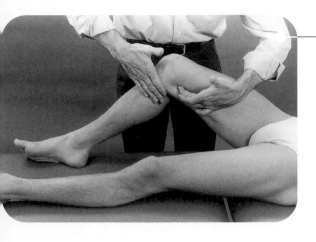

Fig. 10.69 | **The distal tendon of the vertical or inferior bundle of the adductor magnus (*m. adductor magnus, tendo distalis*)**

The main bony landmark is the adductor tubercle (see also Fig. 10.21).

The main muscular landmark is the vastus medialis (see Fig. 10.70).

The tendon you are looking for lies behind this muscle and is felt under your fingers as a solid and relatively thick cylindrical cord (see also Fig. 9.23.)

Note: You can place your distal hand on the medial surface of the knee and push it into abduction against the subject's resistance; your fingers will feel the tendon better.

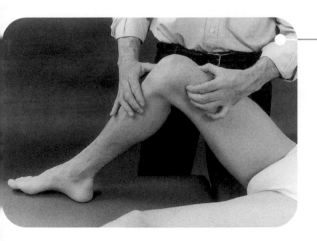

Fig. 10.70 | **The body of the vastus medialis (*m. vastus medialis*)**

To bring out this muscle, if the knee is flexed, ask subjects to dig the heel into the table. If the knee is extended, ask them to contract the quadriceps femoris.

The body of the muscle will stand out above and on the inside of the patella.

Note: This muscle extends farther distally than the vastus lateralis (Fig. 10.52). (See also Fig. 9.10.)

THE POSTERIOR REGION

The muscular and tendinous structures that can be detected by palpation are:
   In the thigh:

- The tendon of the semitendinosus (*m. semitendinosus*) (Fig. 10.72).
- The tendon of the gracilis (*m. gracilis*) (Fig. 10.73).
- The semimembranosus (*m. semimembranosus*) (Fig. 10.74).
- The tendon of the biceps femoris (*m. biceps femoris*) (Fig. 10.75).
- The tendon of the popliteus (*m. popliteus, tendo*) (Fig. 10.76).

   In the leg:

- The medial head of the gastrocnemius (*m. gastrocnemius, caput mediale*) (see Chapter 11).
- The lateral head of the gastrocnemius (*m. gastrocnemius, caput laterale*) (see Chapter 11).

Note: In this chapter only the muscles located in the thigh and the tendon of the popliteus will be dealt with. For the other muscles, refer to Chapter 11.

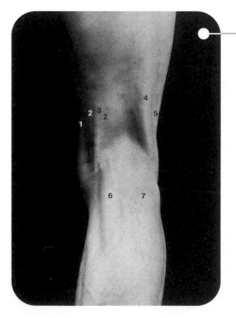

Fig. 10.71

Posterior view of the knee

1. Gracilis.
2. Semimembranosus.
3. Semitendinosus.
4. Biceps femoris.
5. Iliotibial tract.
6. Medial head of the gastrocnemius.
7. Lateral head of the gastrocnemius.

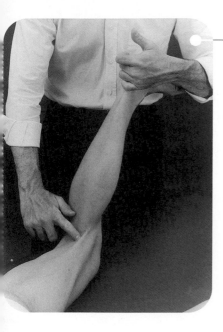

Fig. 10.72 | The tendon of the semitendinosus

With the subject lying on his belly, use your distal hand to take hold of his heel in your palm and resist his knee flexion. You can also resist his medial knee rotation by placing your forearm on the medial border of the foot.

The semitendinosus tendon is the most posterior and lateral of the musculotendinous structures present in the posteromedial aspect of the thigh.

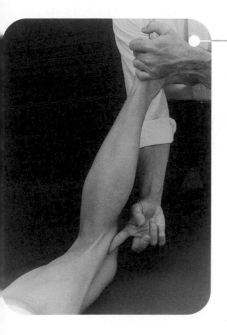

Fig. 10.73 | The tendon of the gracilis

The position of the patient and the resistance applied by the practitioner are the same as those described in Figure 10.72.

The tendon of the gracilis is seen in front and on the inside of the tendon of the semitendinosus.

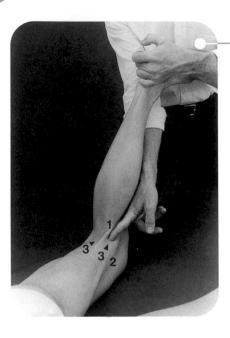

Fig. 10.74 | **The semimembranosus**

The position of the patient and the resistance applied by the practitioner are the same as those described in Figure 10.72.

The semimembranosus (3) is a fleshy muscle felt under the fingers between the tendons of the semitendinosus (1) and the gracilis (2). It is also felt lateral to the tendon of the semitendinosus (1).

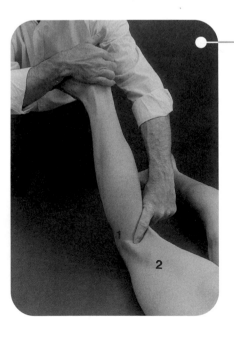

Fig. 10.75 | **Locating the biceps femoris (*m. biceps femoris*) in the popliteal fossa (*fossa poplitea*)**

With subjects lying on their belly, use one hand to take hold of their heel in your palm and place your forearm on the lateral border of their foot so as to be able to resist their knee flexion and lateral knee rotation simultaneously. The tendon appears (see adjacent illustration) (1) in the posterior and lateral part of the popliteal fossa. The body of the muscle (2) is easily visible.

1. Tendon of insertion of the biceps femoris into the fibular head.
2. The body of the long head of the biceps femoris.

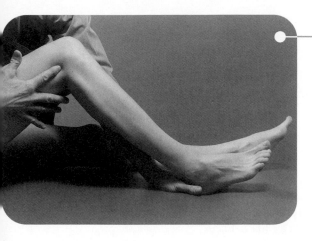

Fig. 10.76 | **The tendon of the popliteus**
(m. popliteus, tendo)

With one hand resist the subject's knee flexion and place your other hand behind the fibular collateral ligament (see also Figs 10.38 and 10.39).

The tendon you are looking for is felt just behind this ligament, but not in every subject. Contraction of the lateral head of the gastrocnemius can also interfere with its detection.

NERVES AND BLOOD VESSELS

THE POPLITEAL FOSSA (*FOSSA POPLITEA*)

The vascular and neural structures that can be detected by palpation are:

- The tibial nerve (*n. tibialis*) (Figs 10.79 and 10.81).
- The common peroneal nerve (*n. peroneus communis*) (Fig. 10.83).
- The lateral sural cutaneous nerve (*n. cutaneus surae lateralis*) (Figs 10.84 and 10.85).
- The popliteal artery (*a. poplitea*) (Figs 10.87–10.89).

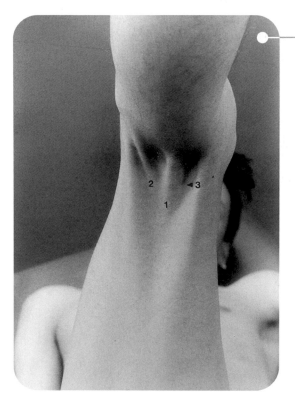

Fig. 10.77

Posterior view of the popliteal fossa (*fossa poplitea*)

The subject is supine with hip and knee flexed.
1. Tibial nerve.
2. Common peroneal nerve.
3. Popliteal artery.

Note: The arrow indicates the recommended point for the optimal approach to the popliteal artery.

THE TIBIAL NERVE (*N. TIBIALIS*)[1]

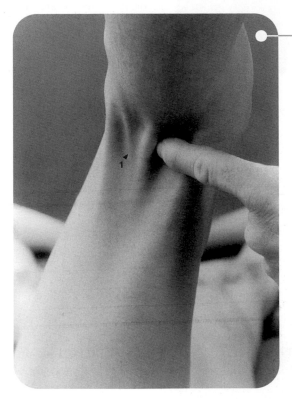

Fig. 10.78

Posterior view of the popliteal fossa

The subject is supine with hip and knee flexed. The index finger points to the tibial nerve.

1. Common peroneal nerve.

[1] The tibial nerve is also called the medial popliteal nerve and the posterior tibial nerve above and below the upper border of the soleus respectively.

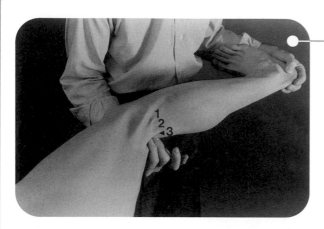

Fig. 10.79 | **Displaying the tibial, common peroneal, and lateral sural cutaneous nerves**

The subject lies on his side with the hip flexed beyond 90°. Flex his knee slightly and also bring his ankle into dorsiflexion.

The index finger in the adjacent illustration is pointing to the structures you are looking for.

Legends for Figures 10.79 and 10.80

1. Common peroneal nerve
2. Lateral sural cutaneous nerve
3. Tibial nerve
4. Tendon of the biceps femoris

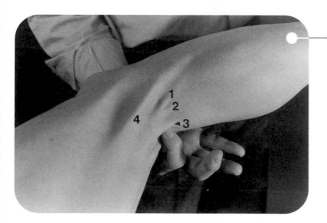

Fig. 10.80 | **Close-up of the popliteal fossa: display of the nerves listed above**

The same technique is used to display the nerves as previously described. With the subject lying on his back, fully dorsiflex his heel passively, slightly flex his knee and progressively flex his hip more or less fully. If this is not enough to bring out the nerve (2) located in the middle of the popliteal fossa, ask the subject to flex his trunk (Fig. 10.81).

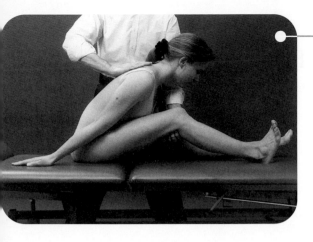

Fig. 10.81 | **Stretching the nerves located in the popliteal fossa**

- The tibial nerve: the subject is seated with the knee flexed between 90° and 40°, and one of the ankles dorsiflexed fully. Place your palpating hand at the centre of the popliteal fossa, and with your other hand placed on the subject's back, bend her trunk in order to stretch farther the sciatic nerve and its terminal branches, including the tibial nerve, further and make them more accessible to palpation. You feel the nerve under your fingers as a full cylindrical cord.
- The common peroneal nerve: while the subject stays in the same position, use your hand to locate the tendon of the biceps femoris; the nerve lies medial to the muscle and runs toward the fibular neck. Ask the subject to invert and dorsiflex the foot in order to stretch the nerve further.
- The lateral sural cutaneous nerve: this is a branch of the common peroneal nerve. To stretch it, use the same method as for the common peroneal nerve.

THE COMMON PERONEAL NERVE

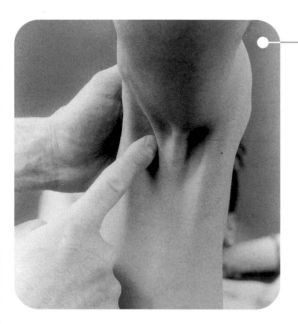

Fig. 10.82 | **Posterior view of the popliteal fossa**

Subjects lie on their back with hip and knee flexed.

In the adjacent illustration the index finger is pointing to the common peroneal nerve.

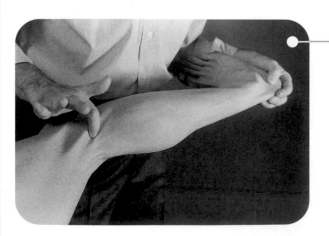

Fig. 10.83 | **Displaying the common peroneal nerve (*n. peroneus/fibularis communis*)**

With subjects lying on their side, use the same technique as described for the nerves of the popliteal fossa (Fig. 10.81).

In the adjacent illustration the index finger is pointing to the nerve.

THE LATERAL SURAL CUTANEOUS NERVE

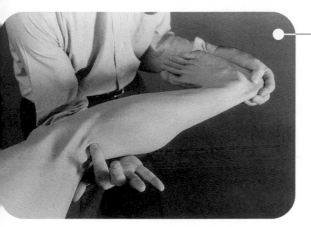

Fig. 10.84 | **Displaying the lateral sural cutaneous nerve (*n. cutaneous surae lateralis*)**

With subjects lying on their side, use the same technique as described for the common peroneal nerve. The practitioner's index finger is indicating the nerve you are looking for.

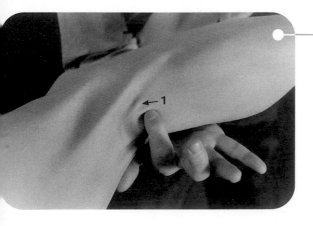

Fig. 10.85 | **Close-up of the popliteal fossa (*fossa poplitea*)**

For the display technique, see Figure 10.81.

The practitioner's index finger is pointing out the structure you are looking for (that is, the lateral sural cutaneous nerve). You can also see the common peroneal nerve (1) lateral to it, as it runs toward the fibular neck.

THE SAPHENOUS NERVE

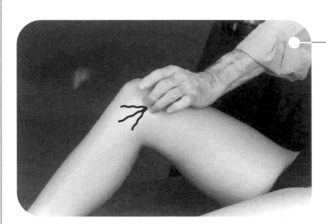

Fig. 10.86 | **The infrapatellar branch of the saphenous nerve (*n. saphenus*)**

This is one of the two terminal branches of the saphenous nerve. All you have to do is roll the nerve under your fingers as soon as it pierces the sartorius. You can thus feel it between the muscle and the patella on the medial tibial condyle, where you can roll it under the pads of two of your fingers.

THE POPLITEAL ARTERY

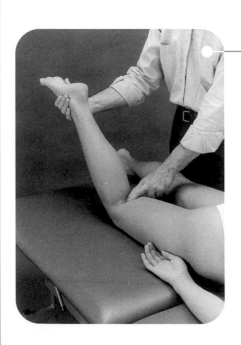

Fig. 10.87 | **Taking the pulse in the popliteal fossa**
Stage 1

Extend the subject's knee almost fully in order to be able to place the pads of two or three of your fingers in the supero-medial part of the popliteal fossa on the tendon of the semitendinosus.

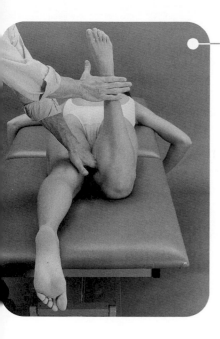

Fig. 10.88 | **Taking the pulse in the popliteal fossa**
Stage 2

Flex the subject's knee progressively and move the pads of your fingers toward the central part of the popliteal fossa as you look for the popliteal pulse, which you will find close to the tibial nerve.

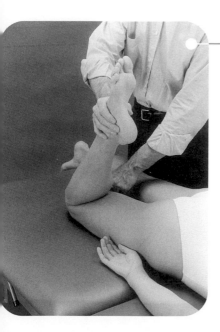

Fig. 10.89 | **Taking the pulse in the popliteal fossa**
Stage 3

When the knee is almost fully flexed, the posterior fascia of the knee is optimally relaxed, and it is easier to gain access to the popliteal artery, which is felt near the medial part of the tibial nerve.

CHAPTER 11

THE LEG

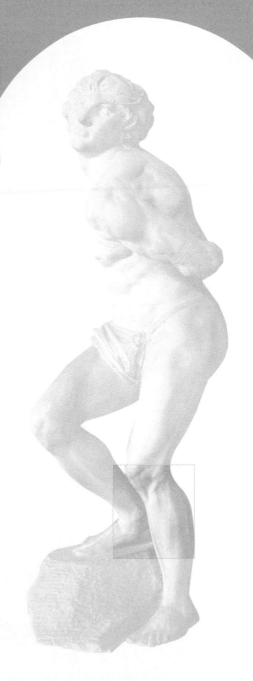

TOPOGRAPHICAL PRESENTATION OF THE LEG (*CRUS*)

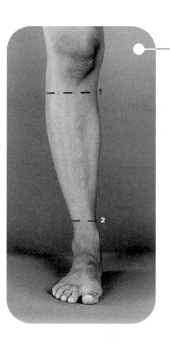

Fig. 11.1 | **Anterior view**

1. Superior boundary.
2. Inferior boundary.

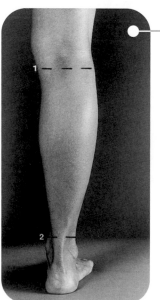

Fig. 11.2 | **Posterior view**

1. Superior boundary.
2. Inferior boundary.

OSTEOLOGY

ATTACHMENTS OF THE LEG MUSCLES

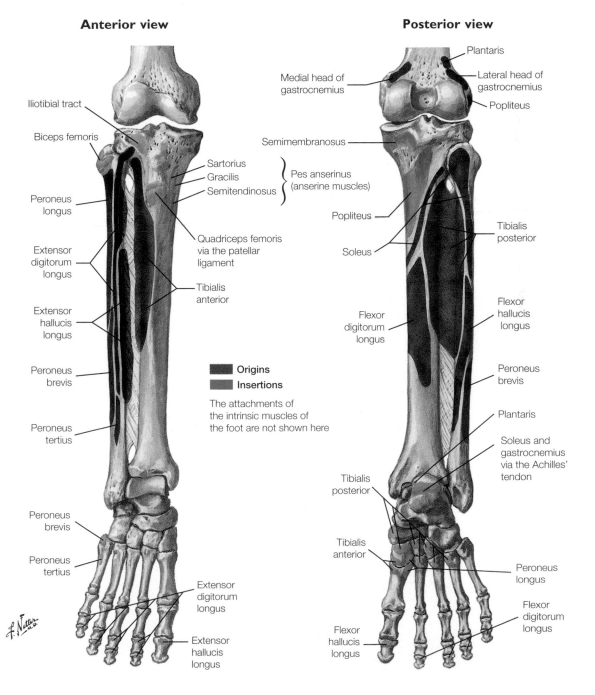

Anterior view

- Iliotibial tract
- Biceps femoris
- Peroneus longus
- Extensor digitorum longus
- Extensor hallucis longus
- Peroneus brevis
- Peroneus tertius
- Peroneus brevis
- Peroneus tertius
- Sartorius
- Gracilis
- Semitendinosus
- } Pes anserinus (anserine muscles)
- Quadriceps femoris via the patellar ligament
- Tibialis anterior
- Extensor digitorum longus
- Extensor hallucis longus

Posterior view

- Medial head of gastrocnemius
- Semimembranosus
- Popliteus
- Soleus
- Flexor digitorum longus
- Tibialis posterior
- Tibialis anterior
- Flexor hallucis longus
- Plantaris
- Lateral head of gastrocnemius
- Popliteus
- Tibialis posterior
- Flexor hallucis longus
- Peroneus brevis
- Plantaris
- Soleus and gastrocnemius via the Achilles' tendon
- Peroneus longus
- Flexor digitorum longus

■ Origins
■ Insertions

The attachments of the intrinsic muscles of the foot are not shown here

F. Netter M.D.

THE LEG

The bony structures that can be detected by palpation are:

- The tibia:
    — The anterior border (*tibia, margo anterior*) (Fig. 11.3).
    — The medial border (*tibia, margo medialis*) (Fig. 11.4).
    — The medial surface (*tibia, facies medialis*) (Fig. 11.5).
    — The posterior border *(tibia, facies posterior)* (Fig. 11.6).
- The fibula (fibula):
    — The lateral surface (*fibula, facies lateralis*) (Fig. 11.7).

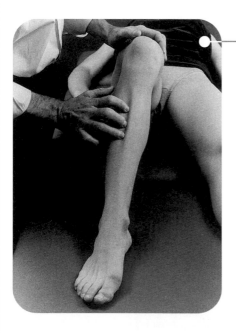

Fig. 11.3 | **The anterior border of the tibia (*tibia, margo anterior*)**

This extends from the tibial tuberosity to the medial malleolus.

In its upper three-quarters it is crest-like: hence the term *tibial crest* (the shin).

In its lower quarter it veers medially towards the medial malleolus and becomes blunt.

As it lies directly under the skin, the anterior border is accessible in its entirety and very easy to investigate.

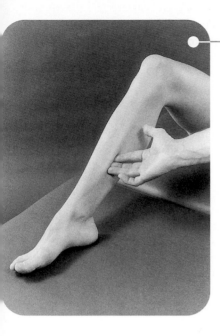

Fig. 11.4 | **The medial border of the tibia**
(tibia, margo medialis)

This stretches from the medial tibial condyle to the medial malleolus, and borders the tibial shaft medially.

It is also accessible to investigation in its entirety.

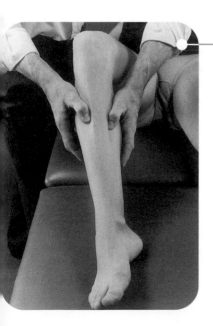

Fig. 11.5 | **The medial surface of the tibia**
(tibia, facies medialis)

This is smooth and flat and lies directly under the skin along its entire length. Its proximal part near the tuberosity receives the insertions of the anserine muscles.

As it lies between the anterior (Fig. 11.3) and the medial border (Fig. 11.4), it is accessible to investigation along its entire length.

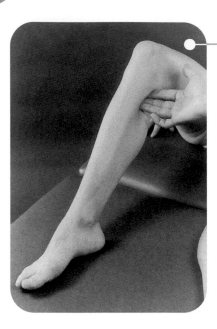

Fig. 11.6 | **The posterior surface of the tibia**
(*tibia, facies posterior*)

This is partly accessible to investigation behind the media
border of the tibia, and particularly at the proximal and dista
ends of the shaft.

In the adjacent illustration the leg is laterally rotated to free
this surface properly for palpation very close to the proxima
end and behind its medial border (see also Fig. 11.4). Take
care to relax the posterior muscles of the leg thoroughly.

Attachments
- The popliteus arises from above the oblique line and its
  upper lip.
- The soleus arises from the oblique line.
- The tibialis posterior and the flexor digitorum longus arise
  from the lower lip of the oblique line.
- Below the oblique line a vertical ridge separates the origin
  of the flexor digitorum longus medially from the tibialis
  posterior laterally.

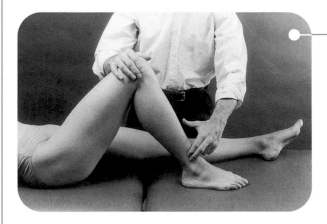

Fig. 11.7 | **The lateral surface of the fibula**
(*tibia, facies lateralis*)

This is directly accessible in its distal part. Its distal end bear
an oblique ridge that runs supero-inferiorly and anteroposte
riorly and divides it into two parts:

- An anterior triangular part, which lies directly under the
  skin and is easily accessible.
- A posterior part, on which the tendons of the peroneu
  brevis and the peroneus longus run.

Attachments
The superiorly convex lateral surface forms a longitudina
gutter in its intermediate part and gives origin to the peroneu
longus and the peroneus brevis.

MYOLOGY

Anterior muscles of the leg

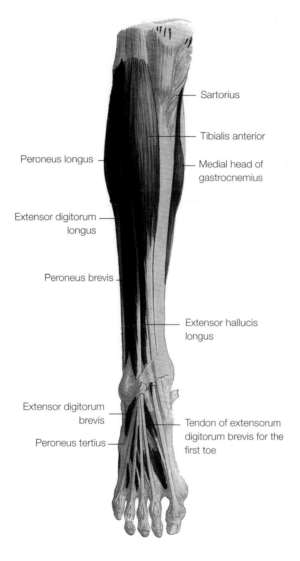

Sartorius

Tibialis anterior

Peroneus longus

Medial head of
gastrocnemius

Extensor digitorum
longus

Peroneus brevis

Extensor hallucis
longus

Extensor digitorum
brevis

Tendon of extensorum
digitorum brevis for the
first toe

Peroneus tertius

THE LEG

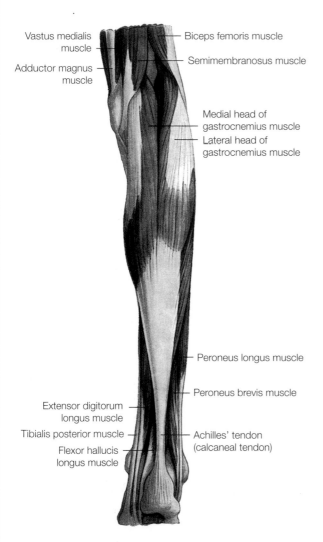

Vastus medialis muscle

Adductor magnus muscle

Biceps femoris muscle

Semimembranosus muscle

Medial head of gastrocnemius muscle

Lateral head of gastrocnemius muscle

Peroneus longus muscle

Peroneus brevis muscle

Extensor digitorum longus muscle

Tibialis posterior muscle

Flexor hallucis longus muscle

Achilles' tendon (calcaneal tendon)

Superficial layer: triceps surae with both heads of the gastrocnemius

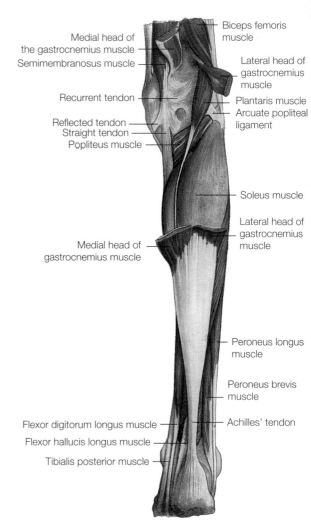

Medial head of the gastrocnemius muscle

Semimembranosus muscle

Recurrent tendon

Reflected tendon
Straight tendon
Popliteus muscle

Medial head of gastrocnemius muscle

Flexor digitorum longus muscle

Flexor hallucis longus muscle

Tibialis posterior muscle

Biceps femoris muscle

Lateral head of gastrocnemius muscle

Plantaris muscle
Arcuate popliteal ligament

Soleus muscle

Lateral head of gastrocnemius muscle

Peroneus longus muscle

Peroneus brevis muscle

Achilles' tendon

Soleus and plantaris:

The two heads of the gastrocnemius have been largely resected and the medial head pulled back.

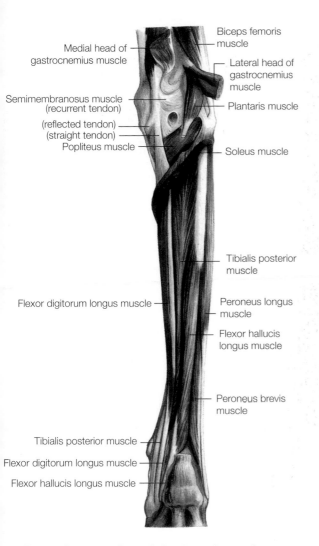

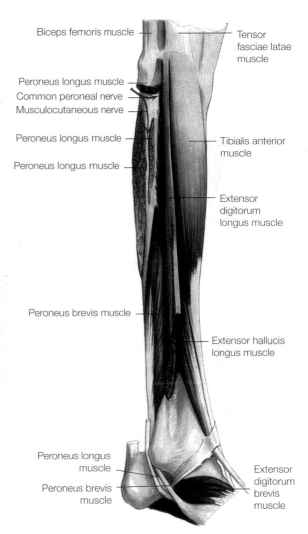

Posterior muscles of the leg, deep plane

Anterior and lateral muscles of the leg

The inferior part of the extensor digitorum longus has been removed, as well as the peroneus longus, which has been resected level with its origin.

THE ANTERIOR MUSCLE GROUP

The muscles are four in number:

- Tibialis anterior (*m. tibialis anterior*) (Figs 11.9–11.12).
- Extensor hallucis longus (*m. extensor hallucis longus*) (Figs 11.15–11.17).
- Extensor digitorum longus (*m. extensor digitorum longus*) (Figs 11.18 and 11.19).
- Peroneus tertius (*m. peroneus tertius*) (Fig. 11.20).

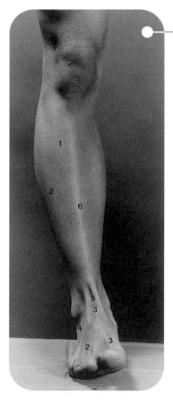

Fig. 11.8

Anterior view of the leg

1. Tibialis anterior.
2. Extensor digitorum longus.
3. Extensor hallucis longus.
4. Peroneus tertius.
5. Inferior extensor retinaculum.
6. Anterior border of the tibia.

*The tibialis anterior (*m. tibialis anterior*)*

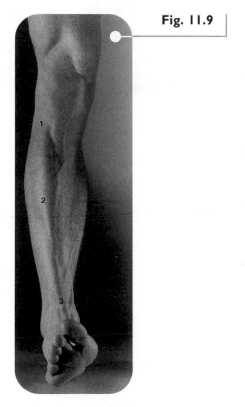

Fig. 11.9

Anterior view of the leg

1. Tibialis anterior: origin.
2. Tibialis anterior: body of muscle.
3. Tibialis anterior: tendon of insertion.

Actions of the tibialis anterior
It adducts, supinates, and dorsiflexes the foot on the leg.

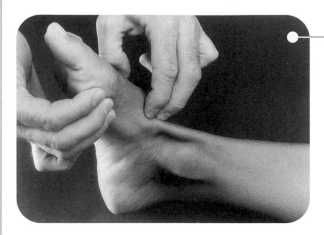

Fig. 11.10 | The distal part of the tibialis anterior tendon (*m. tibialis anterior, tendo distalis*)

First adduct, supinate, and dorsiflex the subject's foot; then place your fingerpads on the medial border of the subject's foot to resist his movements, which are meant to bring out the tendon. This is the most medial of the tendons crossing the ankle and lies just in front of the medial malleolus.

Attachment

In the adjacent illustration the practitioner's fingers face the tendon near its insertion into the medial cuneiform and its expansion into the inferomedial aspect of the base of the first metatarsal.

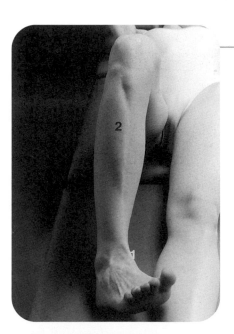

Fig. 11.11 | The tibialis anterior in the leg

This tendon (1) runs laterally along the tibial crest (the anterior border of the tibia). Its body (2) also proceeds lateral to the tibial crest and medial to the extensor digitorum longus.

To bring out the muscle, ask the subject to perform the same movements as described above.

Note: In this figure, the muscle is easily displayed.

Attachment

It arises from the infracondylar tubercle (Gerdy's tubercle), the oblique line (see Fig. 10.34, p. 335), and the upper two-thirds of the anterolateral surface of the tibia.

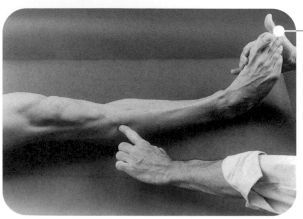

Fig. 11.12 | The origin of the tibialis anterior

(See also Figs 10.56–10.58.)

Ask the subject to move the foot into place as described in Figure 11.10, since these movements are specific for this muscle. At the same time resist these movements by placing your fingers on the medial border of the foot in order to observe the muscle contract under your fingers.

*The extrinsic extensor muscles of the toes and the peroneus tertius (*m. peroneus tertius*)*

This group has three muscles:

- The extensor hallucis longus (*m. extensor hallucis longus*) (Figs 11.15–11.17).
- The extensor digitorum longus (*m. extensor digitorum longus*) (Figs 11.18 and 11.19).
- The peroneus tertius (*m. peroneus tertius*) (Fig. 11.20).

This last muscle, sometimes absent, runs from the inferior third of the fibula to the fifth metatarsal.

Note: The extensor digitorum brevis also extends the toes, but it is an intrinsic muscle of the foot and is dealt with in Chapter 12.

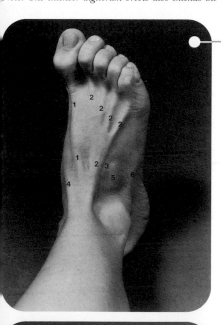

Fig. 11.13 | **Dorsal view of the foot**

1. Extensor hallucis longus.
2. Extensor digitorum longus.
3. Peroneus tertius.
4. Tibialis anterior.
5. Extensor digitorum brevis.
6. Peroneus brevis.

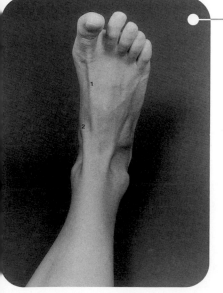

Fig. 11.14 | **Anterior view of the ankle**

1. Extensor hallucis longus.
2. Tibialis anterior.

Actions of the extensor digitorum longus, extensor hallucis longus, and peroneus tertius
- The extensor digitorum longus abducts, pronates, and dorsiflexes the foot on the leg and extends the toes.
- The extensor hallucis longus extends the big toe and takes part in foot dorsiflexion.
- The peroneus tertius dorsiflexes and everts the foot.

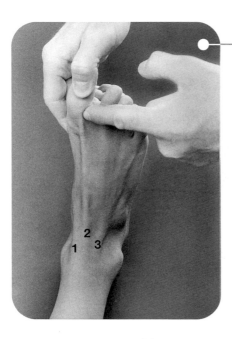

Fig. 11.15 | **The tendon of the extensor hallucis longus (*m. extensor hallucis longus, tendo*) near its insertion**

Ask the subject to extend the big toe and resist this movement by placing your thumb on the dorsum of the distal phalanx of the big toe. This action will tend to flex the distal phalanx.

The practitioner's index finger shows the tendon near its insertion at the base of the dorsum of the distal phalanx of the big toe and the sides of the base of the first phalanx.

Attachments
This muscle arises from the middle part of the medial surface of the fibula in front of the interosseous membrane, and is inserted into the base of the proximal phalanx of the big toe and into its distal phalanx by two lateral expansions.

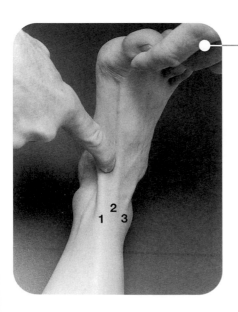

Fig. 11.16 | **The tendon of the extensor hallucis longus**

The subject has made the same movements as described above. The practitioner's index finger shows the tendon as it goes over the instep.

Legends for Figures 11.15–11.17

1. Tibialis anterior.
2. Extensor hallucis longus.
3. Extensor digitorum longus.

Fig. 11.17 | **The body of the extensor hallucis longus in the distal leg**

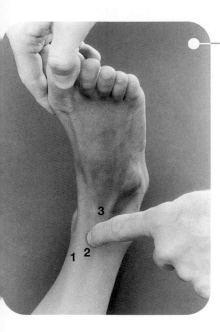

After ascending behind the two extensor retinacula the tendon joins the body of the muscle as it lies between the tibialis anterior on its medial side and the extensor digitorum longus on its lateral side.

See the figures dealing with these last two muscles (Figs 12.119 and 12.122 respectively) in order to observe the location of the muscle in question.

Fig. 11.18 | **The tendons of the extensor digitorum longus (*m. extensor digitorum longus, tendines*) in the dorsum of the foot**

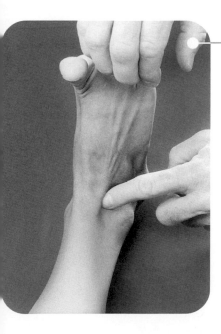

Place your distal hand as shown in the adjacent illustration and resist the extension of the toes.

Run your fingers along the tendons for the four toes from their distal ends to the instep. In the adjacent illustration the tendon is first approached at the instep.

Attachments

- It arises from the lateral tibial condyle lateral to that of the tibialis anterior and the upper two-thirds of the medial surface of the fibula along its anterior border.
- Distally the tendons for each toe separate on the dorsal surfaces of each proximal phalanx before inserting into the bases of the middle and distal phalanges.

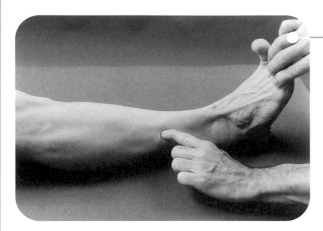

Fig. 11.19 | The extensor digitorum longus in the leg

The body of this muscle, which turns into tendons distally, occupies the full length of the leg and runs supero-inferiorly between the peroneus longus and the peroneus brevis on its lateral side and the tibialis anterior on its medial side.

Carefully locate these last two muscles by taking advantage of their actions; this will allow you to locate the muscle you are looking for better (see also Fig. 11.22).

Moreover, it is useful to ask the subject to keep the foot actively in dorsiflexion, abduction, and "pronation" in order to have a better view of the contracted muscle at this level.

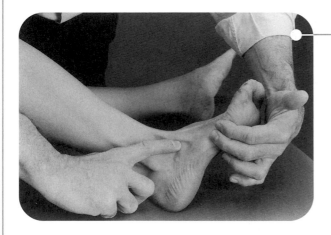

Fig. 11.20 | The peroneus tertius (*m. peroneus tertius*)

This is seen as a tendon on the lateral border of the tendon of the extensor digitorum longus for the fifth toe.

To bring out the tendon you are looking for, simply ask the subject to evert the foot with or without any resistance on your part.

Attachments
- The tendon runs toward the dorsal surface of the base of the fifth metatarsal, where it is inserted.
- It arises from the inferior third of the medial surface of the fibula.

THE LATERAL GROUP OF MUSCLES

This consists of two muscles:

- The peroneus longus (*m. peroneus longus*) (Figs 11.23–11.25).
- The peroneus brevis (*m. peroneus brevis*) (Figs 11.27–11.29).

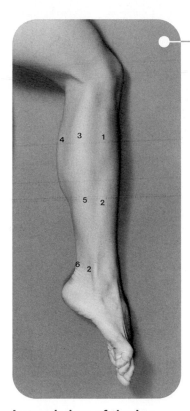

Fig. 11.21

Lateral view of the leg

1. Peroneus longus.
2. Peroneus brevis.
3. Lateral head of gastrocnemius.
4. Medial head of gastrocnemius.
5. Soleus.
6. Achilles' tendon.

*The peroneus longus (*m. peroneus longus*)*

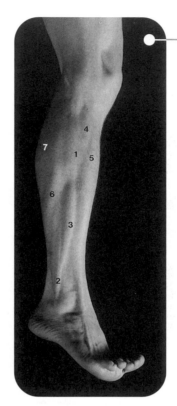

Fig. 11.22

Lateral view of the leg

1. Peroneus longus.
2. Tendon of the peroneus longus.
3. Peroneus brevis.
4. Extensor digitorum longus.
5. Tibialis anterior.
6. Soleus.
7. Lateral head of the gastrocnemius.

Actions of the peroneus longus
- It abducts, pronates, and plantarflexes the foot.
- It lowers the first metatarsal by displacing it laterally and thus unifies the entire metatarsus.
- It is a lateral stabilizer of the foot in the coronal plane in conjunction with the peroneus brevis.

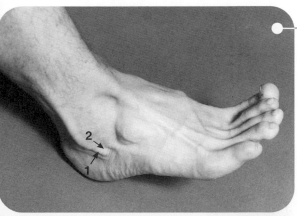

Fig. 11.23 | **The tendon of the peroneus longus on the lateral border of the foot**

Ask the subject to abduct and plantarflex the foot.

After being reflected at the lateral malleolus, the tendon (1) is plastered against the lateral surface of the calcaneus, passes under the peroneal trochlea, and enters the groove on the cuboid bone along the lateral border of the foot.

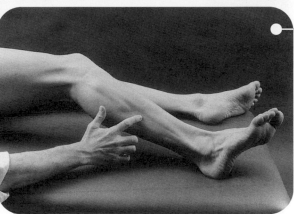

Fig. 11.24 | **The tendon of the peroneus longus in the leg**

Ask the subject to perform the same movements as those described above.

The tendon occupies about half of the lateral surface of the leg and overlies the body of the peroneus brevis, which extends beyond it anteriorly and posteriorly (see Fig. 11.29).

Attachments

- It arises from the lateral tibial condyle lateral to the insertion of the extensor digitorum longus, the anterolateral surface of the fibular head, and the upper third of the lateral surface of the fibular shaft.
- It is inserted into the posterolateral tuberosity on the base of the first metatarsal and very often sends expansions to the medial cuneiform or the second metatarsal and to the first dorsal interosseus.

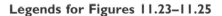

Legends for Figures 11.23–11.25

1. Tendon of the peroneus longus.
2. Peroneus brevis.
3. Extensor digitorum longus.
4. Soleus.

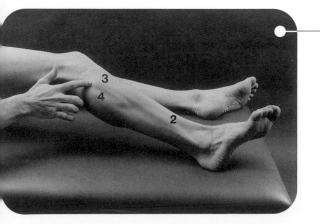

Fig. 11.25 | **The body of the peroneus longus**

Ask the subject to perform the same movements as those described above (Fig. 11.23).

The body of the muscle lies in the upper part of the lateral surface of the leg between the extensor digitorum longus (3) in front and the soleus (4) behind.

The peroneus brevis (m. peroneus brevis)

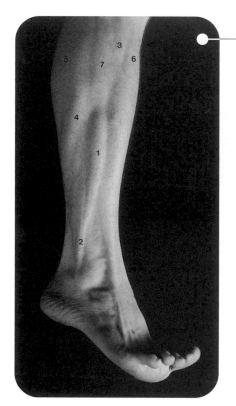

Fig. 11.26

Lateral view of the lower two-thirds of the leg

1. Peroneus brevis.
2. Tendon of the peroneus longus.
3. Extensor digitorum longus.
4. Soleus.
5. The lateral head of the gastrocnemius.
6. Tibialis anterior.
7. Peroneus longus.

Actions of the peroneus brevis
• It pronates and abducts the foot.
• It is a lateral stabilizer of the foot in the coronal plane.

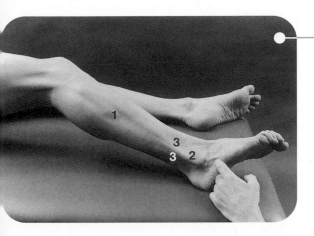

Fig. 11.27 | **The tendon of the peroneus brevis in its most distal part along the lateral border of the foot**

A movement of pure abduction of the foot is enough to bring out the tendon. Then follow its course along the lateral border of the foot to its insertion into the tuberosity of the fifth metatarsal.

Note: In order to observe its passage along the lateral border of the calcaneus above the peroneal tubercle properly, see Chapter 12.

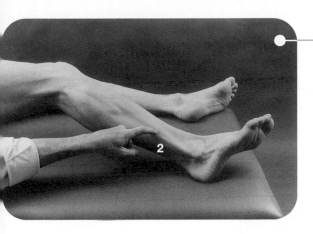

Fig. 11.28 | **The peroneus brevis in the leg**

Ask the subject to abduct the foot as shown above, and the body of the muscle will stand out in front of the tendon of the peroneus longus.

A series of muscular contractions and relaxations is very useful in bringing out the location of this muscle in the relaxed state.

Attachments

It arises from the lower two-thirds of the lateral surface of the fibula and is inserted into the tuberosity of the fifth metatarsal.

Legends for Figures 11.27–11.29

1. Peroneus longus.
2. Tendon of the peroneus longus.
3. Peroneus brevis.

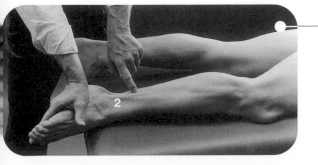

Fig. 11.29 | **The peroneus brevis in the leg**

Ask subjects to abduct the foot as shown above; you can also ask them to plantarflex the foot to bring out the contraction of the muscle even better. You can also feel the body of the muscle behind the tendon of the peroneus longus.

THE POSTERIOR GROUP OF MUSCLES

This consists of:

The superficial plane with:

- The triceps surae (*m. triceps surae*), consisting of:
  — The medial head of gastrocnemius (*m. gastrocnemius, caput mediale*) (Figs 11.32 and 11.33)
  — The lateral head of gastrocnemius (*m. gastrocnemius, caput laterale*) (Figs 11.34 and 11.35)
  — The soleus (*m. soleus*) (Figs 11.36–38)
- The plantaris (*m. plantaris*) (Fig. 11.40).

The deep plane with:

- The popliteus (*m. popliteus*) (Fig. 11.35).
- The tibialis posterior (*m. tibialis posterior*) (Figs 11.42–11.44).
- The flexor digitorum longus (*m. flexor digitorum longus*) (Figs 11.46–11.48).
- The flexor hallucis longus (*m. flexor hallucis longus*) (Figs 11.50–11.52).

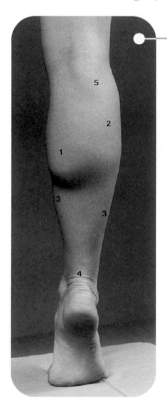

Fig. 11.30

Posterior view of the leg

1. Medial head of gastrocnemius.
2. Lateral head of gastrocnemius.
3. Soleus.
4. Achilles' tendon.
5. Plantaris.

SUPERFICIAL PLANE

*The triceps surae and the plantaris (*m. plantaris*)*

- The triceps surae, consisting of:
    — The medial head of gastrocnemius (*m. gastrocnemius, caput mediale*) (Figs 11.32 and 11.33)
    — The lateral head of gastrocnemius (*m. gastrocnemius, caput laterale*) (Figs 11.34 and 11.35)
    — The soleus (*m. soleus*) (Figs 11.36–38).
    These three muscles are inserted into the calcaneus by a common tendon, the Achilles' tendon (Fig. 11.39).
- The plantaris (*m. plantaris*) (Fig. 11.40).

Note: For teaching purposes the gastrocnemius, the soleus, and the plantaris will be presented separately in this order.

Actions of the triceps surae and of the plantaris
- They plantarflex the foot.
- The gastrocnemius makes a weak contribution to leg flexion on the thigh and is far less active in plantar flexion of the foot when the knee is flexed.
- The plantaris acts like the gastrocnemius. (It is sometimes absent, and its action is at best accessory.)

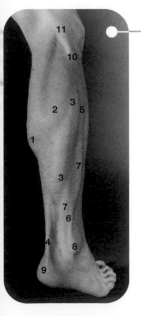

Fig. 11.31 | **Posterolateral view of the leg**

1. Medial head of gastrocnemius.
2. Lateral head of gastrocnemius.
3. Soleus.
4. Achilles' tendon.
5. Peroneus longus.
6. Tendon of peroneus longus.
7. Peroneus brevis.
8. Lateral malleolus.
9. Posterior surface of the calcaneus.
10. Head of the fibula.
11. Tendon of the biceps femoris.

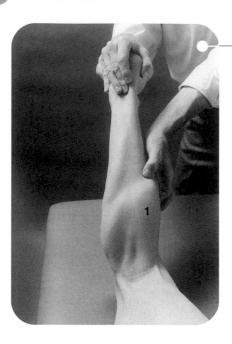

Fig. 11.32 | **The medial head of the gastrocnemius (*m. gastrocnemius, caput mediale*) (1)**

Place your forearm on the sole of the subject's foot and use it to elicit repeated plantar flexions of the foot while you hold the calcaneus in the palm of your hand and prevent the subject from flexing the knee. The movements performed by the subject are those produced by the gastrocnemius. Look for the muscle itself on the posteromedial part of the leg behind the soleus.

Note: The body of the medial head extends further down than that of the lateral head.

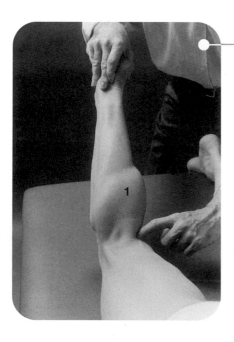

Fig. 11.33 | **The medial head of the gastrocnemius at the knee (1)**

Use the method described above to induce contraction of this muscle.

Attachments

- It arises from the roughened upper border of the medial femoral condyle (which is in fact a reinforcement of the capsule of the knee joint), from the medial supracondylar tubercle, and from the part of the bone adjacent to the capsule and the popliteal surface. You can therefore approach it from the medial aspect of the popliteal fossa, since it forms the inferomedial border of the fossa.
- It is inserted with the lateral head of the gastrocnemius and the soleus into the posterior surface of the calcaneus via the Achilles' tendon (calcaneal tendon).

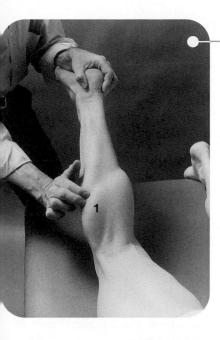

Fig. 11.34 | **The lateral head of the gastrocnemius (*m. gastrocnemius, caput laterale*) (1)**

Here again use your distal hand, which cradles the heel, and your forearm, which lies on the sole of the foot, to resist the subject's plantar flexion of the ankle and flexion of the knee simultaneously. These combined movements bring out the muscle you are looking for. It is always useful to have the subject repeat these movements in order to get a better feel of the contracting muscle.

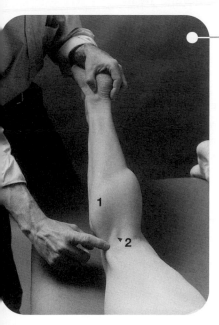

Fig. 11.35 | **The lateral head (1) of the gastrocnemius at the knee and the popliteus (*m. popliteus*)**

Use the above-mentioned method to induce contraction of the muscle.

The proximal part of this muscle is an important region in palpatory anatomy, since it forms the inferolateral border of the popliteal fossa. Its proximal end is flanked medially by the popliteus (2), located in a deeper plane.

Note: The body of the popliteus lies in the proximal and posterior part of the leg, and you can approach it indirectly through the gastrocnemius (palpation not shown). Care is essential in deep palpation of this region because of the presence of the tibial nerve. The tendon of the popliteus is also dealt with in Figure 10.76.

Attachments

- Like the medial head, the lateral head arises from the bony reinforcement of the capsule of the knee joint on the posterior surface of the lateral femoral condyle, from the lateral supracondylar tubercle, and the part of the bone adjacent to the capsule and the popliteal surface.
- It is inserted with the soleus and the medial head into the posterior surface of the calcaneus via the Achilles' tendon.
- The popliteus arises from the popliteal groove located below the lateral epicondyle, and is inserted above the soleal line of the tibia.

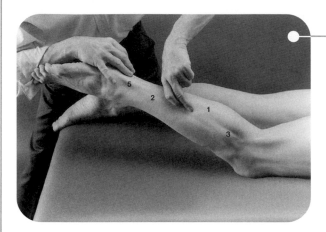

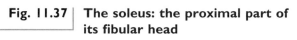

Fig. 11.36 | The soleus (*m. soleus*): the distal part of its fibular head

The most distal part of the fibular head lies superficial to the peroneus brevis (2) and posterior to the tendon of the peroneus longus (3). With the palm of your distal hand take hold of the subject's heel and place your forearm flat on the sole of the foot to resist plantar flexion. The technique of repetitive contraction and relaxation is ideal to bring out the muscle. Look for it along the fibula between the posteriorly located lateral head of the gastrocnemius (1) and the anteriorly located peroneus longus (3) and peroneus brevis (2).

Attachment

The fibular head is the part of the body of the muscle arising from the fibula (that is, the posterior surface of its head and the proximal quarter of its shaft). It extends much more over the lateral surface of the leg than the medial head does on the medial side.

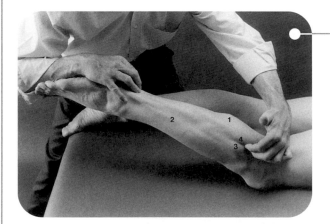

Fig. 11.37 | The soleus: the proximal part of its fibular head

The middle and proximal parts of the fibular head of the soleus (4) lie posterior to the peroneus longus (3) and anterior to the lateral head of the gastrocnemius (1).

Attachments

The two tendinous heads arising from the tibia (Fig. 11.38) and the fibula (Fig. 11.36) fuse into a single expansion that gives rise to fleshy fibers on its posterior and anterior surfaces. This tendinous expansion is thus embedded inside the muscle fibers and is called the intramuscular fascia. It joins the gastrocnemius before inserting into the posterior surface of the calcaneus via the Achilles' tendon.

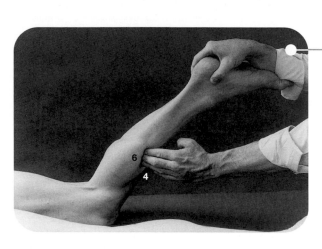

Fig. 11.38 | The soleus: its tibial head

Take hold of the calcaneus in the palm of your distal hand and place your forearm flat on the sole of the foot to resist any plantar flexion of the ankle.

The technique of repetitive contraction and relaxation is ideal for bringing out the tibial head of the soleus. Look for it along the medial border of the fibula down to its middle third as it runs in front of the medial head of the gastrocnemius (6).

Attachment

The tibial head (4) is the part of the muscle arising from the lower lip of the inferomedial half of the soleal line and from the middle third of the medial border of the tibia. It extends much less over the medial surface of the leg than does the fibular head over the lateral surface of the leg.

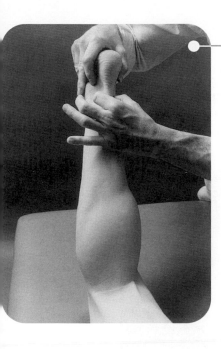

Fig. 11.39 | **The Achilles' tendon (*tendo calcaneus*)**

With the subject's heel held in the palm of your distal hand and your forearm resting on the sole of the subject's foot, you can vary at will the degree of tension in the tendon. This tension can be increased in two ways:

- By exerting pressure on the sole of the foot, to dorsiflex the foot and thus stretch the tendon.
- By using the technique of repetitive contraction and relaxation of the muscle produced by successive plantar flexions of the foot.

Note: Once the tendon is located, you can also approach it in its relaxed state and from its three surfaces (posterior, anterior, and lateral).

Attachment

The tendon is formed by the union of the gastrocnemius and soleus, and is inserted into the lower half of the posterior surface of the calcaneus.

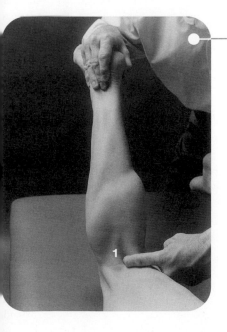

Fig. 11.40 | **The plantaris (*m. plantaris*) in the popliteal fossa (*fossa poplitea*)**

This is located in front of the lateral head of the gastrocnemius, which it borders medially. It is often absent and is difficult to access.

With the palm of your distal hand holding the subject's heel and your forearm lying flat on the sole of the subject's foot, you can simultaneously prevent him from plantarflexing the foot and flexing the knee.

How you feel the contraction of this muscle depends on the subject's build. You can feel it (1) in the popliteal fossa medial to the lateral head of the gastrocnemius.

Note: The number 1 indicates more the course of the muscle than the muscle itself, which lies deep.

Attachments

- It arises from the lateral tibial condyle proximal and medial to the lateral head of the gastrocnemius.
- It is inserted medial to the Achilles' tendon on the posterior surface of the calcaneus.

DEEP PLANE

*The tibialis posterior (*m. tibialis posterior*)*

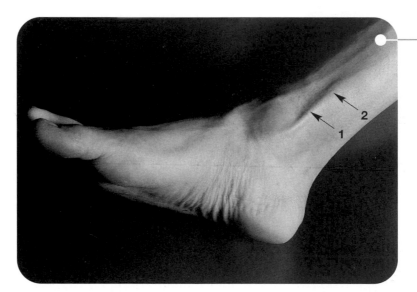

Fig. 11.41

Medial view of the lower third of the leg

1. Tendon of the tibialis posterior.
2. Body of the tibialis posterior.

Note: Refer to page 396 to observe the relations of this muscle with the tendons of the muscles crossing the malleolar groove of the tibia and also belonging to the deep plane of the leg:

• The flexor digitorum longus (*m. flexor digitorum longus*)
• The flexor hallucis longus (*m. flexor hallucis longus*).

Actions
• It adducts and supinates the foot.

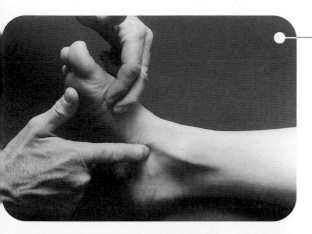

Fig. 11.42 | **The tendon of the tibialis posterior (*m. tibialis posterior, tendo*) between the tuberosity of the navicular bone (*tuberositas ossis navicularis*) and the medial malleolus**

With your distal hand, guide and/or resist the subject's adduction of the foot, which is already in the position of plantar flexion. You will feel the tendon between the above-mentioned structures. In some cases it is helpful to locate the tuberosity of the navicular bone first. See also Chapter 12.

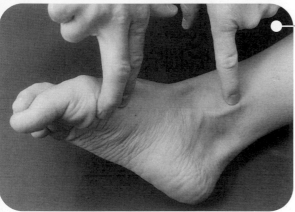

Fig. 11.43 | **The tendon of the tibialis posterior at the ankle**

Your distal hand guides and/or opposes the subject's adduction of the foot, which is already in the position of plantar flexion. The tendon is seen behind the medial malleolus and is felt as a very hard solid cylindrical cord under your fingers.

Attachments
- The tibialis posterior arises from:
  — The upper two-thirds of the posterior surface of the tibia lateral to the medial ridge, which separates it from the flexor digitorum longus
  — The upper two-thirds of the medial surface of the fibula behind the vertical line.
- It is inserted on all the tarsal bones except the talus and on all the metatarsal bones except the last two.

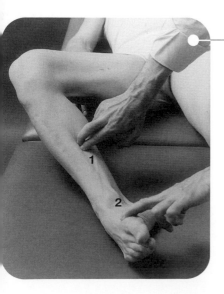

Fig. 11.44 | **The tendon and body of the tibialis posterior**

The subject's leg rests on its lateral surface. To feel the muscle contracting, you simply have to move your fingerpads along the medial tibial border (1). It is easier to feel if you use the technique of repetitive contraction and relaxation. Start with the foot in plantar flexion and ask the subject to adduct repeatedly against resistance. The body of the muscle, which terminates in the tendon of the tibialis posterior (2), runs anterior to the body of the flexor digitorum longus until it reaches the arcade formed at the distal tibial origin of the tendon of the latter muscle (that is, 10 cm (4 in) above the medial malleolus). After passing under this arcade the body of the tibialis posterior comes to lie medial to that of the flexor digitorum longus. At this point it is not directly accessible, as it is concealed by the triceps surae muscle.

*The flexor digitorum longus (*m. flexor digitorum longus*)*

Actions of the flexor digitorum longus
• It flexes the distal phalanx on the middle phalanx, the middle on the proximal, and the proximal on the corresponding metatarsal. This action applies to the last four toes.

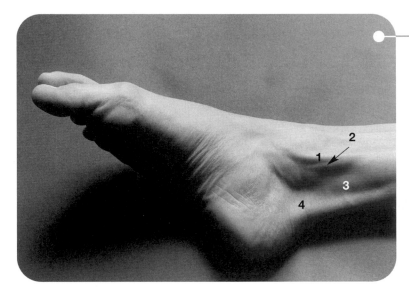

Fig. 11.45

Medial view of the lower third of the leg

1. Tibialis posterior.
2. Flexor digitorum longus.
3. Flexor hallucis longus.
4. Achilles' tendon.

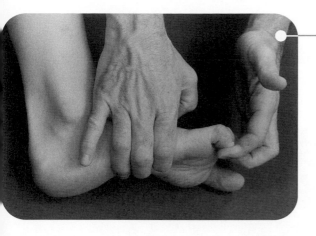

Fig. 11.46 | **The tendons of the flexor digitorum longus (*m. flexor digitorum longus, tendines*) in the sole of the foot**

Your distal hand guides and/or gently resists a succession of rapid flexions of the toes after the ankle has been placed in the neutral position. Place your other hand on the sole of the foot while holding the lateral border of the foot in your palm. Your contact is broad and allows you to feel the contraction of the muscle. You cannot directly feel the tendons under your fingers as they are masked by those of the flexor digitorum brevis.

Note: The contraction of these two muscles will be better felt under your fingers if the proximal phalanges of the toes are already hyperextended.

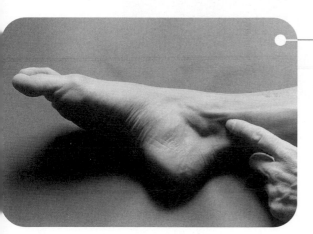

Fig. 11.47 | **The flexor digitorum longus in the medial posterior malleolar groove**

The subject flexes and extends the toes in rapid succession, with the foot resting on its heel or on its lateral border.

You feel the tendon close to the medial malleolus behind the tendon of the tibialis posterior.

Attachments

• It arises:
  — From the medial part of the inferior lip of the oblique line of the tibia
  — From the middle third of the posterior surface of the tibia medial to the vertical line that separates it from the tibialis posterior.
• It inserts into the bases of the distal phalanges of toes II–V.

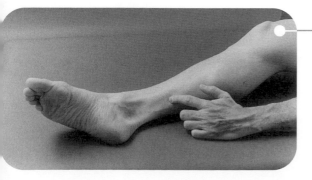

Fig. 11.48 | **The body of the flexor digitorum longus in the lower third of the leg**

The subject's leg rests on its lateral border, and the ankle is fully relaxed.

The practitioner's index finger shows the body of the muscle located behind the tibialis posterior until it reaches the arcade formed at its distal origin from the tibia (that is, 10 cm (4 in) above the medial malleolus). Beyond this arcade the body of the muscle lies lateral to that of the tibialis posterior. You can feel the contraction of the muscle using the technique of alternating contraction and relaxation of the muscle induced by repeated flexions of the toes.

The flexor hallucis longus *(*m. flexor hallucis longus*)*

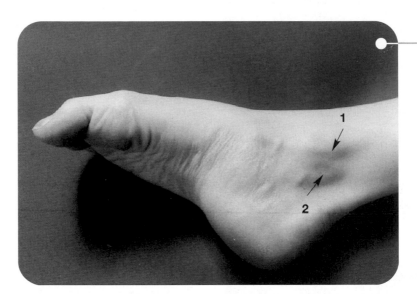

Fig. 11.49

Medial view of the lower third of the leg

1. Tendon of the tibialis posterior.
2. Tendon of the flexor hallucis longus.

Note: Refer to page 396 to observe the relations of this muscle with the other two muscles that cross the medial malleolar groove and also belong to the deep plane of the leg:

- The tibialis posterior.
- The flexor digitorum longus.

Actions of the flexor hallucis longus
- It flexes the middle phalanx on the proximal phalanx, and the proximal phalanx on the firs metatarsal.

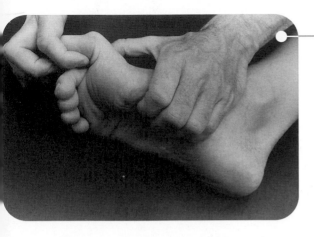

Fig. 11.50 | The flexor hallucis longus in the sole of the foot

With your distal hand guide and/or weakly oppose a rapid succession of flexions of the big toe while the subject's ankle is already in the neutral position and the foot rests on the heel or on its lateral border.

Your other hand lies flat on the plantar surface of the first metatarsal using a wide contact, the better to feel the contraction of the muscle. With this contact you can improve your approach to the tendon, which is felt a little like a cord under your fingers.

Note: You will feel this tendon better if you first hyperextend the proximal phalanx of the big toe.

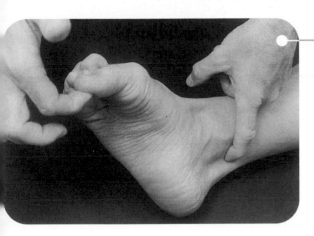

Fig. 11.51 | The flexor hallucis longus in the medial posterior malleolar groove

Your distal hand guides and/or opposes a rapid succession of flexions of the big toe, while the ankle is in the neutral position and the leg rests on its posterolateral surface. You can feel the muscle in the medial malleolar groove between the medial malleolus and the Achilles' tendon and behind the tendon of the flexor digitorum longus. (See also Figure 12.134.)

Attachments

• It arises from the inferior three-quarters of the posterior surface of the fibula.
• It is inserted into the base of the distal phalanx of the big toe after passing between the two sesamoid bones of the metatarsophalangeal joint.

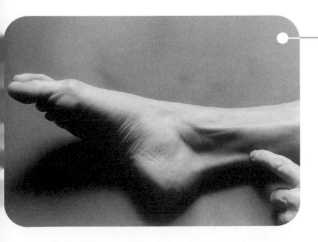

Fig. 11.52 | The flexor hallucis longus in the medial posterior malleolar groove: display of the body of the muscle

This illustration allows a better display of the body of the muscle (indicated by the practitioner's index finger), which has already been studied in the figure above and which lies behind the flexor digitorum longus (see 2 on Fig. 11.45), and on the medial part of the Achilles' tendon. You can feel the contraction of the muscle even better if you ask the subject to flex the big toe repeatedly.

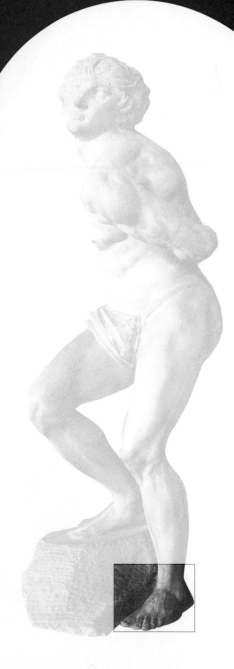

CHAPTER 12

THE ANKLE
AND FOOT

TOPOGRAPHICAL PRESENTATION OF THE FOOT (PES)

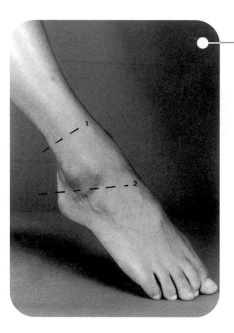

Fig. 12.1 | **Anterolateral view of the ankle and the foot**

1. Upper limit of the ankle region.
2. Lower limit of the ankle region.

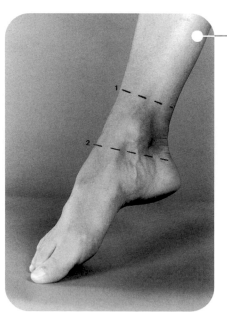

Fig. 12.2 | **Anteromedial view of the ankle and the foot**

1. Upper limit of the ankle region.
2. Lower limit of the ankle region.

OSTEOLOGY

THE BONES OF THE FOOT

LATERAL VIEW

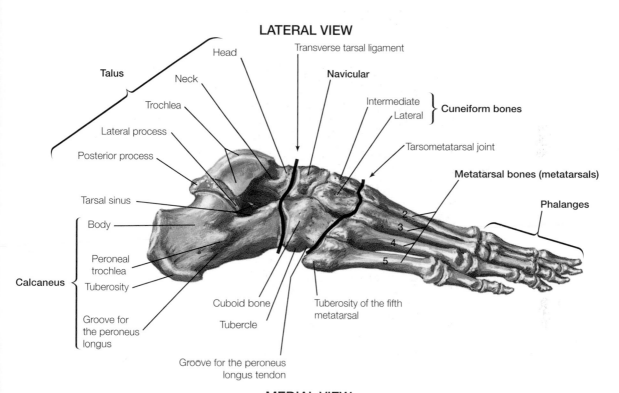

Talus
Head
Neck
Trochlea
Lateral process
Posterior process
Tarsal sinus
Transverse tarsal ligament
Navicular
Intermediate
Lateral
Cuneiform bones
Tarsometatarsal joint
Metatarsal bones (metatarsals)
Phalanges

Calcaneus
Body
Peroneal trochlea
Tuberosity
Groove for the peroneus longus

Cuboid bone
Tubercle
Tuberosity of the fifth metatarsal

Groove for the peroneus longus tendon

MEDIAL VIEW

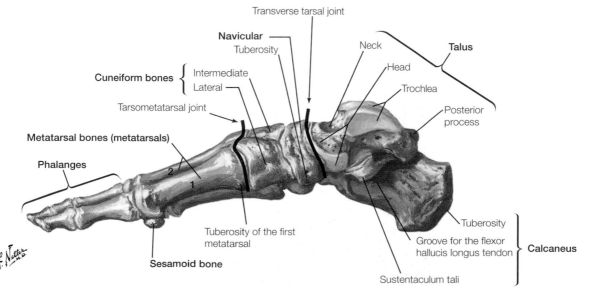

Transverse tarsal joint
Navicular
Tuberosity
Neck
Talus
Head
Trochlea
Posterior process

Cuneiform bones
Intermediate
Lateral
Tarsometatarsal joint
Metatarsal bones (metatarsals)
Phalanges

Tuberosity

Tuberosity of the first metatarsal
Groove for the flexor hallucis longus tendon
Calcaneus

Sesamoid bone
Sustentaculum tali

BONES OF THE FOOT: CALCANEUS

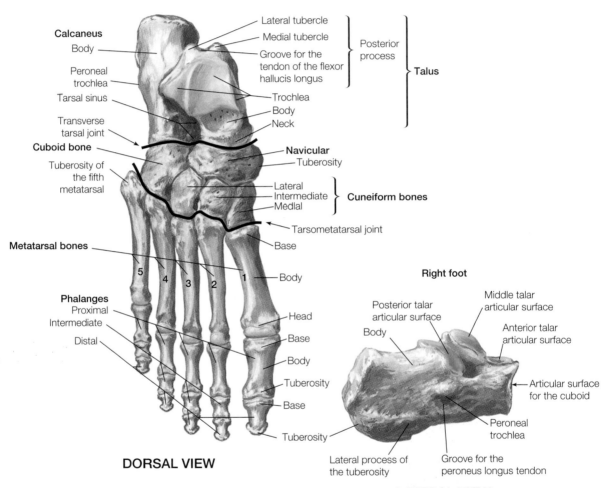

Calcaneus
Body
Peroneal trochlea
Tarsal sinus
Transverse tarsal joint
Cuboid bone
Tuberosity of the fifth metatarsal

Metatarsal bones

5 4 3 2 1

Phalanges
Proximal
Intermediate
Distal

Lateral tubercle
Medial tubercle
Groove for the tendon of the flexor hallucis longus } Posterior process
Trochlea
Body
Neck } Talus

Navicular
Tuberosity

Lateral
Intermediate
Medial } Cuneiform bones

Tarsometatarsal joint
Base

Body

Head
Base
Body
Tuberosity
Base

Tuberosity

DORSAL VIEW

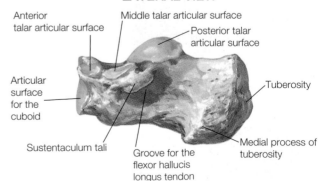

Right foot

Posterior talar articular surface
Body

Middle talar articular surface
Anterior talar articular surface

Articular surface for the cuboid

Peroneal trochlea

Lateral process of the tuberosity

Groove for the peroneus longus tendon

LATERAL VIEW

Anterior talar articular surface

Articular surface for the cuboid

Sustentaculum tali

Middle talar articular surface
Posterior talar articular surface

Tuberosity

Groove for the flexor hallucis longus tendon

Medial process of tuberosity

THE LATERAL BORDER

The bony structures that can be detected by palpation are:

- The fifth metatarsal bone (*os metatarsale V*):
  - — The head (*caput ossis metatarsalis*) (Fig. 12.4)
  - — The lateral surface of the body (*corpus ossis metatarsalis*) (Fig. 12.5)
  - — The inferior surface of the body (Fig. 12.6)
  - — The base of the fifth metatarsal (*basis ossis metatarsalis V*) and the other bones of the lateral border of the foot; overall approach to their location (Fig. 12.7)
  - — The tuberosity (*tuberositas ossis metatarsalis*) (Fig. 12.8).
- The cuboid bone (*os cuboideum*):
  - — The lateral border (Fig. 12.9; also Fig. 12.7)
  - — The dorsal surface (Fig. 12.10)
  - — The plantar surface (Fig. 12.11).
- The calcaneus (*calcaneus*):
  - — The lateral surface (Fig. 12.12)
  - — The greater process or the anterior superolateral angle (Fig. 12.13; also Fig. 12.7)
  - — Articular surface for the cuboid (*facies articularis cuboidea*) (Fig. 12.14)
  - — The floor of the tarsal sinus (*sinus tarsi*) (Fig. 12.15)
  - — The peroneal trochlea (*trochlea peronalis*) (Fig. 12.16)
  - — Tubercle for the insertion of the calcaneofibular ligament (*lig. calcaneofibulare*) (Fig. 12.17)
  - — The posterior part of the lateral surface (Fig. 12.18)
  - — The superior surface: the lateral part of the posterior segment (Fig. 12.19).
- The talus (*talus*):
  - — The lateral surface of the neck (*collum tali*) (Fig. 12.20; see also Fig. 12.7)
  - — The lateral process (*processus lateralis tali*) (Fig. 12.21).
- The lateral malleolus (*malleolus lateralis*):
  - — The anterior border (Fig. 12.22)
  - — The apex (Fig. 12.23)
  - — The posterior border (Fig. 12.24).

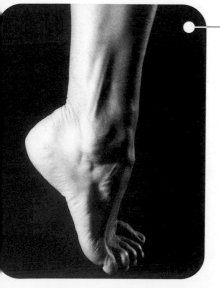

Fig. 12.3 | **Lateral surface of the ankle and the foot**

*The fifth metatarsal (*os metatarsale V*)*

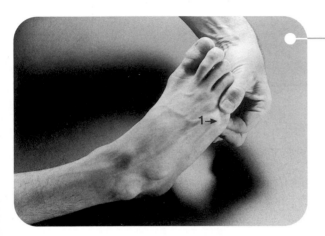

Fig. 12.4 | **The head of the fifth metatarsal (*caput ossis metatarsalis V*)**

You need only plantarflex the fifth toe in order to bring ou[t] the head (1) of the fifth metatarsal on the dorsal part of the lateral border of the foot. This procedure also allows you to locate the metatarsophalangeal joint.

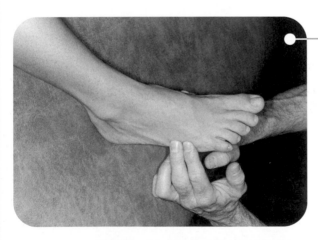

Fig. 12.5 | **The lateral surface of the body of the fifth metatarsal (*corpus ossis metatarsalis V*)**

You can easily run your fingers over this, as it is directly sub[-] cutaneous. It lies just above the abductor digiti minimi.

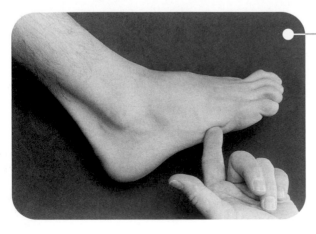

Fig. 12.6 | **The inferior border of the body o[f] the fifth metatarsal**

Your index finger will feel this as a well-defined curved struc[-] ture concave downward.

In the adjacent figure the practitioner's index finger pushe[s] aside the abductor digiti minimi so as to touch the bon[y] structure you are looking for.

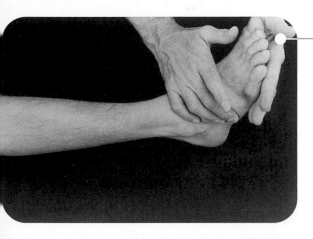

Fig. 12.7 | **The base of the fifth metatarsal (*basis ossis metatarsalis V*) and of the other bones on the lateral side of the foot (cuboid, calcaneus, and talus): localization using an overall approach to the lateral border of the foot**

The foot is relaxed and rests on the table or on the practitioner's knee. The practitioner places his proximal hand on the subject's instep and gently closes it on the lateral side of the foot, with the lateral border of his little finger lying on the lateral malleolus.

The practitioner's little finger is touching the neck of the talus (its dorsal and lateral surfaces), the floor of the tarsal sinus, and the anterior superolateral angle or the greater process of the calcaneus. The practitioner's ring finger faces the cuboid, and the middle finger rests on the base of the fifth metatarsal.

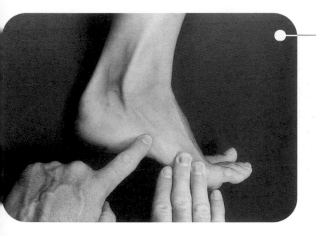

Fig. 12.8 | **The tuberosity of the fifth metatarsal (*tuberositas ossis metatarsalis V*)**

The base articulates with the cuboid and is unusual in having a prominent tuberosity projecting backward, downward, and to the side. This is the bony structure you are looking for, and it carries the insertion of the peroneus brevis. It also overshoots the lateral border of the cuboid.

The cuboid (os cuboideum)

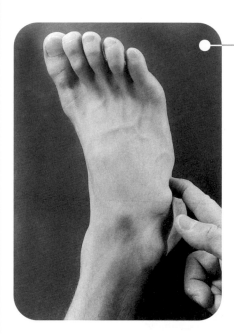

Fig. 12.9 | **The lateral border of the cuboid (*os cuboideum*)**

The cuboid is the bony structure next to the tuberosity of the fifth metacarpal in the hindfoot. Once you locate this tuberosity, you simply need to slide your fingers into the adjacent depression to reach a ridge, which is the structure you are looking for.

Note: The peroneus brevis tendon runs along this border and will stand in the way unless it is relaxed.

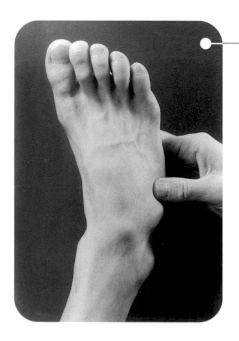

Fig. 12.10 | **The dorsal surface of the cuboid**

Two notable bony structures help you to locate this surface:

- The tuberosity of the fifth metatarsal, already located (Figs 12.7 and 12.8).
- The greater process of the calcaneus (Fig. 12.13).

These two structures are the anterior and posterior bony limits of the structure you are looking for, which lies between the two.

First place your thumb on the lateral border of the cuboid, which you have already located (see figure above), and then move it slightly toward the dorsum of the foot in order to come into contact with the bony structure in question.

Note: This is a rough surface sloping downward and laterally, and is easily investigated, as it lies directly under the skin. The peroneus brevis tendon muscle runs along its border and the extensor digitorum brevis partly covers it.

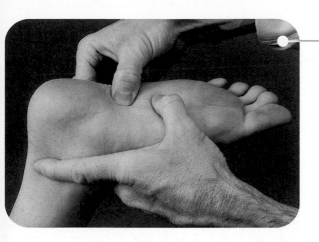

Fig. 12.11 | The plantar surface of the cuboid

Once you have located the tuberosity of the fifth metatarsal (Figs 12.7 and 12.8) and the greater process of the calcaneus (Figs 12.7 and 12.13), you need only put your thumb between these two structures and move it round the lateral border of the foot and consequently round the lateral border of the cuboid to reach the plantar surface of the cuboid.

*The calcaneus (*calcaneus*)*

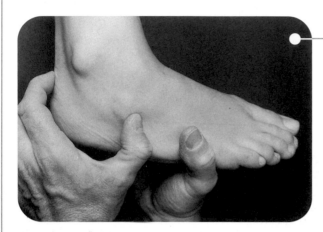

Fig. 12.12 | **The lateral surface of the calcaneus**

Adduct and slightly supinate the forefoot so as to bring out the anterior articular surface of the calcaneus and partially "uncover" it.

Place your thumb on this surface and your index finger on the posterior surface of the calcaneus to obtain a fair estimate of the size of this bone in the foot.

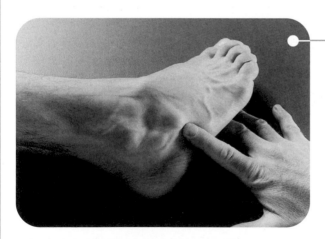

Fig. 12.13 | **The greater process or the anterior superolateral angle of the calcaneus**

This is the posterior border of the lateral part of the calcaneocuboidal joint. It is easy to access if the forefoot is supinated. It can be very prominent in some subjects, as shown in the adjacent figure.

Note: Locating this structure is of interest, since it allows clear assessment of the size of the calcaneus, which is bound to vary from one subject to another.

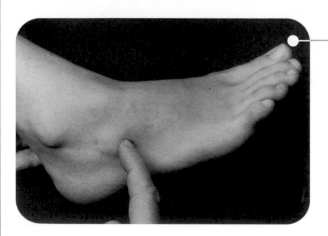

Fig. 12.14 | **The articular surface for the cuboid (*facies articularis cuboidea*)**

To uncover the supero-anterolateral part of this articular surface, it is very often enough to ask subjects to adduct and supinate their already slightly flexed forefoot.

If this is not good enough, you can carry out this passive procedure. Block the calcaneus with one hand and, with the other, bring the forefoot into adduction, supination, and slight plantar flexion (see also Fig. 12.7.)

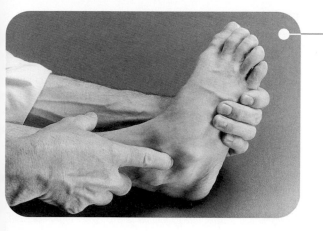

Fig. 12.15 | The floor of the tarsal sinus (*sinus tarsi*)

Anatomical reminder: The tarsal sinus is formed by the interlocking of the calcaneus and the talus. It is a sulcus that progressively widens mediolaterally and postero-anteriorly. Its floor is the calcaneus, and its roof is the talus or, more accurately, the sulcus tali. The superimposition of these two structures forms a canal called the tarsal sinus. Thus the sinus itself is not accessible, but its floor is accessible precisely at the point where it opens on to the superior surface of the anterior part of the calcaneus.

Note: The posterior part of the tarsal sinus is filled by the two bundles of the talocalcaneal interosseous ligament.

Method of approach: With the subject's foot in the neutral position, first place your index finger on the anterior border of the lateral malleolus, and then move it slightly toward the sole of the foot. The pad of your finger will feel it as a depression. The extensor digitorum brevis can be a hindrance as you try to approach this structure. Make sure therefore that it is relaxed or pushed aside. The tendon of the extensor digitorum and the lateral part of the neck of the talus lie on the medial side.

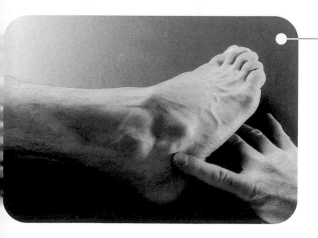

Fig. 12.16 | The peroneal trochlea (*trochlea peronealis*)

This bony projection, which is variable in occurrence, lies about one finger-width below the lateral malleolus. It separates the groove for the peroneus longus below from the groove for the peroneus brevis above (see also Figs 12.12 and 12.13).

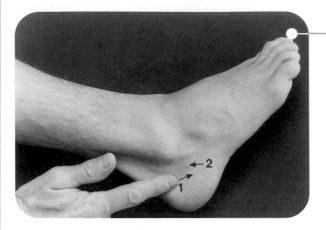

Fig. 12.17 | **The tubercle for the insertion of the calcaneofibular ligament (*lig. calcaneofibulare*)**

This is not always well defined. It receives the insertion of the calcaneofibular ligament (previously called the peroneocalcaneal ligament or the middle bundle of the lateral collateral ligament). When the foot is in the neutral position, the tubercle (1) lies about one finger-width above and behind the peroneal trochlea (2) (Fig. 12.16), and also about one finger-width below the lateral part of the talocalcaneal joint.

Note: The tubercle is not always present. In its absence the calcaneofibular ligament is inserted directly into the lateral surface of the calcaneus.

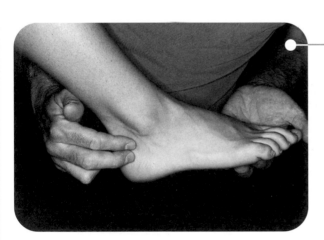

Fig. 12.18 | **The posterior part of the lateral surface of the calcaneus (*calcaneus*)**

This feels flat and rough under the fingers over nearly the whole lateral surface of the calcaneus, which is directly subcutaneous. In the adjacent illustration the contact is placed slightly behind it to allow the best possible view of the bony structure of interest.

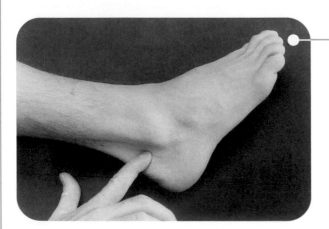

Fig. 12.19 | **The superior and lateral parts of the posterior segment or the dome of the calcaneus**

In the adjacent illustration the practitioner's index finger rests on the bony structure mentioned above (Fig. 12.18), behind the talus and lateral to the Achilles' tendon.

*The talus (*talus*)*

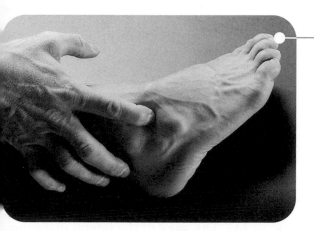

Fig. 12.20 | **The lateral surface of the neck of the talus (*collum tali*)**

First place the subject's foot in the neutral position and your index finger on the anterior border of the lateral malleolus. Then move your index finger slightly anteromedially, and it will face the structure you are looking for. You need simply tilt the forefoot into slight supination to make the lateral surface more accessible.

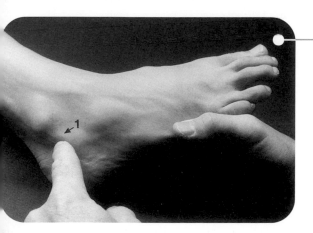

Fig. 12.21 | **The lateral process of the talus (*processus lateralis tali*)**

Invert the subject's foot in order to free the lateral process from the lateral malleolus and you will be in a better position to feel it.

Attachment
This process lies just above the lateral part of the talocalcaneal joint, and receives the insertion of the lateral talocalcaneal ligament.

*The lateral malleolus (*malleolus lateralis*)*

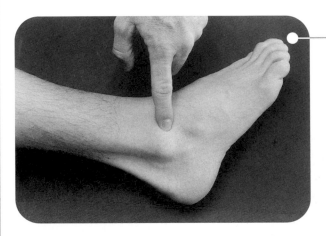

Fig. 12.22 | The anterior border of the lateral malleolus (*malleolus lateralis*)

To its "highest" or most proximal part is attached the anterior tibiofibular ligament, and to its "lowest" or most distal part are attached the anterior talofibular ligament (formerly known as the anterior talofibular ligament or the anterior bundle of the lateral collateral ligament) and the calcaneofibular ligament (Fig. 12.23) (formerly known as the middle bundle of the lateral collateral ligament).

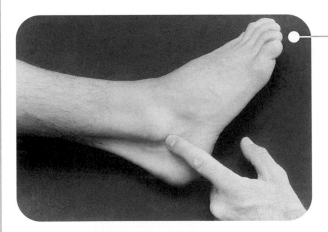

Fig. 12.23 | The apex of the lateral malleolus

This apex has a distinctive feature in that its tip lies just behind a notch to which the calcaneofibular ligament is attached; the rest of the ligament is attached to the most distal part of the anterior border of the fibula.

It is thus an important landmark for the localization of the fibular insertion of this ligament.

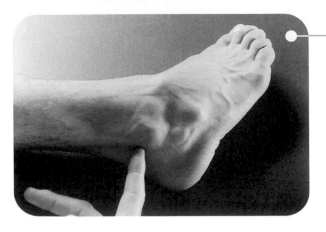

Fig. 12.24 | The posterior border of the lateral malleolus

Simply make sure that your posterior access to this border is not hindered by the tendons of the peroneus longus and peroneus brevis unless these muscles, which run behind this border, have been relaxed or pushed aside.

Note: This border gives attachment to the posterior tibiofibular ligament and to the posterior talofibular ligament.

THE MEDIAL BORDER

The bony structures that can be detected by palpation are:

- The first metatarsal (*os metatarsale I*):
  — The phalanges of the big toe and the head of the first metatarsal (*caput ossis metatarsalis I*): dorsal approach (Fig. 12.26)
  — Its head (*caput ossis metatarsalis I*) (Fig. 12.27)
  — Its body (*corpus ossis metatarsalis I*) (Figs 12.28–12.31)
  — Its base (*basis ossis metatarsalis I*); localization using a global approach to the medial border of the foot (Fig. 12.32)
  — Its posteromedial tuberosity (*basis ossis metatarsalis I, tuberositas medialis*) (Fig. 12.33)
  — Its posterolateral tuberosity (*basis ossis metatarsalis I, tuberositas lateralis*) (Fig. 12.34).
- The medial cuneiform (*cuneiforme mediale*):
  — Its medial surface: its localization with the help of the tibialis anterior (Fig. 12.35; see also Fig. 12.32)
  — Its dorsal surface (Fig. 12.36).
- The navicular (*os naviculare*):
  — Its tuberosity (*tuberositas ossis navicularis*); "direct" approach (Fig. 12.37; see also Fig. 12.32)
  — Its tuberosity: its localization using the tibialis posterior (Fig. 12.38).
- The talus (*talus*):
  — The ligament-related or middle part of its head (*caput tali*) (Fig. 12.39; see also Fig. 12.32)
  — Its neck (*collum tali*) (Figs 12.40 and 12.41; see also Fig. 12.32)
  — Its medial tubercle (*talus, tuberculum mediale*) (Fig. 12.42)
  — Its lateral tubercle (*talus, tuberculum laterale*) (Fig. 12.43).
- The calcaneus (*calcaneus*):
  — The sustentaculum tali (*sustentaculum tali*) (Fig. 12.44)
  — The calcaneal sulcus (*sulcus calcanei*) (Fig. 12.45).
- The medial malleolus (*malleolus medialis*):
  — Its anterior border (Fig. 12.46)
  — Its distal end (Fig. 12.47)
  — Its posterior border (Fig. 12.48).

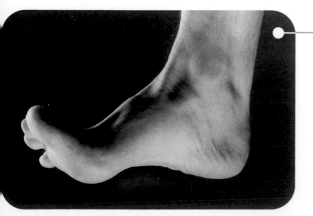

Fig. 12.25 | **The medial border of the foot**

The first metatarsal *(os metatarsale I)*

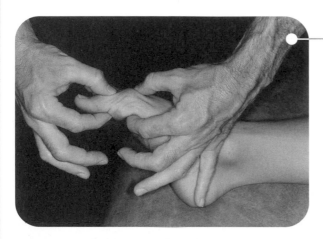

Fig. 12.26 | **The phalanges of the big toe (*hallux*) and the head of the first metatarsal (*caput ossis metatarsalis I*): dorsal approach**

The phalanges are easy to examine, with the reminder that each toe has three, except for the big toe with only two.

By meticulous palpation you can identify the sides, the plantar surfaces, and the dorsal surfaces of the shafts of the two phalanges of the hallux.

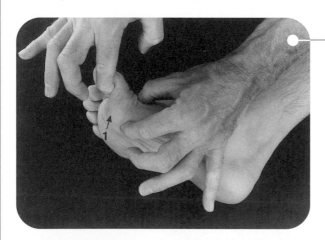

Fig. 12.27 | **The head and the sesamoid bones of the first metatarsal: plantar approach**

Place the pad of the index finger of your distal hand on the proximal phalanx so as to extend it, and you can feel the plantar base of that phalanx. Your other index then feels the plantar articular surface of the head of the first metatarsal and the two sesamoid bones (*ossa sesamoidea*).

Note: The anterior extremity or head of each metatarsal has a convex articular surface more extensive on its plantar (1) than on its dorsal aspect. This hold allows you to free this articular surface adequately.

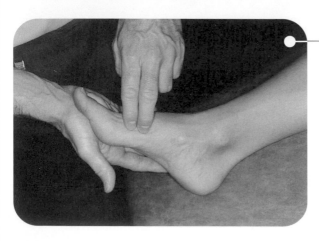

Fig. 12.28 | **The medial surface of the first metatarsal**

This lies in the medial part of the foot.

It is directly under the skin and has the distinction of lying in the dorsal half of the medial border of the foot, whereas the plantar half of this border contains only soft tissue.

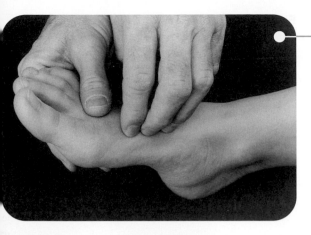

Fig. 12.29 | **The dorsal surface of the first metatarsal**

The shaft of every metatarsal is like a triangular prism. Its dorsal surface is narrow overall, but much wider posteriorly than anteriorly.

Note: A distinctive anatomical feature of the metatarsals is that their dorsal surfaces have two sloping borders, one medial and the other lateral.

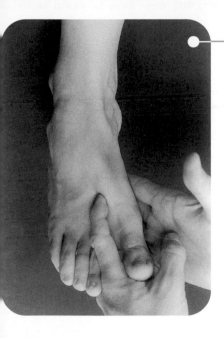

Fig. 12.30 | **The lateral surface of the first metatarsal**

With the medial surfaces of the adjacent metatarsals, the lateral surfaces of the metatarsals form a special space called the intermetatarsal or interosseous space.

Attachments

- Each of the four dorsal interossei arises from the lateral and dorsal surfaces of the two metatarsals that demarcate the corresponding interosseous space.
- The three plantar interossei arise from the plantar aspect of the sides of the metatarsals facing the axis of the foot, which passes through the second toe, and also from the inferior borders and bases of these metatarsals.

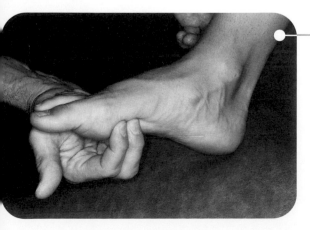

Fig. 12.31 | **The inferior or plantar border of the shaft of the first metatarsal (*corpus ossis metatarsalis I*)**

You can see very clearly the inferior or plantar border of the shaft, which you can feel under your fingers as a curved structure concave inferiorly (Figs 12.4 and 12.7).

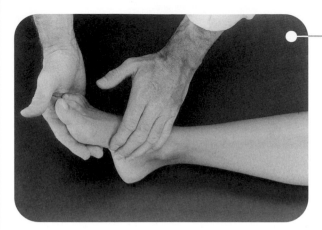

Fig. 12.32 **The base of the first metatarsal (*basis ossis metatarsalis I*) and the other bones of the medial border of the foot: localization by a global approach to the medial border of the foot.**

The subject's foot is relaxed and rests on a table or on the practitioner's knee.

The latter places his proximal hand on the instep and closes it gently over the medial border of the foot, while keeping the ulnar border of the little finger on the anterior border of the subject's medial malleolus.

In this case:

- The practitioner's little finger faces the medial surface of the neck of the talus.
- The ring finger faces the navicular.
- The middle finger faces the medial cuneiform.
- The index finger faces the base of the first metatarsal.

Note: This global approach to the bony structures on the medial border of the foot can be considered as reliable in the majority of subjects—except, of course, for extreme cases.

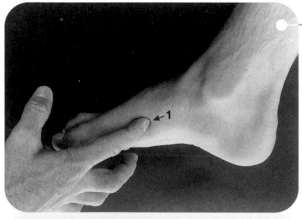

Fig. 12.33 **The posteromedial tuberosity of the first metatarsal (*tuberositas medialis ossis metatarsalis I*)**

This tuberosity receives the metatarsal insertion of the tibialis anterior, while the medial part of the medial cuneiform (1) (Fig. 12.35) receives the other insertion.

Slide your index finger between the body of the abductor hallucis and the plantar border of the first metatarsal, which feels curved under your fingers. Follow the medial border of the metatarsal shaft and you will find the tuberosity on its base near the joint space.

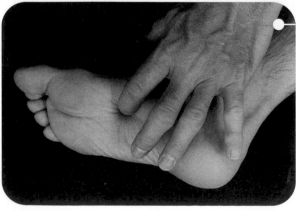

Fig. 12.34 **The posterolateral tuberosity of the base of the first metatarsal (*tuberositas lateralis ossis metatarsalis I*)**

This lies on the plantar surface, lateral and posterior to the posteromedial tuberosity, and receives the main insertion of the peroneus longus.

It is clear that this bony projection, buried as it is under soft tissues, will be more easily recognized after some muscle loss, as in the case of a subject bedridden for a long time. Otherwise you must apply a strong enough pressure to detect this structure.

*The medial cuneiform (*cuneiforme mediale*)*

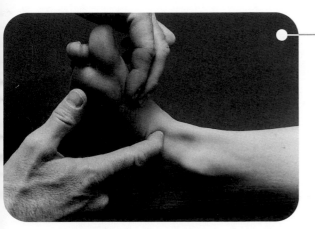

Fig. 12.35 | **The medial surface of the medial cuneiform: localization using the tibialis anterior**

An efficient way of localizing this medial surface is to make the tibialis anterior contract by asking the subject to supinate and dorsiflex the foot with or without resistance on your part. As the muscle is inserted into the medial part of the medial surface, you can easily locate it.

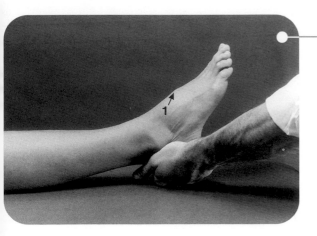

Fig. 12.36 | **Lateral view of the dorsal border of the medial cuneiform**

This lies on the medial border of the foot between the navicular and the first metatarsal, and has a fairly sharp ridge-like superior dorsal (1) border, particularly in its posterior part.

Note: This feature is displayed in the adjacent illustration featuring a lateral view, especially chosen to underscore this feature of the medial cuneiform.

The navicular bone (os naviculare)

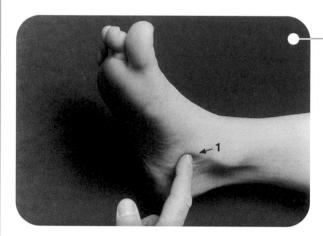

Fig. 12.37 **The tuberosity of the navicular (*tuberositas ossis navicularis*): direct approach**

This tuberosity juts out on the plantar part of the medial surface of the navicular (1), and is the site of the insertion of the tibialis posterior.

It is accessible behind the tendon of the tibialis anterior (see this muscle, Fig. 12.119). In many subjects it is clearly visible, as in the adjacent illustration.

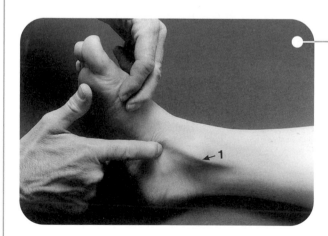

Fig. 12.38 **The tuberosity of the navicular: localization using the tibialis posterior**

Throwing the tibialis posterior (1) into contraction is an efficient way of localizing the tuberosity when it is less apparent.

First place the subject's foot in plantar flexion, and then simply ask him or her to adduct the foot.

Starting from the medial malleolus, follow the tibialis posterior down to the tuberosity you are looking for.

The talus (talus)

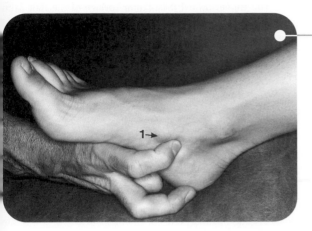

Fig. 12.39 | **The ligament-related or middle portion of the head of the talus (*caput tali*)**

As its name indicates, this structure is related to the plantar calcaneonavicular ligament, and lies behind the anterosuperior region of the head of the talus, which articulates with the navicular. Just put your fingers behind the tuberosity of the navicular (1) on the medial and plantar border of the foot and you will feel it as a smooth surface.

Note: Depending on the subject, it is sometimes useful to position the forefoot in abduction and pronation, the better to feel this structure under your fingers as they rest on the midline of the sole of the foot between the navicular tuberosity and the sustentaculum tali.

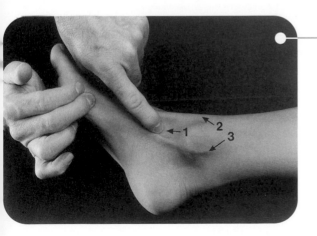

Fig. 12.40 | **The medial part of the talar neck (*collum tali*) (see also Fig. 12.32)**

The approach to this structure (1) lies mainly between the tendons of the tibialis anterior (2) laterally and of the tibialis posterior (3) medially.

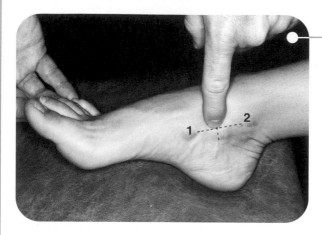

Fig. 12.41 | **The medial surface of the talar neck (second method)**

In addition to the approach using the tendons (figure above), you can also locate this structure using an imaginary line running from the navicular tuberosity (1) to the medial malleolus (2).

As you move toward the malleolus from the midpoint of this line, you will face the talar neck, which you will feel as a rough surface under your fingers.

As you move toward the plantar surface of the foot from the midpoint of this line, you will face the ligament-related portion of the talar head, which your fingers will feel as a smooth surface (Fig. 12.39).

Note: A rough ridge, more or less prominent depending on the subject, separates these two parts of the talus: the ligament-related portion of the head and the neck of the talus.

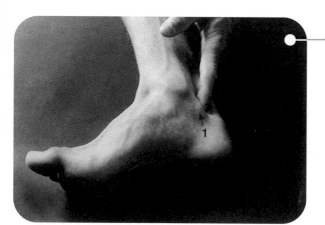

Fig. 12.42 | **The medial tubercle of the talus (*talus, tuberculum mediale*)**

It is important to remember that this bony structure (1) belongs to the posterior surface of the talus and that it provides insertion to the posterior tibiotalar or the deep bundle of the deltoid ligament.

From this bony structure the talocalcaneal ligament also runs toward the posterior border of the sustentaculum tali.

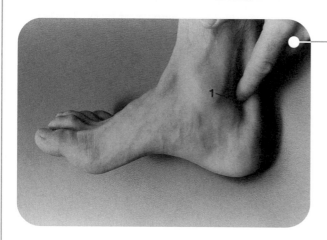

Fig. 12.43 | **The lateral tubercle of the talus (*talus, tuberculum laterale*)**

This tubercle (1) also belongs to the posterior surface of the talus. Place your fingers on the medial part of the Achilles' tendon and look for it at the level of the posterior border of the talus, where it is accessible.

Note: In most subjects it is not easily accessible but it is a notable bony structure as it is the site of insertion of the posterior talofibular ligament (formerly known as the posterior astragaloperoneal ligament or the lateral collateral ligament).

Attachment

Also inserted into this tubercle is the posterior talocalcaneal ligament, which terminates on the posterosuperior surface of the calcaneus.

Between these posteromedial and posterolateral tubercles lies a groove for the tendon of the flexor hallucis longus.

The calcaneus (calcaneus)

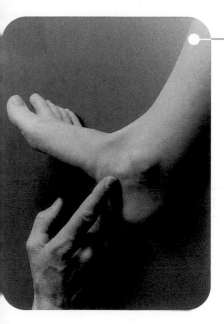

Fig. 12.44 | The sustentaculum tali (*sustentaculum tali*)

This lies about a finger-width below the medial malleolus. Its upper part supports the middle talar articular facet.

The medial part of the talocalcaneal joint is quite close and lies between the sustentaculum tali and the talus.

Attachments

- From the anterior border of the sustentaculum the plantar calcaneonavicular ligament runs toward the middle portion of the head of the talus.
- From its posterior border the talocalcaneal ligament runs toward the posteromedial tubercle of the talus.
- A groove runs along its top and is traversed by the tendon of the flexor digitorum longus.
- Another groove lying below the sustentaculum tali is traversed by the tendon of the flexor hallucis longus
- It also receives the insertion of the tibialis posterior.

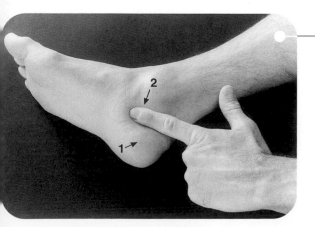

Fig. 12.45 | The calcaneal sulcus (*sulcus calcanei*)

This runs supero-inferiorly and postero-anteriorly, and occupies most of the medial surface of the calcaneus. It is bordered posteriorly and inferiorly by the posteromedial tubercle of the calcaneus (1), and anteriorly and superiorly by a variably prominent projection (that is, the sustentaculum tali, 2).

THE ANKLE AND FOOT

*The medial malleolus (*malleolus medialis*)*

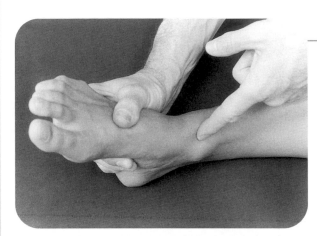

Fig. 12.46 | **The anterior border of the medial malleolus (*malleolus medialis*)**

This is thick and rough, and provides insertion to the superficial fibers of the deltoid ligament.

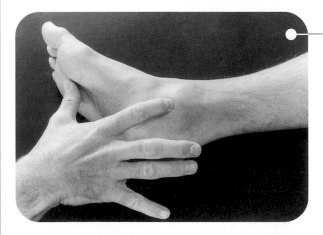

Fig. 12.47 | **The distal end of the medial malleolus**

This consists of two tubercles (anterior and posterior) separated by a notch, which gives attachment to the superficial and deep layers of the deltoid ligament.

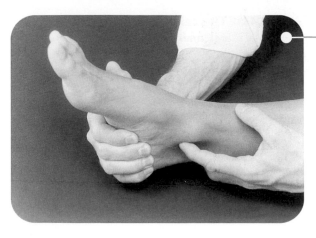

Fig. 12.48 | **The posterior border of the medial malleolus**

This contains an oblique groove, which runs supero-inferiorly and lateromedially. You can easily approach this groove by relaxing the tendons of the muscles in the area: that of the tibialis posterior, which is the most anteriorly located, and that of the flexor digitorum longus, which lies behind the former.

Note: In reality these two tendons run behind the malleolus, each in its own osteofibrous sheath.

THE ANTERIOR SURFACE OF THE ANKLE AND THE DORSAL SURFACE OF THE FOOT

The notable structures that can be detected by palpation are:

- The dorsal aspects of the metatarsal heads (*ossa metatarsalia, capita*) (Fig. 12.50).
- The fifth metatarsal (*os metatarsale V*) (Fig. 12.51).
- The fourth metatarsal (*os metatarsale IV*) (Fig. 12.52).
- The third metatarsal (*os metatarsale III*) (Fig. 12.53).
- The second metatarsal (*os metatarsale II*) (Fig. 12.54).
- The first metatarsal (*os metatarsale I*) (Fig. 12.55).
- The neck of the talus (*collum tali*) (Fig. 12.56).
- The anterior border of the tibia (*tibia, epiphysis distalis*) (Fig. 12.57).
- Other techniques of approach (Figs 12.58–12.61).

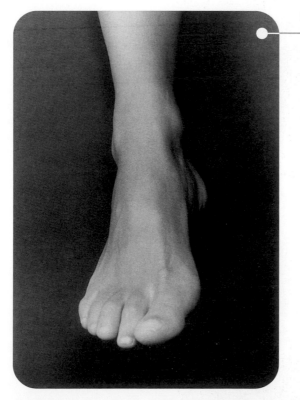

Fig. 12.49

Anterior view of the ankle and dorsal view of the foot

THE ANKLE AND FOOT

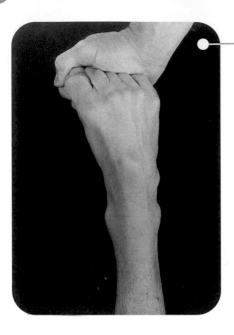

Fig. 12.50 | The metatarsal heads: dorsal view

Use a global approach, with the palm of your hand holding all the subject's toes, and then apply a sufficiently strong pressure to plantarflex the toes and bring out the metatarsal heads. You can also proceed metatarsal by metatarsal individually.

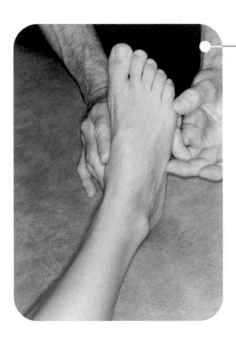

Fig. 12.51 | The fifth metatarsal (*os metatarsale V*)

First locate its head (see Fig. 12.4) and its base (Figs 12.7 and 12.8), and then place your fingers in the spaces of the appropriate joints (Figs 12.89 and 12.92). You will then hold this bone between your thumb and your index finger.

It is interesting to note the location and size of this bone with respect to the other metatarsals. Its base articulates posteriorly with the cuboid and medially with the fourth metatarsal. Its posterolateral surface bears a styloid process known as the tuberosity of the fifth metatarsal.

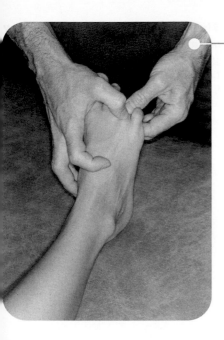

Fig. 12.52 | **The fourth metatarsal (*os metatarsale IV*)**

Locate its head and base after locating the appropriate joints (Figs 12.89 and 12.93).

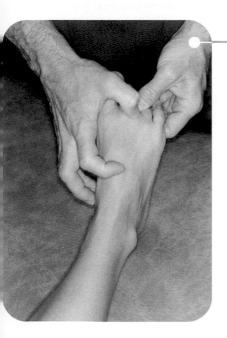

Fig. 12.53 | **The third metatarsal (*os metatarsale III*)**

Locate its head and base after locating the appropriate joints (Figs 12.89 and 12.94).

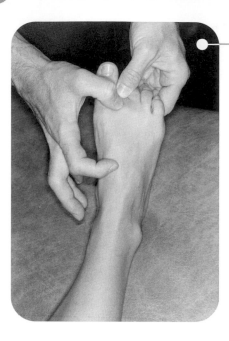

Fig. 12.54 | **The second metatarsal (os metatarsale II)**

Locate the head and the base after locating the appropriate joints (Figs 12.89 and 12.95).

Note: This is the longest of all the metatarsals.

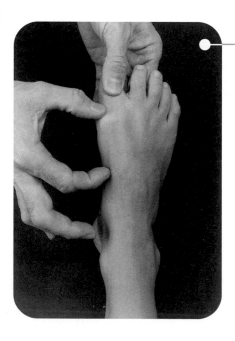

Fig. 12.55 | **The first metatarsal (os metatarsale I)**

Locate its head (Fig. 12.26) and its base (Figs 12.32 and 12.33) after locating the appropriate joints (Figs 12.89 and 12.96).

Note: This is the shortest and the biggest of all the metatarsals.

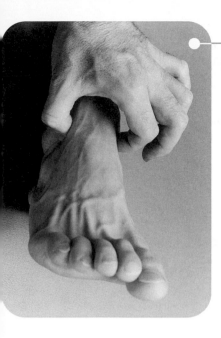

Fig. 12.56 | The neck of the talus (*collum tali*)

In the adjacent illustration the practitioner is holding the lateral and medial sides of the talar neck with his index finger resting on its medial side. These two parts of the neck have already been seen when the lateral (Figs 12.7 and 12.20) and the medial (Figs 12.32, 12.40 and 12.41) borders of the foot were studied.

The dorsal surface of the talar neck lies between the practitioner's thumb and index finger.

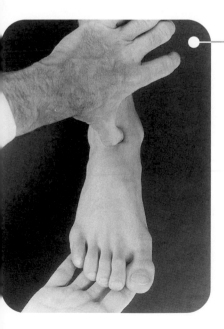

Fig. 12.57 | The anterior border of the distal end of the tibia (*tibia, epiphysis distalis*)

Note: This border is the one that is pulled into the transverse groove on the dorsal surface of the talar neck when the ankle is dorsiflexed.

OTHER TECHNIQUES OF APPROACH

The palpatory approaches described below are meant to make it easier to learn the articular techniques for this region.

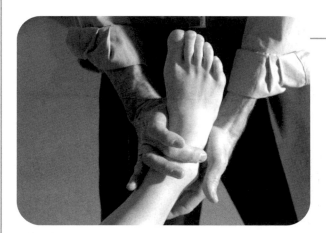

Fig. 12.58 | **The dorsal surface of the talar neck**

The practitioner's ring finger rests on the dorsal surface of the talar neck behind the navicular tubercle.

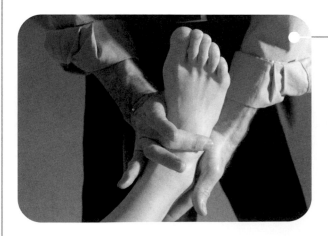

Fig. 12.59 | **The dorsal surface of the navicular bone**

Its easily palpable tuberosity is a helpful landmark for the localization of the dorsal surface of the navicular.

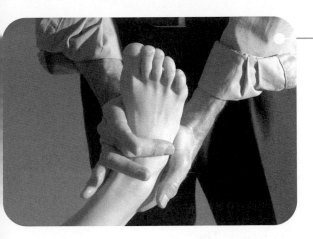

Fig. 12.60 | The dorsal surfaces of the three cuneiforms

Starting from the dorsal surface of the navicular, the practitioner slides the middle finger ahead of the navicular tuberosity, and it will come to lie on the dorsal surfaces of the three cuneiforms.

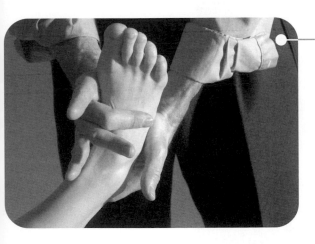

Fig. 12.61 | The dorsal surface of the base of the first metatarsal

This is always approached by sliding the middle finger from the dorsal surface of the three cuneiforms down to the dorsal surface of the base of the first metatarsal.

THE POSTERIOR SURFACE OF THE ANKLE AND FOOT

The bony structures that can be detected by palpation are:

- The medial malleolus (*malleolus medialis*) (Fig. 12.63).
- The sustentaculum tali (*sustentaculum tali*) (Fig. 12.64).
- The posterior surface of the calcaneus (*calcaneus, facies posterior*) (Fig. 12.65).
- The posterior segment of the dorsal surface of the calcaneus (*calcaneus*) (Fig. 12.66).
- The lateral malleolus (*malleolus lateralis*) (Fig. 12.67).
- The peroneal trochlea (*trochlea fibularis*) (Fig. 12.68).

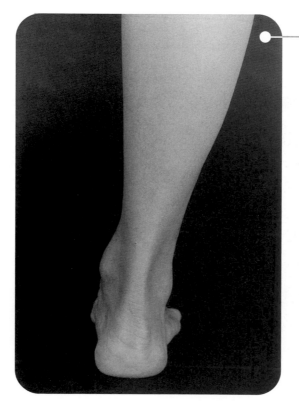

Fig. 12.62

Posterior view of the ankle and foot

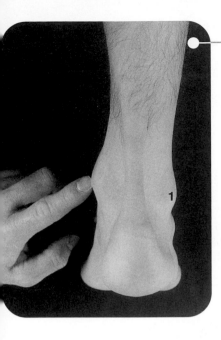

Fig. 12.63 | **The medial malleolus (*malleolus medialis*)**

You have already located the structure indicated by the practitioner's index finger while dealing with the approach to the medial border of the foot. This is a different view, meant to highlight its topographical location with respect to the other anatomical structures of the region.

Note: This view underscores the "high" position of the medial malleolus relative to the lateral malleolus (1).

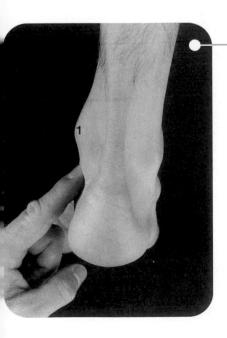

Fig. 12.64 | **The sustentaculum tali (*sustentaculum tali*)**

This structure, also indicated by the practitioner's index finger, was also dealt with when the medial border of the foot was presented. This posterior view confirms its topographical location with respect to the medial malleolus (1) (that is, one finger-width below it).

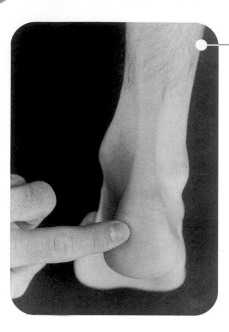

Fig. 12.65 | **The posterior surface of the calcaneus (*calcaneus*)**

This is narrow and smooth superiorly and wide and rough inferiorly, where the Achilles' tendon is inserted. Your fingers will feel it more or less as a triangle with a wide inferior base.

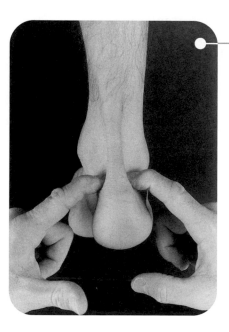

Fig. 12.66 | **The posterior part of the dorsal surface of the calcaneus**

This is concave in the sagittal plane and convex in the horizontal plane. You can approach it on both sides of the Achilles' tendon.

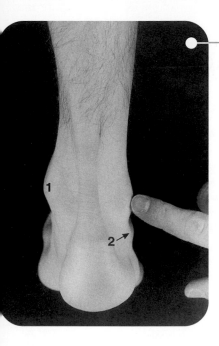

Fig. 12.67 | **The lateral malleolus (malleolus lateralis)**

We have already dealt with this structure (indicated here by the practitioner's index finger) while studying the lateral border of the foot. This different view allows the underscoring of its "low" position relative to the medial malleolus (1), and of its location with respect to the peroneal trochlea (2) (see figure below).

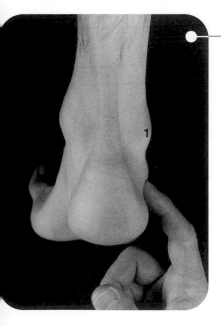

Fig. 12.68 | **The peroneal trochlea (*trochlea peronealis fibularis*)**

This has already been dealt with when the lateral border of the foot was presented. This view underscores its position relative to the apex of the lateral malleolus (1), which lies about one finger-width above it.

THE PLANTAR SURFACE

The structures that can be detected by palpation are:

- The heads of the five metatarsals (*ossa metatarsalia I–V, capita*) (Fig. 12.70).
- The plantar surface of the cuboid (*os cuboideum, facies plantaris*) (Fig. 12.71).
- The medial and lateral sesamoid bones (*ossa sesamoidea*) (Figs 12.72 and 12.73).
- The posterolateral tuberosity of the first metatarsal (Fig. 12.74) (*tuberositas ossis metatarsalis I*)
- The anterior tubercle of the plantar surface of the calcaneus (*tuberculum calcanei*), plantar view (Fig. 12.75).
- The posterior part of the plantar surface of the calcaneus (*calcaneus*) (Fig. 12.76).
- The medial process of the calcaneal tuberosity (*processus medialis tuberis calcanei*) (Fig. 12.77).
- The lateral process of the calcaneal tuberosity (*processus lateralis tuberis calcanei*) (Fig. 12.78).
- Other methods of approach (Figs 12.79–12.85).

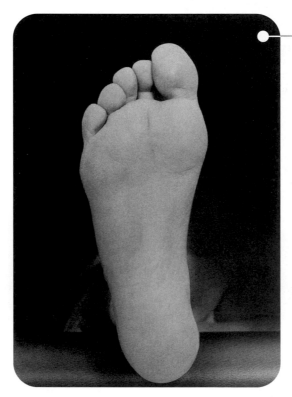

Fig. 12.69

Plantar view of the foot

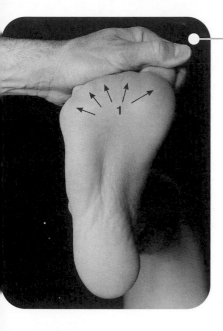

| Fig. 12.70 | **The heads of the five metatarsals** (*ossa metatarsalia I–V, capita*) |

Each metatarsal is characterized by having its head covered by a convex articular surface that is peculiar in being much more extensive on its plantar side than on its dorsal side.

You can therefore recognize this specific feature by palpating a large, smooth convex surface (1) just behind the metatarsophalangeal joints for each of the five metatarsals.

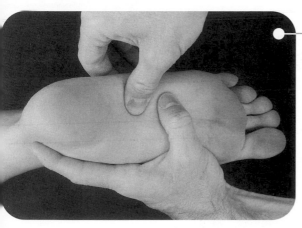

| Fig. 12.71 | **The plantar surface of the cuboid** (*os cuboideum*) |

We have already dealt with this bone while studying the lateral border of the foot. Once you have located the tuberosity of the fifth metatarsal (Figs 12.7 and 12.8) and the greater process of the calcaneus (Figs 12.7 and 12.13), simply put your thumb between these two structures and then slide it around the lateral border of the foot and therefore round the lateral border of the cuboid until it comes to lie on the plantar surface of the cuboid.

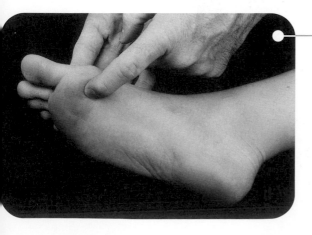

| Fig. 12.72 | **The medial sesamoid bone** (*os sesamoideum mediale*) |

You need only place the pads of two fingers on the plantar surface of the head of the first metatarsal and rub it from side to side. With this method you can feel under your fingers two "tubercles" separated by a groove. In the adjacent illustration the practitioner's index finger curves under the medial sesamoid bone.

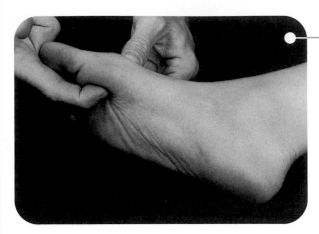

Fig. 12.73 | The lateral sesamoid bone (*os sesamoideum laterale*)

Use the same method as above. You simply move your index finger toward the lateral border of the foot so your finger can feel the lateral sesamoid bone after it crosses the above-mentioned groove.

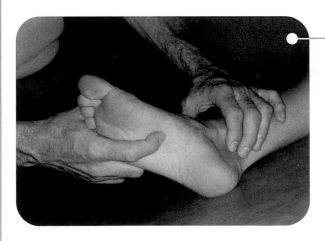

Fig. 12.74 | The posterolateral tuberosity of the first metatarsal (*tuberositas ossis metatarsalis I*)

First locate the base of the first metatarsal and then move to the plantar surface of the foot, toward its lateral border. The adjacent illustration shows the location of the tuberosity (see also Fig. 12.34).

Note: As this structure lies deep, you should apply sufficiently strong pressure to find it. Using your thumb may turn out to be more efficient.

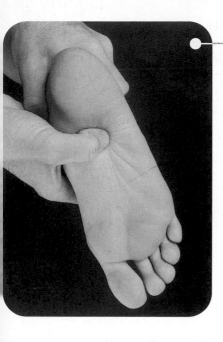

Fig. 12.75 | **The anterior tubercle of the plantar surface of the calcaneus (*tuberculum calcanei*)**

The adjacent illustration shows the plantar surface of the foot, which allows a more precise topographical localization of the tubercle.

If you start from the medial border, use the talar neck (Figs 12.56 and 12.58) as a landmark for your thumb. Then go round the medial border of the foot until you reach the tubercle.

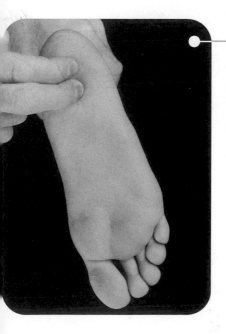

Fig. 12.76 | **The posterior part of the plantar surface of the calcaneus**

This is also called the calcaneal tuberosity. It occupies the posterior third of the bone, and forms the part of the calcaneus that rests on the ground (Fig. 12.7).

The tuberosity contains two processes: the medial (Fig. 12.77) and the lateral processes (Fig. 12.78).

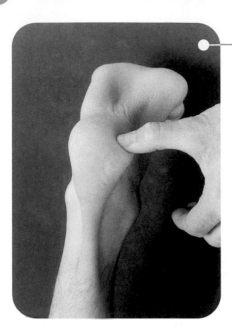

Fig. 12.77 | **The medial process of the calcaneal tuberosity (*processus medialis tuberis calcanei*)**

This is the bulkier of the two posterior processes.

Attachment
It gives origin to the flexor digitorum brevis and the abductor hallucis.

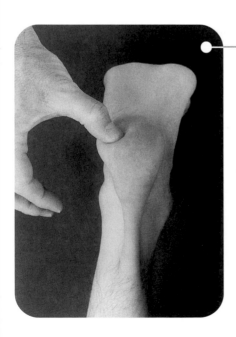

Fig. 12.78 | **The lateral process of the calcaneal tuberosity (*processus lateralis tuberis calcanei*)**

This is the less bulky of the two posterior processes.

Attachment
It gives origin to the abductor digiti minimi.

OTHER METHODS OF APPROACH

The methods of approach to palpation described below are meant to make it easier to learn the articular techniques for this region.

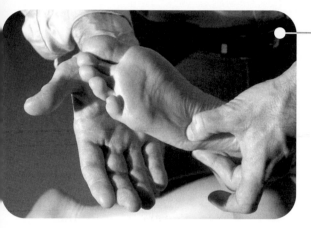

Fig. 12.79 | The plantar surface of the base of the fifth metatarsal

While the subject lies prone, the practitioner flexes the knee, takes hold of the foot, and blocks the posterior aspect of the calcaneus between the middle and ring fingers. With the thumb the practitioner can then palpate the plantar surface of the fifth metatarsal and its tuberosity. The practitioner's other hand rests on the dorsal surface of the subject's foot.

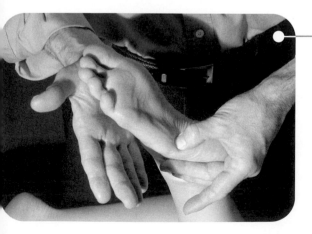

Fig. 12.80 | The plantar surface of the cuboid

The subject and the practitioner adopt the same positions as described in Figure 12.79. The practitioner places the thumb on the plantar surface of the cuboid.

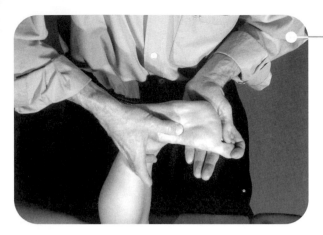

Fig. 12.81 | **The plantar surface of the first metatarsal**

The practitioner's thumb rests on the plantar surface of the first metatarsal, and can feel its posteromedial tuberosity on the inside and its posterolateral tuberosity on the outside.

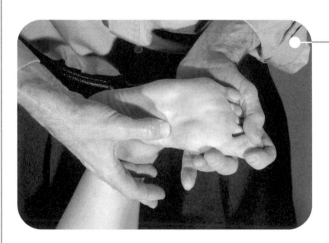

Fig. 12.82 | **The plantar surface of the medial cuneiform**

The practitioner moves the thumb on the plantar surface of the foot toward the calcaneus to palpate the plantar surface of the medial cuneiform.

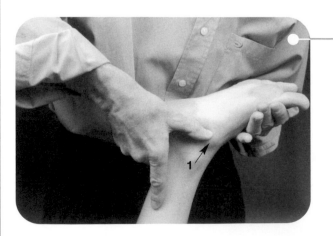

Fig. 12.83 | **The plantar surface of the tuberosity of the navicular**

You have already encountered this structure (1) while studying the medial border of the foot (Figs 12.37 and 12.38). You can also palpate it by this plantar approach, as shown in the adjacent illustration.

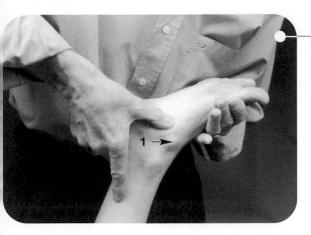

Fig. 12.84 | **The plantar surface of the navicular**

Starting from the plantar surface of the navicular tuberosity (1), move your thumb laterally to reach the plantar surface of the navicular.

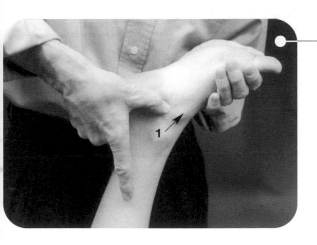

Fig. 12.85 | **The plantar approach to the ligament-related part or middle part of the head of the talus**

You can touch the talar head between the navicular tuberosity (1) and the sustentaculum tali, which lies a finger-width from the medial malleolus. Your fingers will feel a smooth surface.

This structure can be palpated by a medial and a plantar approach, since this part of the talar head is quite free on the plantar side of the foot.

ARTHROLOGY

LIGAMENTS AND TENDONS OF THE ANKLE

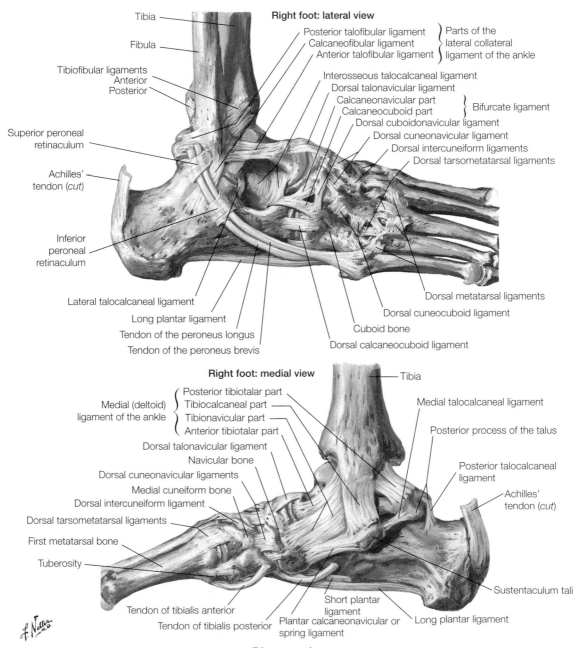

Right foot: lateral view

Tibia

Fibula

Tibiofibular ligaments
Anterior
Posterior

Superior peroneal retinaculum

Achilles' tendon (cut)

Inferior peroneal retinaculum

Lateral talocalcaneal ligament

Long plantar ligament

Tendon of the peroneus longus

Tendon of the peroneus brevis

Posterior talofibular ligament ⎫
Calcaneofibular ligament   ⎬ Parts of the lateral collateral ligament of the ankle
Anterior talofibular ligament ⎭

Interosseous talocalcaneal ligament

Dorsal talonavicular ligament

Calcaneonavicular part ⎫
Calcaneocuboid part   ⎬ Bifurcate ligament

Dorsal cuboidonavicular ligament

Dorsal cuneonavicular ligament

Dorsal intercuneiform ligaments

Dorsal tarsometatarsal ligaments

Dorsal metatarsal ligaments

Dorsal cuneocuboid ligament

Cuboid bone

Dorsal calcaneocuboid ligament

Right foot: medial view

Medial (deltoid) ligament of the ankle
{
Posterior tibiotalar part
Tibiocalcaneal part
Tibionavicular part
Anterior tibiotalar part
}

Dorsal talonavicular ligament

Navicular bone

Dorsal cuneonavicular ligaments

Medial cuneiform bone

Dorsal intercuneiform ligament

Dorsal tarsometatarsal ligaments

First metatarsal bone

Tuberosity

Tibia

Medial talocalcaneal ligament

Posterior process of the talus

Posterior talocalcaneal ligament

Achilles' tendon (cut)

Sustentaculum tali

Tendon of tibialis anterior

Tendon of tibialis posterior

Short plantar ligament

Plantar calcaneonavicular or spring ligament

Long plantar ligament

Plantar view

LIGAMENTS AND TENDONS OF THE FOOT

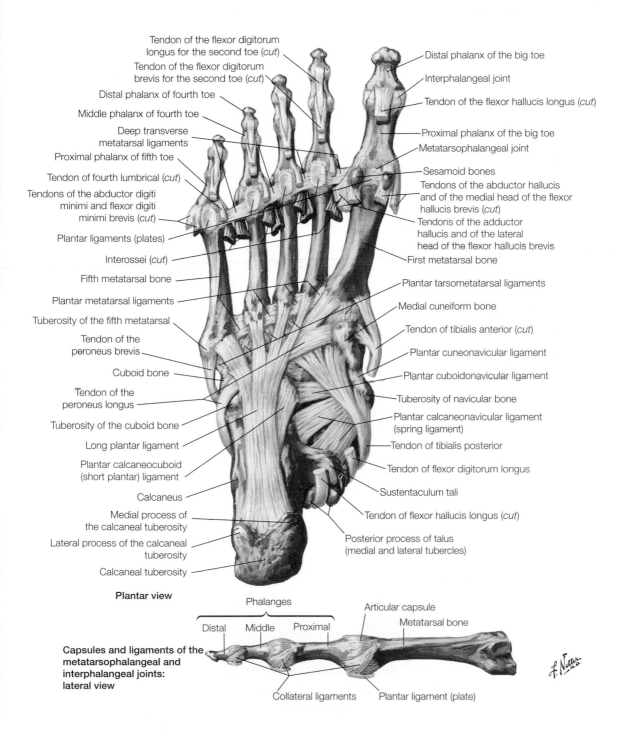

Tendon of the flexor digitorum longus for the second toe (*cut*)

Tendon of the flexor digitorum brevis for the second toe (*cut*)

Distal phalanx of fourth toe

Middle phalanx of fourth toe

Deep transverse metatarsal ligaments

Proximal phalanx of fifth toe

Tendon of fourth lumbrical (*cut*)

Tendons of the abductor digiti minimi and flexor digiti minimi brevis (*cut*)

Plantar ligaments (plates)

Interossei (*cut*)

Fifth metatarsal bone

Plantar metatarsal ligaments

Tuberosity of the fifth metatarsal

Tendon of the peroneus brevis

Cuboid bone

Tendon of the peroneus longus

Tuberosity of the cuboid bone

Long plantar ligament

Plantar calcaneocuboid (short plantar) ligament

Calcaneus

Medial process of the calcaneal tuberosity

Lateral process of the calcaneal tuberosity

Calcaneal tuberosity

Distal phalanx of the big toe

Interphalangeal joint

Tendon of the flexor hallucis longus (*cut*)

Proximal phalanx of the big toe

Metatarsophalangeal joint

Sesamoid bones

Tendons of the abductor hallucis and of the medial head of the flexor hallucis brevis (*cut*)

Tendons of the adductor hallucis and of the lateral head of the flexor hallucis brevis

First metatarsal bone

Plantar tarsometatarsal ligaments

Medial cuneiform bone

Tendon of tibialis anterior (*cut*)

Plantar cuneonavicular ligament

Plantar cuboidonavicular ligament

Tuberosity of navicular bone

Plantar calcaneonavicular ligament (spring ligament)

Tendon of tibialis posterior

Tendon of flexor digitorum longus

Sustentaculum tali

Tendon of flexor hallucis longus (*cut*)

Posterior process of talus (medial and lateral tubercles)

Plantar view

Phalanges

Distal Middle Proximal

Articular capsule

Metatarsal bone

Capsules and ligaments of the metatarsophalangeal and interphalangeal joints: lateral view

Collateral ligaments

Plantar ligament (plate)

THE JOINTS AND LIGAMENTS OF THE FOOT

The joints accessible to manual surface exploration are (from the tips of the toes to the ankle):

- Interphalangeal joints (*articulationes interphalangeae*) (Figs 12.87 and 12.88).
- Metatarsophalangeal joints (*articulationes metatarsophalangeae*) (Figs 12.89–12.91).
- The tarsometatarsal joints (*articulationes tarsometatarseae*) (Lisfranc's joint) (Figs 12.92–12.96).
- The transverse tarsal joint (*articulatio tarsi transversa*) (Chopart's joint) (Figs 12.97–12.99), including the bifurcate ligament and the talocalcaneonavicular joint (*lig. bifurcatum*) (Fig. 12.99).
- The subtalar joint (*art. subtalaris*) (Figs 12.100–101).
- The ankle joint (*art. talocruralis*) (Figs 12.102–12.107).
- The ligaments of the ankle joint (*art. talocruralis*) (Figs 12.108–12.113).
- The posterior tibiofibular ligament (*lig. tibiofibulare posterius*) (Fig. 12.114).
- The superior peroneal retinaculum (*retinaculum, mm. fibularium superius*) (Fig. 12.115).
- The inferior and superior extensor retinacula (*retinacula mm. extensorum superius et inferius*) (Fig. 12.116).
- The dorsal fascia of the foot (*fascia dorsalis pedis*) (Fig. 12.117).

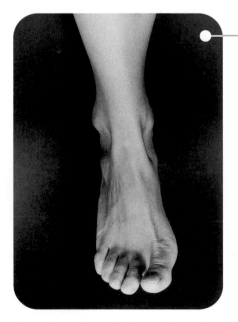

Fig. 12.86

Anterior view of the ankle and dorsal view of the foot

*The interphalangeal joints (*articulationes interphalangeae*)*

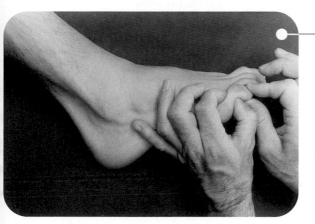

Fig. 12.87 | **The interphalangeal joints of the little toe (*articulationes interphalangeae digiti minimi*)**

These two joints are easily identified.

In the adjacent illustration, the practitioner's proximal hand fixes the proximal phalanx, while the distal hand plantarflexes the distal phalanx.

Note: These are hinge joints or ginglymi. The articular surfaces are: the articular surface of the pulley-shaped head of the immediately posterior phalanx, and the articular surface of the base of the immediately anterior phalanx with an ill-defined median crest as its special feature.

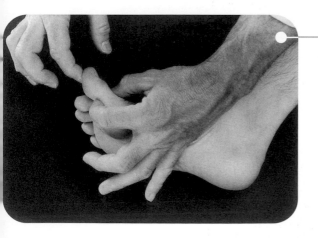

Fig. 12.88 | **The interphalangeal joint of the big toe (*hallux*) in dorsiflexion**

The big toe has the distinction of having only one interphalangeal joint.

In the adjacent illustration the proximal head fixes the proximal phalanx, while the distal hand dorsiflexes the second phalanx.

*The metatarsophalangeal joints (*articulationes metatarsophalangeae*)*

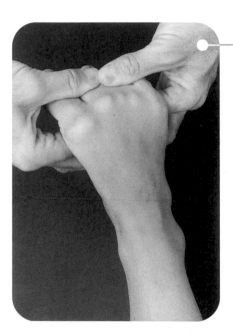

Fig. 12.89 | **The metatarsophalangeal joints (*articulationes metatarsophalangeae*): dorsal view**

In the adjacent illustration, as the practitioner's hands take hold of the toes and plantarflex them, the posterior and dorsal articular surfaces of the metatarsal heads are revealed.

Note: Your fingers will feel the articular surface as a smooth one; the most accessible one is that of the big toe.

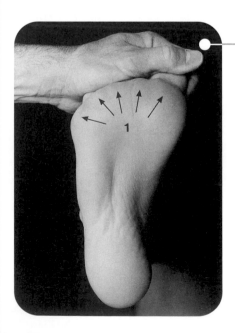

Fig. 12.90 | **The metatarsophalangeal joints: plantar view**

In the adjacent figure, as the practitioner's hand takes hold of the toes and dorsiflexes them, the anterior and plantar articular surfaces of the metatarsal heads (1) are revealed.

Note: The articular surface of each metatarsal head "overshoots" extensively on the plantar side.

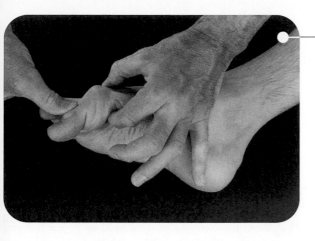

Fig. 12.91 | **The metatarsophalangeal joint of the big toe**

As you examine this joint, you will feel the sesamoid bones on its plantar aspect (see Figs 12.72 and 12.73).

The tarsometatarsal joints (Lisfranc's joint, articulationes tarsometatarseae*)*

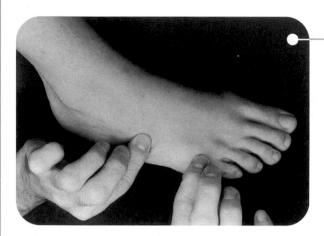

Fig. 12.92 | **The joint between the cuboid (os cuboideum) and the fifth metatarsal (os metatarsale V)**

Place the index finger of your distal hand on the anterolateral surface of the cuboid (Figs 12.7, and 12.9–12.11) and touch the base of the fifth metatarsal (Figs 12.7 and 12.8). In order to feel the joint better you need only take hold of the head of the fifth metatarsal and move it up and down repeatedly. Your index finger will feel the joint you are looking for.

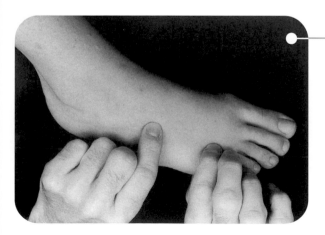

Fig. 12.93 | **The joint between the cuboid and the fourth metatarsal (os metatarsale IV)**

Move the index finger of your proximal hand slightly medially to face the anteromedial surface of the cuboid while staying in contact with the base of the fourth metatarsal.

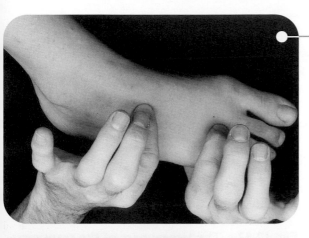

Fig. 12.94 | The joint between the lateral cuneiform (*os cuneiforme laterale*) and the third metatarsal (*os metatarsale III*)

Starting from the position described in Fig. 12.93 for your proximal hand, move your index finger one finger-width toward the inside of the foot and at the same time you will come into contact with the anterior border of the lateral cuneiform and the base of the third metatarsal.

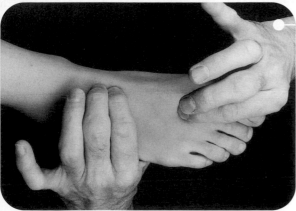

Fig. 12.95 | The joint between the intermediate cuneiform (*os cuneiforme intermedium*) and the second metatarsal (*os metatarsale II*)

Again starting from the position described in Figure 12.94 for your proximal hand, you need only move it one finger-width toward the inside of the foot, while keeping in mind that the anterior border of the intermediate cuneiform lies deep to those of the other two cuneiforms, which flank it, one on either side. Then move your index finger toward the hindfoot to contact the intermediate cuneiform and the base of the second metatarsal.

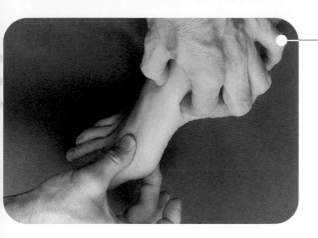

Fig. 12.96 | The joint between the medial cuneiform (*os cuneiforme mediale*) and the first metatarsal (*os metatarsale I*)

To locate the medial cuneiform, see Figures 12.7 and 12.32.

In the adjacent illustration the practitioner's proximal hand lies at the level of the joint of interest. The distal hand holds the head of the first metatarsal.

Note: The tarsometatarsal joints (articulationes metatarseae) or Lisfranc's joint link the three cuneiforms and the cuboid with the five metatarsals. They consist of three tarsometatarsal joints:

- A medial joint between the medial cuneiform and the first metatarsal.
- An intermediate joint between the intermediate and lateral cuneiforms and the second and third metatarsals.
- A lateral joint between the cuboid and the fourth and fifth metatarsals.

THE ANKLE AND FOOT

The transverse tarsal joint (Chopart's joint) (art. tarsi transversa)

This links the distal and proximal parts of the tarsus. Functionally, it consists of a single unit made up of the talocalcaneonavicular and calcaneocuboid joints. The bifurcate ligament is shared by these two joints.

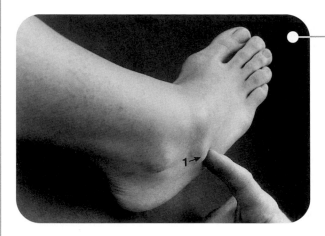

Fig. 12.97 | **The lateral part of the transverse tarsal joint (Chopart's lateral joint)**

This is the calcaneocuboid joint. Place your index finger on the anteriorly located cuboid facet of the calcaneus, which articulates anteriorly with the cuboid. Invert the subject's foot to make it easier for you to reach the lateral part of this surface.

   The greater process of the calcaneus is also shown (1).
   (See *Note*, p. 411.)

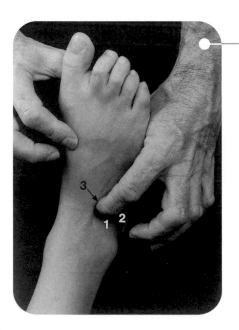

Fig. 12.98 | **The bifurcate ligament (*lig. bifurcatum*) of the transverse tarsal joint**

This is attached posteriorly to the dorsal surface of the greater process of the calcaneus (1) and divides into two limbs:

* A lateral limb inserted into the dorsal surface of the cuboid (2).
* A medial limb inserted into the entire lateral surface of the navicular (3).

Note: The bifurcate is considered to be the key ligament of this joint.

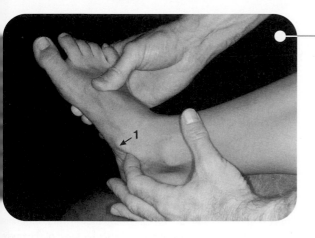

Fig. 12.99 | **The medial part of the transverse tarsal joint (Chopart's medial joint)**

This is the talocalcaneonavicular joint. Evert the foot the better to free up the talar head, which articulates with the navicular (1).

In the adjacent illustration, the practitioner's index finger frees the middle part of the talar head, which is related to the plantar calcaneonavicular ligament. Your index finger will feel a smooth surface.

*The subtalar joint (*art. subtalaris*)*

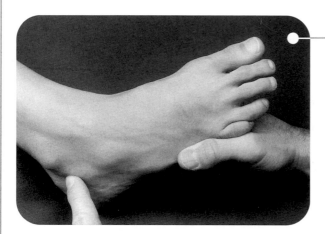

Fig. 12.100 | The subtalar joint: lateral view

The practitioner's index finger is pointing to the lateral part of the subtalar joint. The bony prominence facing the index finger is in fact the lateral tubercle of the talus, which supports the most lateral part of the peroneal articular facet of the body of the talus.

Note: The lateral talocalcaneal ligament is attached to this lateral tubercle.

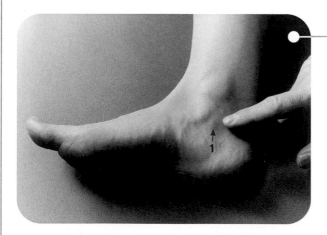

Fig. 12.101 | The subtalar joint: medial view

The practitioner's index finger is pointing to the medial part of the subtalar joint. The bony prominence facing the index finger is the sustentaculum tali (1). It supports the middle talar articular surface of the calcaneus, which is directly continuous with the anterior talar articular surface of the calcaneus.

The ankle joint (art. talocruralis)

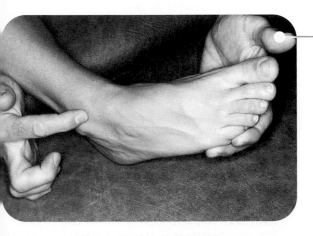

Fig. 12.102 | The lateral border of the lateral side of the talar trochlea (*trochlea tali*)

Place the index finger of your proximal hand on the anterior border of the distal end of the fibula, with the foot in the neutral position. You need only plantarflex the foot slightly for your finger to feel this border.

By slightly adducting the foot at the same time you can get a better feel of this structure.

Note: This border is felt as both "smooth" (since it is coated with cartilage) and "sharp."

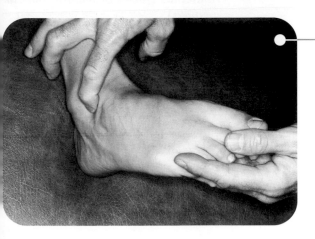

Fig. 12.103 | The articular facet of the lateral malleolus (*facies articularis malleoli lateralis*)

First place the subject's foot in the neutral position, and then place the index finger of your proximal hand just in front of the anterior border of the distal end of the fibula.

With your distal hand invert the foot while plantarflexing it slightly. The articular facet you are interested in is palpable under your index finger as a smooth surface.

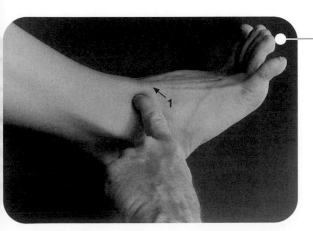

Fig. 12.104 | The lateral surface of the talar trochlea (*trochlea tali*)

Starting from the lateral border that has already been located (Fig. 12.102), you need only slide your index finger behind the tendon of the extensor digitorum longus (1) toward the medial border of the foot.

Inverting and plantarflexing the foot will cause the talar trochlea to jut out and make it easier for you to gain access to the articular surface you are interested in.

THE ANKLE AND FOOT

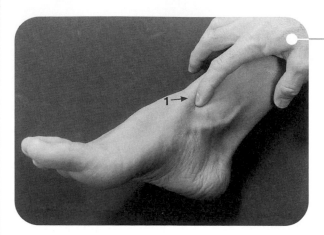

Fig. 12.105 | The medial border of the medial surface of the talar trochlea

The index finger of your distal hand rests on the anterior border of the medial malleolus, where it joins the anterior border of the distal end of the tibia.

With the foot in the neutral position, you need only plantarflex it slightly in order to be able to feel this border under your finger. It is better to evert the foot a little at the same time in order to avoid any hindrance from the tendon of the tibialis anterior (1).

Note: This border, which your finger feels as a smooth surface, is much less prominent on its medial side.

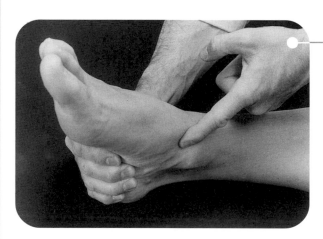

Fig. 12.106 | The articular facet of the medial malleolus (*facies articularis malleoli medialis*)

First place the index finger of your distal hand in front of the anterior border of the medial malleolus, and then completely uncover the articular facet by everting the foot and slightly plantarfexing it at the same time.

Your finger will feel the articular facet as a smooth surface.

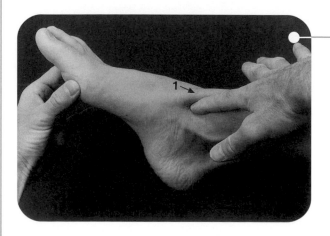

Fig. 12.107 | The medial surface of the talar trochlea

Starting from the medial border that has already been located (Fig. 12.105), you simply slide your finger behind the tendon of the tibialis anterior (1) toward the lateral border of the foot.

From this starting point it is preferable to follow this maneuver with eversion and slight plantarflexion of the foot in order to make the trochlea stick out on the medial border of the foot. You will then find it easier to gain access to the structure you are interested in.

*The ligaments of the ankle joint (*art. talocruralis*)*

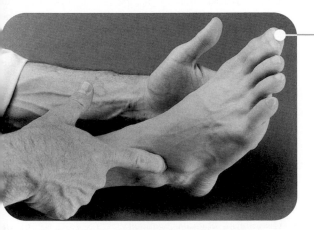

Fig. 12.108 | The anterior talofibular ligament (*lig. talofibulare anterius*)

In order to approach this ligament you must have a clear idea of its proximal insertion into the middle part of the anterior border of the lateral malleolus, and its distal insertion just in front of the lateral malleolar facet on the lateral surface of the talar neck. It is often useful to adduct, supinate, and slightly plantarflex the foot to have better access to this ligament.

Note: These three ligaments (Figs 12.108–12.110) were formerly called the anterior, middle, and posterior slips of the lateral collateral ligament.

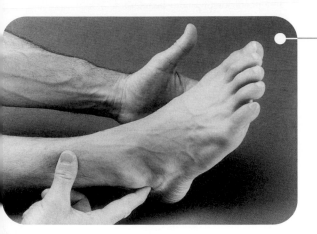

Fig. 12.109 | The calcaneofibular ligament (*lig. calcaneofibulare*)

In order to approach it correctly, you must be able to envisage the course of this ligament clearly, along with its proximal insertion into the anterior border of the lateral malleolus below the ligament mentioned above, and its distal insertion into the lateral surface of the calcaneus.

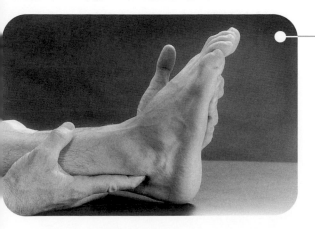

Fig. 12.110 | The posterior talofibular ligament (*lig. talofibulare posterius*)

To approach this ligament correctly it is also essential to have a clear idea of its lateral insertion into the medial surface of the lateral process of the posterior border of the talus. It runs almost horizontally between these two structures.

Note: It lies below the posterior tibiofibular ligament of the inferior tibiofibular joint.

THE ANKLE AND FOOT

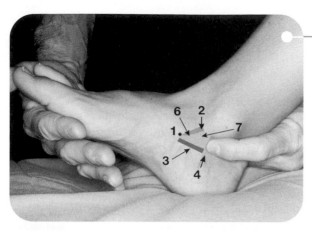

Fig. 12.111 | The superficial layer of the medial or deltoid ligament

This consists of two bundles:

- A tibionavicular bundle (6) (that is, the superficial and anterior part of the deltoid ligament), stretching from the tibial malleolus to the navicular (1).
- A tibiocalcaneal bundle (7) stretching from the tibial malleolus to the sustentaculum tali (4) and to the plantar calcaneonavicular or the spring ligament (3).

Note: The practitioner's index finger is pointing to the entire superficial bundle of this ligament.

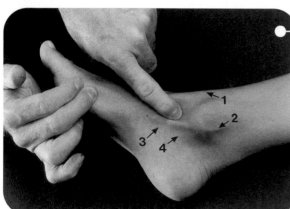

Fig. 12.112 | The deep layer of the medial or deltoid ligament

This consists of two bundles:

- The anterior tibiotalar ligament.
- The posterior tibiotalar ligament.

Note: The practitioner's index finger is pointing to the anterior tibiotalar ligament stretching from the tibial malleolus to the talar neck.

Legends for Figures 12.111–12.113

1. Navicular bundle.
2. Anterior tibiotalar ligament.
3. Plantar calcaneonavicular ligament.
4. Sustentaculum tali.
5. Posterior tibiotalar ligament.
6. Tibionavicular ligament.
7. Tibiocalcaneal ligament.

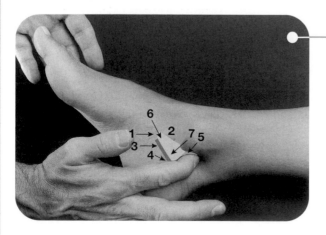

Fig. 12.113 | The deep layer of the medial or deltoid ligament (posterior portion)

The posterior tibiotalar ligament (5) is inserted into the medial surface of the body of the talus below the articular surface right up to its posteromedial tubercle.

Note: In the adjacent illustration, it is the posterior portion of the ligament that is being approached near its insertion into the posteromedial tubercle of the talus.

*The posterior tibiofibular ligament (*lig. tibiofibulare posterius*)*

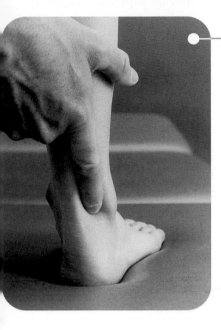

Fig. 12.114 | The posterior tibiofibular ligament

As you slide your index finger superomedially along the lateral malleolar grove, the first ligament you feel is the posterior tibiofibular ligament. Below it you come across a bundle of fibers that reinforce the articular capsule, and then you come into contact farther down with the posterior talofibular ligament (the posterior part of the lateral collateral ligament).

The extensor retinacula and the dorsal fascia of the foot

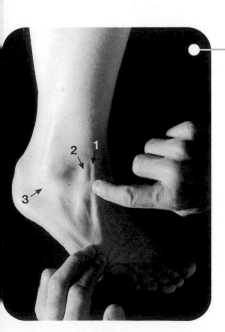

Fig. 12.115 | The superior peroneal retinaculum (*retinaculum mm. peroneorum/fibularium superius*)

In this illustration you can see clearly the lateral part of the inferior extensor retinaculum (indicated by the practitioner's index finger). It covers the tendons of the extensor digitorum longus (1) and of the peroneus tertius (2), and extends upward along the lateral border of the foot to blend with the superior peroneal retinaculum (3).

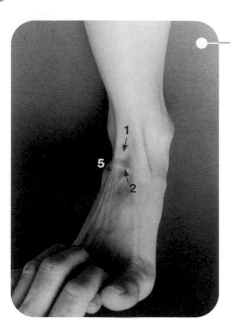

Fig. 12.116 | **The superior and inferior extensor retinacula (*retinacula extensorum superius et inferius*)**

In this illustration you can clearly make out the superior (1) and the inferior (2) extensor retinacula at the point where they split after providing cover for the extensor digitorum longus (5).

*The dorsal fascia of the foot (*fascia dorsalis pedis*)*

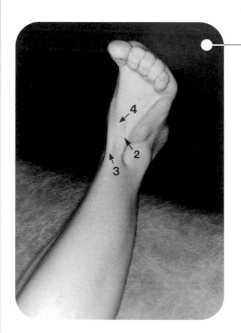

Fig. 12.117 | **The dorsal fascia of the foot**

In this illustration you can see the dorsal fascia of the foot (2) particularly well, covering the tendons of the extensor hallucis longus (4) and the tibialis anterior (3).

MYOLOGY

DORSAL MUSCLES OF THE FOOT: SUPERFICIAL PLANE

Superficial peroneal nerve (*cut*)

Peroneus brevis muscle

Tendon of the peroneus longus

Extensor digitorum muscle and its tendon

Superior extensor retinaculum

Fibula

Perforating branch of the peroneal artery

Lateral malleolus and anterior lateral malleolar artery

Inferior extensor retinaculum

Lateral tarsal artery and lateral branch of the deep peroneal nerve (going to the dorsal muscles of the foot)

Tendon of the peroneus brevis

Tuberosity of the fifth metatarsal

Tendon of the peroneus tertius

Extensor digitorum brevis and extensor hallucis brevis muscles

Tendons of the extensor digitorum longus

Lateral dorsal cutaneous nerve (continuation of the sural nerve) (*cut*)

Dorsal metatarsal arteries

Dorsal digital arteries

Dorsal branches of the proper plantar digital arteries and nerves

Tendon of the tibialis anterior

Anterior tibial artery and deep peroneal nerve

Tibia

Tendon of the extensor hallucis longus

Synovial sheath of the tendons of the extensor digitorum longus

Medial malleolus

Synovial sheath of tibialis anterior

Synovial sheath of the tendon of the extensor hallucis longus

Anterior medial malleolar artery

Dorsalis pedis artery and medial branch of the deep peroneal nerve

Medial tarsal artery

Arcuate artery

Deep plantar artery running between the two heads of the first dorsal interosseus to join the deep plantar arch

Tendon of the extensor hallucis longus

Expansions of the extensor muscles

Dorsal digital branches of the deep peroneal nerve

Dorsal digital branches of the superficial peroneal nerve

MUSCULOTENDINOUS STRUCTURES OF THE ANKLE AND THE FOOT

As you go round the ankle you can see the following structures:

- The tendon of the tibialis anterior (*m. tibialis anterior*) (Fig. 12.119).
- The tendon of the extensor hallucis longus (*m. extensor hallucis longus*) (Fig. 12.120).
- The extensor hallucis brevis muscle (*m. extensor hallucis brevis*) (Figs 12.121 and 12.124).
- The tendon of the extensor digitorum longus (*m. extensor digitorum longus*) (Fig. 12.122).
- The tendon of the peroneus tertius (*m. peroneus tertius*) (Fig. 12.123).
- The body of the extensor digitorum brevis (*m. extensor digitorum brevis*) (Fig. 12.124).
- The tendon of the peroneus brevis (*m. peroneus brevis*) (Fig. 12.125).
- The tendon of the peroneus longus (*m. peroneus longus)* (Fig. 12.126).
- The posterior part of the body of the peroneus brevis (Fig. 12.127).
- The Achilles' tendon (*tendo calcanei*) (Figs 12.128–12.129).
- The tendon of the tibialis posterior (*m. tibialis posterior*) at the medial malleolus (*malleolus medialis*) (Fig. 12.130).
- The tendon of the tibialis posterior (*m. tibialis posterior*) on the medial border of the foot (Fig. 12.131).
- The tendon of the flexor digitorum longus (*m. flexor digitorum longus*) at the medial malleolus (Fig. 12.132).
- The tendon of the flexor digitorum longus (Fig. 12.133) at the medial border of the foot.
- The tendon of the flexor hallucis longus (*m. flexor hallucis longus*) (Fig. 12.134) in the medial malleolar groove.
- The tendon of the flexor hallucis longus (Fig. 12.135) at the medial border of the foot.

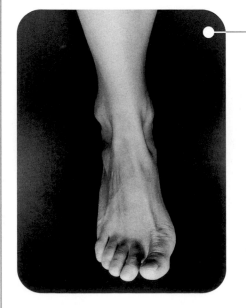

Fig. 12.118 | **Anterior view of the ankle and dorsal view of the foot**

Note: This topographical region must not be taken in the strict sense of the term. It is only a teaching tool for the method of approach to structures that extend well beyond them in the foot.

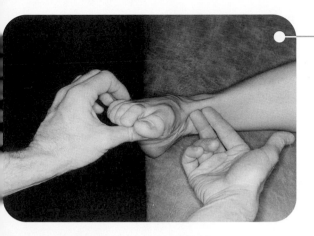

Fig. 12.119 | The tendon of the tibialis anterior (*m. tibialis anterior, tendo*)

This is a big strong tendon shaped like a cylindrical cord and it lies just in front of the medial malleolus as it runs toward the medial border of the foot to insert principally into the medial cuneiform; it also sends an expansion to the postero-medial tuberosity at the base of the first metatarsal. In the adjacent illustration the practitioner's distal hand inverts and dorsiflexes the foot. The subject is then asked to maintain this foot position.

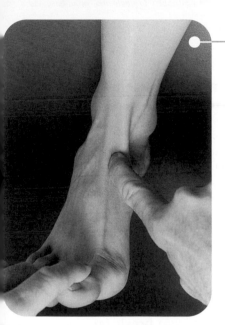

Fig. 12.120 | The tendon of the extensor hallucis longus (*m. extensor hallucis longus, tendo*)

Ask the subject to extend both the interphalangeal and the metatarsophalangeal joints of the big toe. You can put your thumb on the dorsal aspect of the big toe to resist these movements and make the subject aware of them. The tendon stands out just outside the tendon you located above.

Note: The tendon of this muscle also contributes to adduction, supination, and dorsiflexion of the ankle. It is inserted into both phalanges of the big toe.

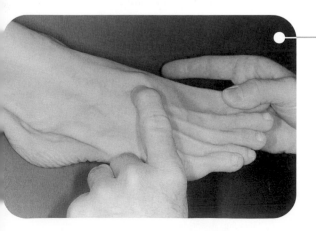

Fig. 12.121 | The body of the extensor hallucis brevis (*m. extensor hallucis brevis*)

This is not always present. It is the most medial part of the extensor digitorum brevis since it is meant for the big toe.

Ask the subject to extend the first metatarsophalangeal joint repeatedly to allow you to locate this muscle on the dorsal surface of the foot just lateral to the tendon of the extensor hallucis longus you located above.

Note: It comes to lie deep to the tendons of the extensor digitorum longus and is inserted into the base of the proximal phalanx of the big toe.

THE ANKLE AND FOOT

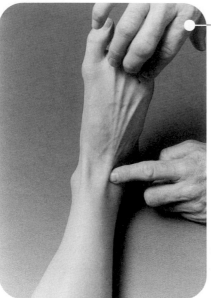

Fig. 12.122 | The tendon of the extensor digitorum longus (*m. extensor digitorum longus, tendo*)

Since it contributes to dorsiflexion of the ankle and abduction of the foot, you simply ask the subject to perform these movements and the tendon will stand out at the ankle lateral to the tendon of the extensor hallucis longus (Fig. 12.120).

You can bring out the dorsal tendons of the foot by placing your hand on the dorsal surfaces of the phalanges of the last four toes and applying an overall resistance to the extension of the interphalangeal and metatarsophalangeal joints of the same toes.

Note: This muscle also contributes to abduction, pronation, and dorsiflexion of the foot.

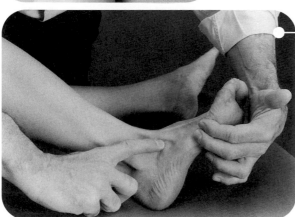

Fig. 12.123 | The tendon of the peroneus tertius (*m. peroneus tertius, tendo*)

Ask the subject to abduct, pronate, and dorsiflex the foot, and you can resist these movements or not by placing a contact on the lateral border of the foot, as shown in the adjacent illustration.

The tendon stands out lateral to the tendon of the extensor digitorum longus for the fifth toe. It runs toward the dorsal surface of the base of the fifth metatarsal, where it is inserted.

Note: It is not always present.

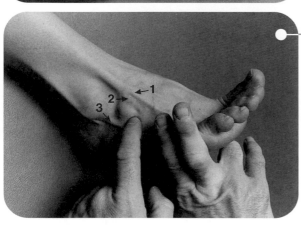

Fig. 12.124 | The body of the extensor digitorum brevis (*m. extensor digitorum brevis*)

Ask the subject to extend the interphalangeal and metatarsophalangeal joints of all the toes simultaneously (The fifth toe is not supplied by this muscle.)

The body of the muscle will stand out lateral to the tendons of the extensor digitorum longus (1) and the peroneus tertius (2), anterior to the medial malleolus and medial to the tendon of the peroneus brevis (3).

Note: Resistance applied to the lateral border of the foot by your distal hand will bring out the tendons that "frame" this muscle, which is indicated by the practitioner's index finger. Most of the time it presents as a globular structure inserted into the anterior part of the dorsal surface of the calcaneus.

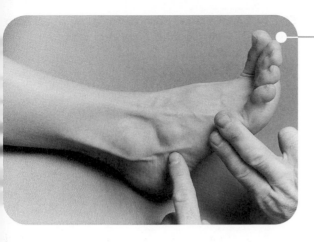

Fig. 12.125 | The tendon of the peroneus brevis (*m. peroneus brevis, tendo*)

With the subject's foot in the neutral position, ask him or her to perform a pure abduction of the foot. You can resist this movement with your distal hand resting on the lateral border of the foot.

The index finger of the practitioner's proximal hand indicates the structure you are looking for.

Note: This tendon passes above the peroneal trochlea and is inserted into the base of the tuberosity of the fifth metatarsal.

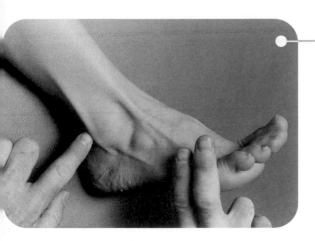

Fig. 12.126 | The tendon of the peroneus longus (*m. peroneus longus, tendo*)

You can ask the subject to perform the same movements as described above. This may be enough to bring out the tendon on the lateral border of the foot just before it enters its groove on the cuboid (*sulcus tendinosus m. peronei longi*). You can also ask for pronation and plantar flexion of the foot.

Note: This tendon passes below the peroneal trochlea and is inserted into the posterolateral tuberosity on the base of the first metatarsal. It very often sends slips to the medial cuneiform, the second metatarsal, and the first dorsal interosseus.

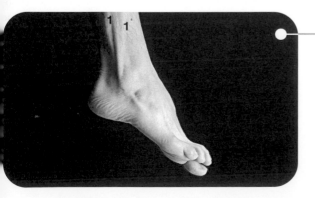

Fig. 12.127 | The body of the peroneus brevis (*m. peroneus brevis*)

The subject is asked to perform the same movements as those described in Figure 12.125. The body of the muscle (1) is accessible slightly above the lateral malleolus, behind and in front of the tendon of the peroneus longus.

Depending on the subject, the body of this muscle may be more noticeable in front of or behind the tendon of the peroneus longus.

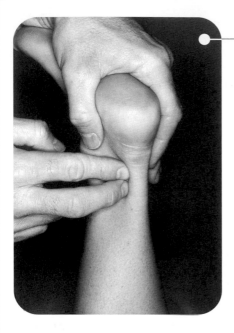

Fig. 12.128 **Lateral and posterior approach to the Achilles' tendon (*tendo calcanei*)**

This tendon is superficial and is easily accessible.

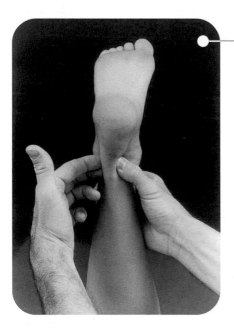

Fig. 12.129 **Anterolateral and anteromedial approach to the Achilles' tendon**

You only need use your thumb to push the tendon laterally in order to gain access to the anterolateral part of this tendon, which you can examine by sliding your finger pads up and down. Likewise, simply push the tendon medially with your thumb to gain access to the anteromedial part of this tendon.

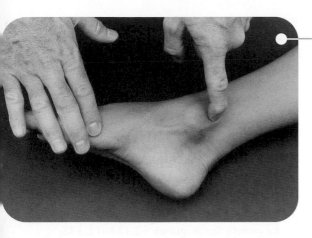

Fig. 12.130 The tendon of the tibialis posterior (*m. tibialis posterior, tendo*) at the medial malleolus

With the foot plantarflexed, ask the subject to adduct the foot against resistance applied to the medial border of the foot.

The tendon stands out on the posterior border of the medial malleolus.

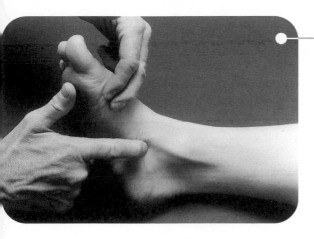

Fig. 12.131 The tendon of the tibialis posterior at the navicular bone (*os naviculare*)

To make the muscle contract, use the technique described above.

After skirting the medial malleolus, the tendon runs along the medial border of the foot and is inserted into the tuberosity of the navicular (indicated by the practitioner's index finger in the adjacent illustration), into all the tarsal bones except the talus and the metatarsals except the first and the fifth.

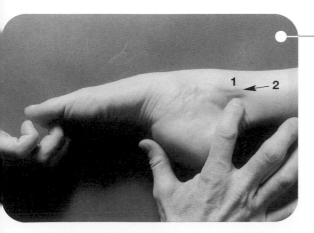

Fig. 12.132 The tendon of the flexor digitorum longus (*m. flexor digitorum longus, tendo*) at the medial malleolus (*malleolus medialis*)

Place one hand on the plantar surface of the last four toes and ask the subject to plantarflex them repeatedly and rapidly. Your other hand, placed behind the posterior tibialis (1), will feel these repeated movements of the toes. The practitioner's index finger shows the tendon of the flexor digitorum longus (2), which also lies behind the medial malleolus.

THE ANKLE AND FOOT

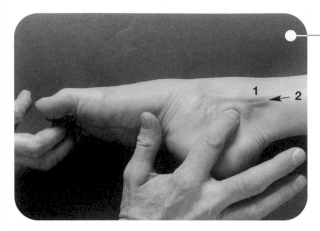

Fig. 12.133 | **The tendon of the flexor digitorum longus on the medial border of the foot**

After skirting the medial malleolus in a special osteofibrous sheath, the tendon crosses the deltoid ligament of the ankle and runs along its groove on the upper surface of the sustentaculum tali.

In the adjacent illustration the practitioner's index finger rests on this groove. Thereafter the tendon (2) enters the plantar surface of the foot.

Legends for Figures 12.133–12.135

1. Tibialis posterior.
2. Flexor digitorum longus.
3. Flexor hallucis longus.

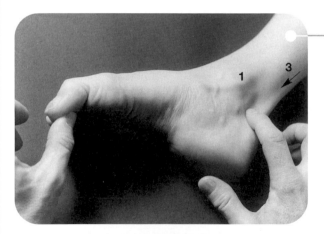

Fig. 12.134 | **The tendon of the flexor hallucis longus (*m. flexor hallucis longus, tendo*) in the medial posterior malleolar groove**

Place one hand on the plantar surface of the big toe and ask the subject to flex it repeatedly and rapidly.

Your other hand will feel these repeated movements in the medial posterior malleolar groove at a distance from the medial malleolus and quite close to the Achilles' tendon.

Note: This tendon (3), which stands out in the adjacent illustration, is not visible in all subjects.

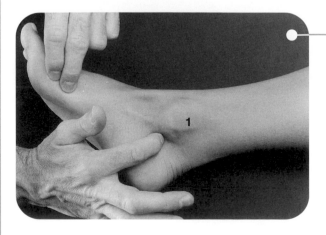

Fig. 12.135 | **The tendon of the flexor hallucis longus on the medial border of the foot**

Beyond the ankle joint the tendon slides into the groove on the posterior surface of the talus between its posterolateral and posteromedial tubercles, and comes to lie below the tendon of the flexor digitorum longus (Fig. 12.133) (2) in a special groove on the medial surface of the calcaneus underneath the sustentaculum tali.

Note: It may be useful, as shown in the adjacent illustration, to tighten the tendon of the tibialis muscle (1), as it is a landmark in your search for the tendon you are interested in.

THE INTRINSIC MUSCLES OF THE FOOT

The muscular structures that can be detected by palpation are:

- The extensor digitorum brevis (*m. extensor digitorum brevis*) (Figs 12.138–12.142).

Action

It extends the proximal phalanges of the first four toes and flexes them laterally.

- The abductor digiti minimi (*m. abductor digiti minimi*) (Fig. 12.143).

Action

It abducts the little toe.

- The opponens digiti minimi: display of its action (*m. opponens digiti minimi*) (Fig. 12.145).

Action

It pulls the fifth metatarsal medially.

- The abductor hallucis (*m. abductor hallucis*) (Fig. 12.146).

Action

— It abducts the proximal phalanx of the big toe on the first metatarsal.
— It flexes and abducts the big toe.

- The flexor hallucis brevis (*m. flexor hallucis brevis*) (Fig. 12.147).

Action

It flexes the big toe.

- The adductor hallucis (*m. adductor hallucis*) (Fig. 12.148).

Action

It adducts and flexes the big toe.

- The quadratus plantae or the flexor accessorius (*m. quadratus plantae*): display of its action (Fig. 12.149).

Action

It stabilizes the flexor digitorum longus by pulling it medially.

- The flexor digitorum brevis (*m. flexor digitorum brevis*): display of its action (Fig. 12.150).

Action

It flexes the middle phalanges of the last four toes on their proximal phalanges and flexes their first phalanges on the corresponding metatarsals.

- The plantar and dorsal interossei (*mm. interossei plantares et dorsales*): display of their actions (Fig. 12.151–153).

Action

— They flex the proximal phalanx of the toes.
— The dorsal interossei move the toes away from the axis of the foot (that is, the second toe) (Figs 12.152 and 12.153).
— The plantar interossei move the last three toes toward the axis of the foot (Figs 12.151).

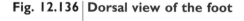

Fig. 12.136 Dorsal view of the foot

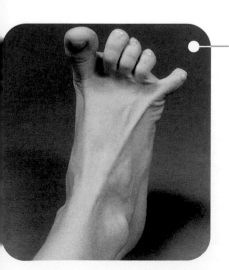

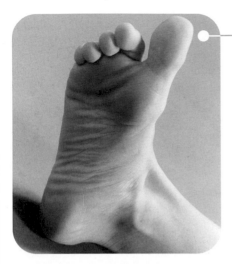

Fig. 12.137 | **Plantar view of the foot**

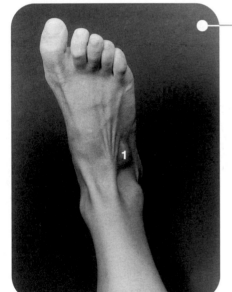

Fig. 12.138 | **The extensor digitorum brevis (*m. extensor digitorum brevis*): display and topographical location**

This is the only fleshy muscle (1) forming part of the dorsal region of the foot.

Attachments
- It arises from the anterior part of the dorsal surface of the greater process of the calcaneus.
- It terminates in four tendons:
    — The first is inserted into the dorsal surface of the base of the proximal phalanx of the big toe.
    — The three lateral tendons for the second, third, and fourth toes are inserted separately into the lateral borders of the tendons of the extensor digitorum longus for the second, third, and fourth toes.

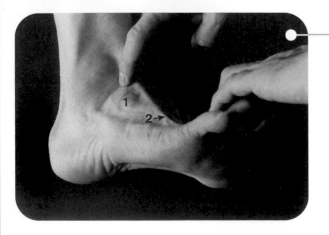

Fig. 12.139 | **The extensor digitorum brevis**

You simply have to ask the subject to extend the proximal phalanges of the first four toes against or without resistance to feel the body of the muscle (1) in front of the lateral malleolus and lateral to the tendon of the extensor digitorum longus (2). Beyond this point it is more difficult to feel, as it is covered by the extensor digitorum longus.

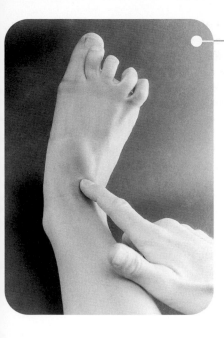

Fig. 12.140 | **The extensor hallucis brevis (*m. extensor hallucis brevis*)**

This is part of the extensor digitorum brevis. Ask the subject to perform the same movements as described in Figure 12.139. You can feel the body of the muscle distal to the inferior extensor retinaculum (Figs 12.116 and 12.117) and medial to the extensor digitorum longus (Fig. 12.123).

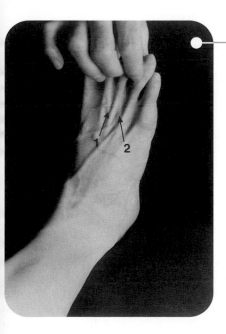

Fig. 12.141 | **Termination of the tendons of the extensor digitorum brevis on the second and third toes**

Ask the subject to perform the movements described in Figure 12.139. Place the pads of three of your fingers on the dorsal surfaces of the toes and gently plantarflex them in order to make the tendons stand out as follows: the tendon inserting into the tendon of the extensor digitorum longus for the second toe (1), and the tendon inserted into the tendon of the extensor digitorum longus for the third toe (2).

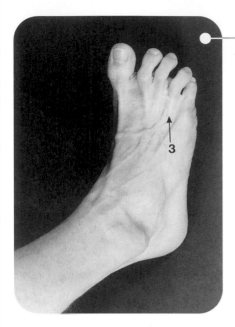

Fig. 12.142 **Termination of the tendon of the extensor digitorum brevis on the fourth toe**

The figure displays the tendon of the extensor digitorum brevis inserted into the tendon of the extensor digitorum for the fourth toe (3).

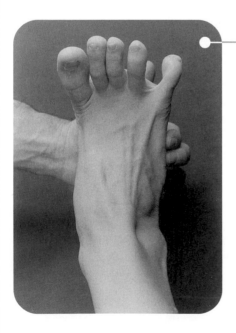

Fig. 12.143 **The abductor digiti minimi (*m. abductor digiti minimi*)**

Place the pads of two of your fingers on the lateral border of the foot and ask the subject to abduct the fifth toe repeatedly. You will easily feel the muscle contracting under your fingers.

Attachments
It arises from:

- The posterolateral process of the calcaneal tuberosity.
- The plantar aponeurosis.
- The tuberosity of the fifth metatarsal.

It is inserted into:

- The lateral border of the plantar surface of the base of the proximal phalanx of the big toe.

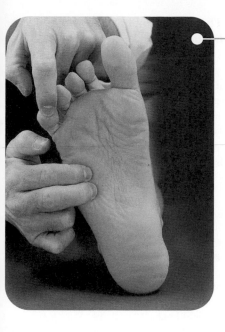

Fig. 12.144 | The flexor digiti minimi brevis (*m. flexor digiti minimi brevis*)

Place the pads of two of your fingers on the plantar surface of the fifth metatarsal and then move them toward the medial border of the foot. The body of the muscle is covered laterally by the abductor digiti minimi.

Attachments

It arises from:

- The lateral part of the crest of the cuboid.
- The synovial sheath of the peroneus longus.
- The base of the fifth metatarsal.

It is inserted into:

- The plantar surface of the base of the proximal phalanx of the fifth toe.

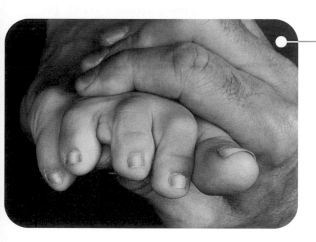

Fig. 12.145 | Display of the action of the opponens digiti minimi (*m. opponens digiti minimi*)

Its action is to pull the fifth metatarsal medially.

Note: Like the two muscles mentioned above, this one belongs to the lateral group of muscles. It cannot be palpated on its own and may be absent.

Attachments

It arises from:

- The lateral part of the crest of the cuboid.
- The plantar sheath of the peroneus longus.

It is inserted into the entire lateral border of the fifth metatarsal.

THE ANKLE AND FOOT

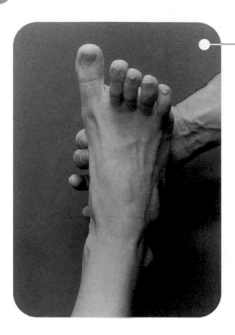

Fig. 12.146 | The abductor hallucis (*m. abductor hallucis*)

Use the pads of your fingers to place a broad contact on the medial border of the foot and ask the subject to abduct the big toe on the first metatarsal. However, if subjects are unable to do so, ask them to flex their big toe on the first metatarsal instead. You will easily feel the muscle contract on the medial border of the foot, especially on the plantar surfaces of the medial cuneiform and of the navicular.

Attachments

It arises from:

- The posteromedial process of the calcaneal tuberosity.
- The plantar aponeurosis.

It is inserted into:

- The medial sesamoid bone.
- The medial border of the base of the proximal phalanx of the big toe.

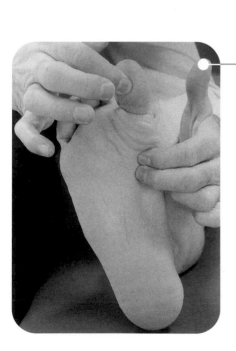

Fig. 12.147 | The flexor hallucis brevis (*m. flexor hallucis brevis*)

Place the pads of two of your fingers in such as way to make the widest possible contact on the plantar surface of the first metatarsal behind the sesamoid bones. Then move slightly toward the medial border of the foot in order to feel its medial tendon. To feel the lateral tendon, move your fingers toward the lateral border of the foot, remembering that this tendon is partly covered by the tendon of the flexor hallucis longus. Ask the subject to flex the big toe on the first metatarsal.

Attachments

It arises from:

- The plantar surfaces of the intermediate and lateral cuneiforms.
- The calcaneocuboid ligament.
- The expansions of the tendon of the tibialis posterior.

It is inserted as follows:

- The medial tendon into the tendon of the abductor hallucis.
- The lateral tendon into the tendon of the adductor hallucis.

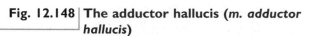

Fig. 12.148 | The adductor hallucis (*m. adductor hallucis*)

Place your whole thumb over the plantar surface of the first intermetatarsal space, more on its lateral border. Then ask the subject to flex the big toe on the first metatarsal in order to feel under your fingers the contraction of the oblique bundle of the muscle as it blends with the lateral head of the flexor hallucis brevis. It is difficult to feel the contraction of this muscle.

Attachments

It arises by two heads:

- The oblique head from:
    - The crest of the cuboid
    - The plantar surface of the lateral cuneiform and the bases of the third and fourth metatarsals
    - The calcaneocuboid ligament
    - The expansions of the tendon of the tibialis posterior.
- The transverse head from:
    - The capsules of the third, fourth, and fifth metatarsophalangeal joints.

It is inserted into:

- The lateral sesamoid bone.
- The lateral border of the base of the proximal phalanx of the big toe.

Fig. 12.149 | Display of the action of the quadratus plantae (m. *quadratus plantae*)

As in the adjacent illustration, place your fingers roughly where the muscle joins the lateral border of the tendon of the flexor digitorum longus.

Note: Because of its obliquity the tendon of the flexor digitorum longus tends to produce some "deviation" of the foot and the toes. The raison d'être of the muscle under consideration is to correct this deviation. Hence it helps to flex the last four toes.

Attachments

It arises by two heads:

- The lateral head from the plantar surface of the calcaneus and the plantar calcaneocuboid ligament.
- The medial head from the concave part of the medial surface of the calcaneus.

It is inserted into the lateral border of the tendon of the flexor digitorum longus.

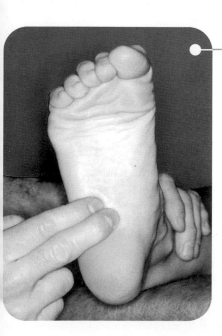

THE ANKLE AND FOOT

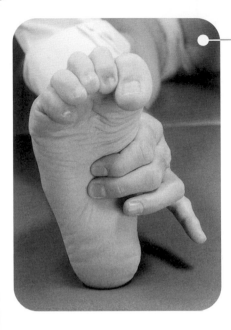

Fig. 12.150 | Display of the flexor digitorum brevis (*m. flexor digitorum brevis*)

Take hold of the medial or lateral border of the foot in your palm; this will allow you to get a wide grip on the median and plantar parts of the foot. You need only ask the subject to flex the toes on the metatarsals repeatedly in order to feel the muscle contracting under your fingers.

Note: The tendons of this muscle lie superficial to those of the flexor digitorum longus.

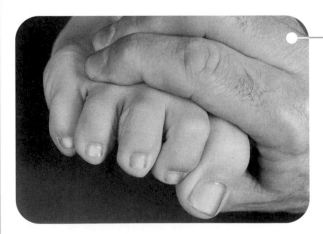

Fig. 12.151 | Display of one of the actions of the plantar interossei (*mm. interossei plantares*) and of the lumbricals (*mm. lumbricales*)

The adjacent illustration displays the proximal phalanges flexed over the metatarsals of the last four toes. The big toe, contrary to what is shown in the figure, is not involved in this action. The plantar interossei flex the proximal phalanx of the last four toes and move the last three toes closer to the axis of the foot (which passes through the second toe). The lumbricals flex the proximal phalanges of the last four toes and extend the other two phalanges on the proximal one.

Attachments
- The three plantar interossei arise from the medial surfaces and the plantar borders of the third, fourth, and fifth metatarsals and are inserted into the medial part of the bases of the proximal phalanx of the corresponding toes.
- The four lumbricals arise from both borders of the third, fourth, and fifth tendons of the flexor digitorum longus, except for the first lumbrical, which arises from the medial border of the tendon for the second toe. They are inserted into the medial parts of the bases of the proximal phalanges of the last four toes, and each sends an expansion to the corresponding extensor tendon.

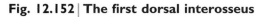

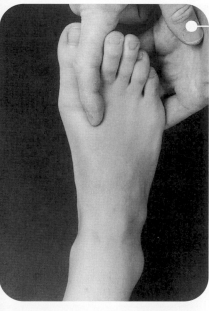

Fig. 12.152 | The first dorsal interosseus

The general approach to these muscles is made through the four intermetatarsal spaces. When placed on the lateral surfaces of the metatarsals, your fingers will find them directly accessible.

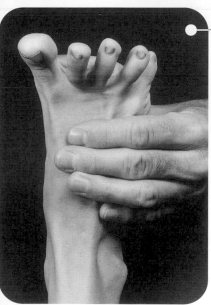

Fig. 12.153 | Display of one of the main actions of the dorsal interossei (*mm. interossei dorsales*)

The adjacent illustration shows abduction of the second, third, and fourth toes relative to the main axis of the foot, which passes through the second toe.

Note: These muscles also flex the proximal phalanges of the last four toes.

Attachments

- These four interossei arise from the lateral and medial surfaces of the second, third, and fourth metatarsals and from the medial surface of the fifth metatarsal.
- The second, third, and fourth interossei are inserted into the lateral surfaces of the second, third, and fourth toes. The first interosseus is also inserted into the medial surface of the proximal phalanx of the second toe.
- The second interosseus is inserted into the lateral surface of the base of the proximal phalanx of the second toe.
- The third and fourth interossei are inserted into the lateral surfaces of the bases of the proximal phalanges of the third and fourth toes.

Note: It is clear that the different actions of the intrinsic muscles, when viewed individually, are less important than their overall action when viewed as a functional indissoluble unit.

If they are viewed from this angle, you can imagine their considerable role in walking and in standing upright, without forgetting their extraordinary ability to adapt when the subject moves over diverse and variable surfaces, such as sandy or rocky terrain.

NERVES AND BLOOD VESSELS

The notable structures that can be detected by palpation are:

- The superficial peroneal nerve (*n. peroneus superficialis*) (Fig. 12.156).
- The lateral dorsal cutaneous nerve (*n. cutaneus dorsalis lateralis*) (Fig. 12.157).
- The anastomosis of the intermediate dorsal cutaneous nerve (*n. cutaneus dorsalis intermedius*) and the lateral dorsal cutaneous nerve (Fig. 12.157).
- The intermediate dorsal cutaneous nerve (Fig. 12.158).
- The tibial nerve (*n. tibialis*) (Figs 12.160 and 12.161).
- The posterior tibial artery (*a. tibialis posterior*) (Figs 12.160 and 12.161).
- The dorsalis pedis artery (*a. dorsalis pedis*) (Fig. 12.162).

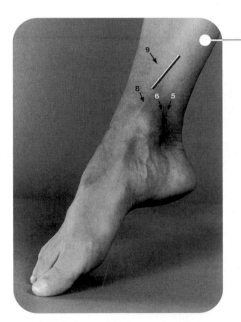

Fig. 12.154

Medial view of the ankle and foot

1. The superficial peroneal nerve.
2. The intermediate dorsal cutaneous nerve.
3. The lateral dorsal cutaneous nerve.
4. The anastomosis of the intermediate dorsal cutaneous nerve and the lateral cutaneous nerve.
5. The tibial nerve.
6. The posterior tibial artery.
7. The dorsalis pedis artery.
8. The great saphenous vein.
9. The saphenous nerve.

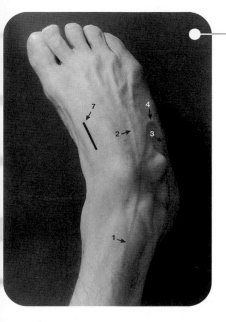

Fig. 12.155 Anterior view of the ankle and foot

1. The superficial peroneal nerve.
2. The intermediate dorsal cutaneous nerve.
3. The lateral dorsal cutaneous nerve.
4. The anastomosis of the intermediate dorsal cutaneous nerve and the lateral cutaneous nerve.
5. The tibial nerve.
6. The posterior tibial artery.
7. The dorsalis pedis artery.
8. The great saphenous vein.
9. The saphenous nerve.

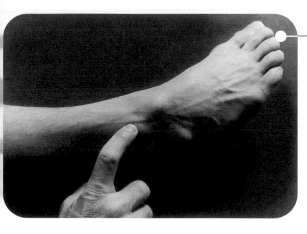

Fig. 12.156 The superficial peroneal nerve (*n. peroneus/fibularis superficialis*)

There are two ways of investigating this nerve:

- Either look for it very high in the leg (that is, roughly at the junction of the proximal two-thirds and the distal third of the anterolateral part of the leg).
- Or look much more distally at the instep.

Note: In Figs 12.155 and 12.156 it becomes subcutaneous after perforating the deep fascia of the leg.

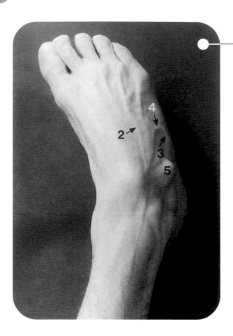

Fig. 12.157 **The lateral dorsal cutaneous nerve (branch of the sural nerve) (*n. cutaneus dorsalis lateralis*) (3) and the anastomosis (4) between the intermediate dorsal cutaneous nerve (*n. cutaneus dorsalis intermedius*) (2) and the lateral dorsal cutaneous nerve (*n. cutaneus dorsalis lateralis*)(3)**

This figure clearly shows the superficial peroneal nerve in the distal and anterolateral part of the leg. Beyond the lateral malleolus it turns into the intermediate dorsal cutaneous nerve (2), which runs in the third intermetatarsal space.

You can also see both the lateral dorsal cutaneous nerve (3), which is the continuation of the lateral saphenous nerve and runs along the lateral border of the foot, and the anastomosis (4) between the above-mentioned nerves, as it lies well beyond the greater process of the calcaneus (5).

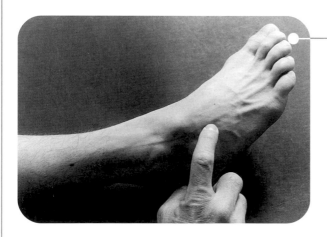

Fig. 12.158 **The intermediate dorsal cutaneous nerve (*n. cutaneus dorsalis intermedius*)**

This is a lateral view of the nerve, whose topographical relations with the other nervous elements have been described above (Fig. 12.157).

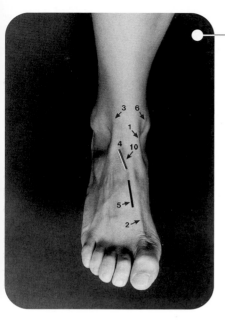

Fig. 12.159 | Anterior view of the ankle and foot

1. The tendon of the tibialis anterior.
2. The tendon of the extensor hallucis longus.
3. The tendon of the extensor digitorum longus.
4. The inferior extensor retinaculum.
5. The dorsalis pedis artery.
6. The great saphenous vein.
7. The posterior tibial artery.
8. The tibial nerve.
9. The saphenous nerve.
10. The deep peroneal nerve.

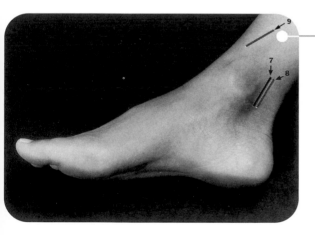

Fig. 12.160 | Medial view of the ankle and foot

1. The tendon of the tibialis anterior.
2. The tendon of the extensor hallucis longus.
3. The tendon of the extensor digitorum longus.
4. The inferior extensor retinaculum.
5. The dorsalis pedis artery.
6. The great saphenous vein.
7. The posterior tibial artery.
8. The tibial nerve.
9. The saphenous nerve.
10. The deep peroneal nerve.

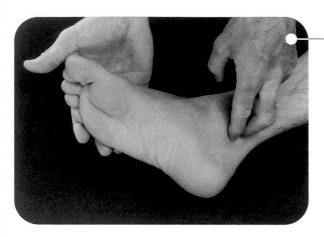

Fig. 12.161 | **The posterior tibial artery (*a. tibialis posterior*) and the tibial nerve (*n. tibialis*)**

The artery enters the medial posterior malleolar groove between the flexor digitorum longus lying in front and the flexor hallucis longus lying behind.

To make it easier to locate and take the arterial pulse, first invert the foot slightly in order to relax the various soft tissues in the region. Palpate the tibial nerve just behind the artery and your fingers will feel it as a solid cylindrical cord.

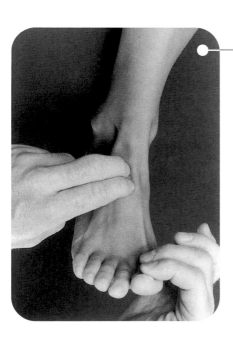

Fig. 12.162 | **The dorsalis pedis artery (*a. dorsalis pedis*) and the medial branch of the deep peroneal nerve**

The dorsalis pedis artery is the continuation of the anterior tibial artery distal to the inferior extensor retinaculum (Figs 12.115 and 12.116).

It descends on the dorsal surface of the foot down to the posterior end of the first interosseous space, which it crosses vertically to anastomose with the lateral plantar artery.

Your essential landmark on the dorsum of the foot is the tendon of the extensor hallucis longus. Using the pads of two fingers, look for the dorsalis pedis arterial pulse on the dorsum of the foot just lateral to this tendon and medial to the tendon of the extensor digitorum communis for the second toe.

The essential landmarks on the instep are the inferior extensor retinaculum and the tendons of the extensor hallucis longus medially, and the extensor digitorum communis laterally. You will feel the pulse under your fingertips between these two tendons and below or through the retinaculum.

You can palpate the medial branch of the deep peroneal nerve in the same space as the dorsalis pedis artery, but remember that it lies lateral to the artery.

BIBLIOGRAPHY

Beauthier JP, Lefèvre P. Traité d'anatomie, de la théorie à la pratique palpatoire. Brussels: De Boeck University.

    Vol. 2: Membre supérieur, ceinture scapulaire; 1991.

    Vol. 3: Tête et tronc, propédeutique viscérale; 1993.

Bonnel F, Chevrel JP, Outrequin G (series edited by J.P. Chevrel). Anatomie clinique, Vol. 1: Les Membres. Paris: Springer; 1991.

Bouchet A, Cuilleret J. Anatomie topographique, descriptive et fonctionnelle. Paris: SIMEP.

    Vol. 2: Le Cou, le thorax. 2nd edn; 1992.

    Vol. 3 (A): Le membre supérieur. 3rd edn; 1996.

    Vol. 3 (B): Le membre inférieur. 3rd edn; 1996.

Guntz M. Nomenclature anatomique illustrée. Paris: Masson; 1975.

Hislop H, Montgomery J. Daniels and Worthingham's Muscle Testing. Philadelphia, PA: Elsevier Health Sciences; 2002.

Hoppenfeld S. Physical Examination of the Spine and Extremities. New Jersey: Prentice Hall; 1979.

Kamina P. Dictionnaire atlas d'anatomie. Paris: Maloine; 1983.

Kamina P. Ostéologie des membres, Vol. 2. Paris: Maloine; 1986.

Kamina P. Tête et cou. Vol. 1: Muscles, vaisseaux, nerfs et viscères. Paris: Maloine; 1996.

Kamina P. Dos et thorax. Paris: Maloine; 1997.

Kamina P, Francke J-P. Arthrologie des membres. Paris: Maloine; 1994.

Kamina P, Rideau Y. Myologie des membres, Vol. 3. 2nd edn. Paris: Maloine; 1992.

Kamina P, Santini JJ. Anatomie, introduction à la clinique, nerfs des membres. Paris: Maloine; 1989.

Kendall HO, Peterson Kendall F, Wadsworth GE. Muscles, Testing and Function. Baltimore, MD: Williams & Wilkins; 1971.

Lacote M, Chevalier AM, Miranda A, Bleton JP, Stevenin P. Évaluation clinique de la fonction musculaire. Paris: Maloine; 2005.

Lazorthes G. Le système nerveux périphérique. Paris: Masson; 1981.

Lockhart RD. Living Anatomy. 3rd edn. London: Faber & Faber; 1951.

Lumley JS. Surface Anatomy. Edinburgh: Churchill Livingstone; 1990.

McMinn RMH, Hutchings RT, Marks SC, Abrahams PH. Color Atlas of Human Anatomy. Edinburgh: Mosby; 1998.

Mollier S. Plastische Anatomie. 2nd edn. Munich: JF Bergmann; 1967.

Netter FH. Atlas of Human Anatomy. 4th edn. Philadelphia, PA: Elsevier Health Sciences; 2006.

Netter FH. Atlas d'anatomie palpatoire. 3rd edn. Paris: Masson; 2005.

Pierron G, Leroy A, Peninou G, Dufour M, Genot C. Kinésithérapie. Paris: Flammarion Médecine-Sciences.

    Vol. 2: Membre inférieur; 1984.

    Vol. 3: Membre supérieur, bilans, techniques passives et actives; 1997.

    Vol. 4: Tronc et tête; 1997.

Bibliography

Rouvière H, Delmas A. Anatomie humaine, descriptive, topographique et fonctionnelle. Paris: Masson.

    Vol. 1: Tête et cou. 15th edn; 2002.

    Vol. 2: Tronc. 15th edn; 2002.

    Vol. 3: Membres. 15th edn; 2002.

Royce J. Surface Anatomy. Philadelphia, PA: F.A. Davis; 1965.

Sobotta J. (ed. J. Staubesand) Sobotta Atlas of Human Anatomy. Munich: Urban & Schwarzenberg.

    Vol 1: Head, Neck, Upper Limbs, Skin. 11th English edn; 1989.

    Vol 2: Thorax, Abdomen, Pelvis, Lower Limbs. 11th English edn; 1989.

Testut L, Jacob O. Traité d'anatomie topographique. Paris: Octave Douin; 1914.

Toby C. Methodische Palpation. Berlin: S. Karger; 1905.

Wolf-Heidegger G. Atlas der systematischen Anatomie des Menschen, vol. III. Basel: S. Karger; 1972.

INDEX

English term	Latin (Terminologia Anatomica) (TA)	Parisiensia Nomina Anatomica (PNA)	
Arthrology			
Joint(s)	*Articulatio(iones)*	**Articulatio(iones)**	
ankle joint	***talocruralis***	**talocruralis**	**446, 455, 457**
articular facet of medial malleolus	*facies articularis malleoli medialis*	facies malleolaris medialis	455,
articular facet of lateral malleolus	*facies articularis malleoli lateralis*	facies malleolaris lateralis	456
talar trochlea	*trochlea tali*	trochlea tali	455, 456
⇒ lateral border	——————————	——————————	455
⇒ medial border	——————————	——————————	456
Ankle joint and joints of the foot			
ligament(s)	***ligamentum(a)***	**ligamentum(a)**	
bifurcate	*bifurcatum*	bifurcatum, calcaneocuboideum	444, 446, 452
calcaneofibular	*calcaneofibulare*	calcaneofibulare	444
⇒ anterior talofibular	*talofibulare anterius*	talofibular anterius	444
⇒ posterior talofibular	*talofibulare posterius*	talofibulare posterius	444
extensor retinacula	*retinacula musculorum extensorum*	retinacula mm. extensorum	381, 446, 459, 460
medial or deltoid	*collaterale mediale/deltoideum*	mediale/deltoideum	422, 424, 458, 468
⇒ anterior tibiotalar	*pars tibiotalaris anterior*	pars tibiotalaris anterior	444, 458
⇒ posterior tibiotalar	*pars tibiotalaris posterior*	pars tibiotalaris posterior	422, 444, 458
⇒ tibiocalcaneal	*pars tibiocalcanea*	pars tibiocalcanea	458
⇒ tibionavicular	*pars tibionavicularis*	pars tibionavicularis	458
peroneal retinacula	*retinacula musculorum fibularium; retinacula musculorum peroneorum*	retinacula mm. peroneorum (fibularium)	444
plantar calcaneonavicular (spring ligament)	*calcaneonaviculare plantare*	calcaneonaviculare plantare	421, 423, 444, 445, 453, 458
posterior tibiofibular	*tibiofibulare posterius*	tibiofibulare posterius	457
talocalcaneal	*talocalcaneum interosseum*	talocalcaneare	413, 422, 423, 444
subsidiary structure:			
dorsal fascia of the foot	*fascia dorsalis pedis*	fascia dorsalis pedis	446, 460
interphalangeal joints	***interphalangeae***	**interphalangeae**	**445, 446, 447**
⇒ of the big toe	*hallucis*	hallucis	447
⇒ of the little toe	*digiti minimi*	digiti minimi	447
Knee joint	**Genus**		
ligament(s)	***ligamentum(a)***	**ligamentum(a)**	
fibular collateral	*collaterale fibulare*	collaterale fibulare	332
lateral patellar retinaculum	*retinaculum patellae laterale*	retinaculum patellae laterale	338, 339, 340
medial patellar retinaculum	*retinaculum patellae mediale*	retinaculum patellae mediale	338, 342, 343
patellar ligament	*ligamentum patellae*	ligamentum patellae	247, 290, 292, 294, 321, 323, 324, 333, 336, 337, 343, 344, 369

INDEX

English terms with a Latin TA equivalent alongside are those of the Terminologia Anatomica.

*The tibial nerve is also called the medial popliteal nerve and the posterior tibial nerve, above and below the upper border of the soleus respectively.